Treating Obesity with Personalized Cognitive Behavioral Therapy

Riccardo Dalle Grave • Massimiliano Sartirana
Marwan El Ghoch • Simona Calugi

Treating Obesity with Personalized Cognitive Behavioral Therapy

Springer

Riccardo Dalle Grave
Department of Eating and Weight Disorders
Villa Garda Hospital
Garda (VR)
Italy

Massimiliano Sartirana
Department of Eating and Weight Disorders
Villa Garda Hospital
Garda (VR)
Italy

Marwan El Ghoch
Department of Eating and Weight Disorders
Villa Garda Hospital
Garda (VR)
Italy

Simona Calugi
Department of Eating and Weight Disorders
Villa Garda Hospital
Garda (VR)
Italy

ISBN 978-3-030-08261-1 ISBN 978-3-319-91497-8 (eBook)
https://doi.org/10.1007/978-3-319-91497-8

Softcover re-print of the Hardcover 1st edition 2018

Printed on acid-free paper

This Springer imprint is published by the registered company Springer International Publishing AG part of Springer Nature.
The registered company address is: Gewerbestrasse 11, 6330 Cham, Switzerland

Preface

This book provides a detailed description of a new personalised cognitive behavioural therapy for obesity, termed "CBT-OB". The treatment has been developed to help patients reach and maintain a healthy weight loss by combining strategies and procedures derived from traditional behavioural therapy for obesity (BT-OB) with others targeting the cognitive processes that our research has found to influence attrition, weight loss and weight-loss maintenance.

CBT-OB has been primarily designed for outpatient settings in which patients with obesity are treated on a one-to-one basis, but it has subsequently also been adapted for delivery in a group setting, as well as for patients with binge-eating disorders (BED) associated with obesity. This versatile treatment can be delivered within a multistep approach that can be applied, with appropriate adaptation, at three levels of care—outpatient, day hospital and residential settings. What is more, it can be effectively used to treat all classes of obesity, including patients with severe comorbidities and obesity-associated disabilities—who are not generally recruited for lifestyle modification trials, and therefore have limited non-surgical evidence-based treatment options. Importantly, however, it can be used in conjunction with other proven treatment strategies such as weight-loss drugs and bariatric surgery.

CBT-OB adopts some principles of the so-called enhanced cognitive behavioural therapy (CBT-E)—an evidence-based treatment for all eating disorders. Indeed, our consolidated clinical experience of treating many patients with eating disorders has shown that many problems that CBT-E enables us to successfully address in patients with bulimia nervosa and other eating disorders overlap with those seen in patients with obesity. Specifically, these include the difficulties patients have in playing an active role in their own treatment, their loss of control over eating, dissatisfaction with shape and weight and unhealthy preoccupation with eating. As such, many principles of CBT-E were exploited in the design of CBT-OB, in particular the collaborative style of treatment, the general structure of the sessions, the strategies used to encourage patients' active participation in their own treatment and lifestyle change and to overturn their negative body image, as well as procedures to address episodes of binge eating where appropriate (in patients with BED). Like CBT-E, CBT-OB is also flexible, modular and personalised.

The book has been written in the form of a clinician's manual. The major contributors come from different clinical backgrounds—specifically two medical doctors and two clinical psychologists—but all can be described as experts in delivering

CBT-OB in real-world clinical settings, from outpatient to residential. In order to aid the practitioner, the treatment is described in detail, from the first assessment session through to the post-treatment review. Clinical vignettes are included to illustrate important points, and strategies for personalising the intervention and adapting it to an individual patient's needs and particular settings are discussed.

We have endeavoured to make this book of interest to all professionals working with patients with obesity, whether physicians, dieticians, nutritionists, psychologists, psychiatrists, nurses or physical educators and more. It is particularly suitable for healthcare professionals working as part of a multidisciplinary team that wishes to adopt an evidence-based, non-eclectic, stepped-care approach to the treatment of obesity, grounded in cognitive behavioural theory.

Although no specific professional qualifications are required to practice CBT-OB, potential therapists should ideally have had some training in cognitive behavioural therapy, as well as clinical experience of treating patients with obesity. Most therapists with these two prerequisites will be able to practice CBT-OB successfully using the strategies and procedures described in this book.

That being said, and though extensive cross-referencing has been included to help readers navigate the concepts with ease, it is advisable for readers to approach the book as a whole, as each sequential chapter assumes knowledge of the content of those which have come before. As such, the book is structured as follows:

- Chapter 1 describes the problems associated with the current treatments for obesity, in particular the neglected role of cognitive processes. It then goes on to summarise the data obtained from our extensive clinical research on the cognitive factors associated with attrition, weight loss and weight maintenance.
- Chapter 2 provides a general overview of CBT-OB. It outlines its goals, general strategies and specific procedures designed to promote weight loss and minimise attrition. It also describes the different versions of CBT-OB, highlights certain points regarding the respective roles of patient and therapist in the treatment and explains how the environment in which treatment is provided can best be organised.
- Chapter 3 explains how patients should be assessed and prepared for treatment. It also provides some advice to non-medical therapists on the medical management of patients.
- Chapters 4–9 describe the core protocols of CBT-OB and details of how to implement the six programme modules.
- Chapter 10 illustrates the importance of the involvement of significant others in the sessions and how to help patients receive support from family members and others in their social circle.
- Chapters 11–14 describe, respectively, how to adapt CBT-OB for group treatment, intensive levels of care, and patients with BED and how CBT-OB can be combined with weight-loss drugs and bariatric surgery.
- Chapter 15 provides suggestions on how to exploit modern technology in delivering treatment and training CBT-OB therapists.

- Appendices A–E provide useful handouts for clinicians, including the CBT-OB Monitoring Record and the Personal Formulation template, as well as CBT-OB menus and food group information sheets, and the latest versions of the Weight-Loss Obstacles Questionnaire and Weight and Primary Goals Questionnaire (see Chaps. 6–10 for details).

Before moving on, we would like to take this opportunity to thank our brilliant colleagues whose ideas inspired us to write this book. In particular, we thank Kelly Brownell for his pioneering work incorporating the principle of behaviour modification in the treatment of obesity in a comprehensive manual, Giulio Marchesini for his fundamental role in the research we performed together on the cognitive factors influencing the treatment of obesity and, especially Zafra Cooper and Christopher Fairburn, who were the first not only to underscore the importance of cognitive processes in hindering the treatment of obesity, but also to propose a treatment based on the cognitive behavioural precepts from which we derived many of the principles described in this book. We also wish to thank all of the colleagues—too numerous to mention—who work with us in our outpatient and intensive CBT-OB clinics for their enthusiasm, the passion and dedication with which they help patients with obesity to address their individual problems and for their continuous precious feedback, much of which has helped to improve the treatment. Particular thanks are also due to Anna Forster for her assistance and competence in editing the English text and to Elena Mischiatti for her help in producing the figures. Last but not least, we would like to extend special thanks to the patients we have had the privilege to treat; they also made invaluable suggestions that enabled us to become better therapists and to perfect the treatment that we present in this book.

Garda (VR), Italy

Riccardo Dalle Grave
Massimiliano Sartirana
Marwan El Ghoch
Simona Calugi

Contents

Abbreviations

6MWT	Six-minute walk test
BED	Binge-eating disorder
BMI	Body Mass Index
BSI	Brief Symptom Inventory
BT-OB	Behavioural therapy for obesity
CASCO-R	Comprehensive Appropriateness Scale for the Care of Obesity in Rehabilitation
CBT-E	Enhanced cognitive behavioural therapy
CBT-OB	Cognitive behavioural therapy for obesity
CVD	Cardiovascular disease
DEXA	Dual Energy X-ray Absorptiometry
EDE	Eating Disorder Examination
EDE-Q	Eating Disorder Examination Questionnaire
FFM	Fat-free mass
MET	Metabolic Equivalent Task

Introduction

1

The main goals of CBT-OB—and obesity treatment in general—are first and foremost to create a persistent negative energy balance that will enable patients to reach a healthy weight. This is usually achieved by combining specific recommendations on diet and exercise—an approach that is generally successful in producing some degree of weight loss in a large subgroup of patients. However, a neutral energy balance—in which the calorie intake equals the calories expended—is necessary for patients to maintain the weight lost, and many obesity treatments fail in this regard, making them ineffective in the long term.

Indeed, by focusing only on the biological and behavioural factors regulating food intake and energy expenditure, traditional treatments for obesity ignore the distinctive cognitive processes that can affect an individual's ability to adhere to lifestyle modification over time. In contrast, treatments that are specifically designed to target such cognitive processes and permanently change a person's "mindset" with respect to control of eating and the adoption of an active lifestyle may have more success.

In this chapter, we briefly describe the limitations of the available treatments for obesity in more detail and then discuss the main obstacles to weight loss and weight maintenance; we explore the cognitive processes associated with attrition, weight loss and weight-loss maintenance that have emerged from our research and the rationale behind the development of CBT-OB. Finally, we give a brief description of the main characteristics that distinguish cognitive behavioural treatments from purely behavioural approaches and the features that set CBT-OB apart.

1.1 Current Treatments for Obesity

1.1.1 Biomedical Treatment

Traditionally, treatment of obesity has been based on a biomedical model which includes three major elements: (1) the diagnosis of obesity and associated medical,

R. Dalle Grave et al., *Treating Obesity with Personalized Cognitive Behavioral Therapy*, https://doi.org/10.1007/978-3-319-91497-8_1

psychiatric and psychosocial complications; (2) the prescription of a hypocaloric diet associated with physical activity recommendations and, in some cases, weight-loss drugs; and (3) the patient's "willpower", which will affect their ability to adhere to the behavioural changes required to lose weight.

Nonetheless, more than 150 years has passed since William Banting wrote his seminal booklet, *Letter on Corpulence, Addressed to the Public* [1]. This contained a low-carbohydrate diet plan—an idea that was adopted and has since been expanded by clinicians and researchers suggesting diets with different nutrient compositions (e.g. low-fat or low-carbohydrate diet) with a view to increasing the amount of weight lost. However, data from several randomised trials over the past 10 years have demonstrated that, in the long term (1–2 years), there is little difference between such diets as regards the weight loss achieved, which is in any case modest [2]. In fact, the latest research indicates that the key to significant weight loss is adherence to diet, rather than the composition of the diet itself [3].

Similarly, all the drugs for the treatment of obesity that have been tested over the last half-century have produced discouragingly little weight loss on the whole, and many have had to be withdrawn from the market due to unacceptably severe side effects [4]. Although combinations of slimming drugs might substantially increase weight loss and may therefore be an avenue worth pursuing, to date the success of antiobesity drugs has been limited. As recently summed up by Rodgers et al., "the history of anti-obesity drug development is far from glorious, with transient magic bullets and only a handful of agents currently licensed for clinical use" [5].

Furthermore, in addition to poor weight loss (about 5%) and a high rate of long-term failure, the biomedical model of obesity treatment is burdened by a very high dropout rate (about 50%) [6]. Indeed, it promotes feelings of guilt and failure in patients [7], who likely attribute slow progress to their lack of willpower, rather than the unsuitability of treatment to their particular biopsychosocial makeup. That being said, perhaps because they are relatively easy to learn and disseminate, biomedical treatments still comprise the approach most commonly offered to patients with obesity.

1.1.2 Behavioural Therapy

BT-OB, a specific form of behavioural therapy for obesity, was developed in the late 1960s with a view to overcoming the abovementioned limitations of the biomedical model [8]. BT-OB was based on the principles of learning theory (behaviourism) and on the observation that the key behaviours involved in the development of obesity (i.e. overeating and sedentary lifestyle) are mainly determined by education, environmental stimuli and their consequences. This prompted the development of specific education programmes for patients with obesity, and the design of strategies and procedures to facilitate changes in dietary and physical activity habits through recognition and modification of environmental stimuli (antecedents) and consequences of food intake (reinforcements) [9]. Later on, procedures derived from social cognitive theory and cognitive therapy, as well as specific dietary recommendations and physical activity, were integrated into the approach, and this multifaceted combination is what we commonly refer to today as "weight-loss lifestyle modification" [9].

Although today's BT-OB has benefited from the introduction of some generic cognitive procedures for tackling obstacles to losing weight (e.g. problem solving and basic cognitive restructuring techniques), its main focus is still on changing eating habits rather than producing cognitive change [10]. Moreover, even nowadays there is little focus on the individual, as the treatment tends to be administered to groups following a prescribed order of sessions, irrespective of the relative progress of each group member [10]. Finally, outcomes appear to indicate that the traditional once-a-week session frequency of BT-OB may be inadequate, especially in terms of the management of patients with severe obesity and associated comorbidities, disability and poor quality of life. Instead, these patients often require intensive rehabilitation protocols, which need to be administered in appropriate environments by purpose-trained staff.

That being said, data from randomised controlled trials of structured group BT-OB indicate that, on average, 80% of participants of such programmes complete the treatment, achieving a mean weight loss of 8–10% of their initial body weight within roughly 30 weeks, and some even losing as much as 15–20% [11]. According to the 2013 AHA/ACC/TOS Guideline for the Management of Overweight and Obesity in Adults (produced jointly by the American Heart Association, the American College of Cardiology and The Obesity Society), the amount of weight loss generally achieved by BT-OB can be considered successful (i.e. in line with a 5–10% reduction of initial weight), as it is associated with a significant reduction in the incidence of type 2 diabetes, as well as clinical improvements in weight-related medical comorbidities such as sleep apnoea, diabetes, hypertension and hyperlipidaemia. A 5–10% reduction in body weight also has a positive effect on psychosocial outcomes like mood, and body image, which can improve overall quality of life [12].

Nonetheless, there is great variability in the amount of weight loss achieved through BT-OB, and about 20–30% of participants fail to lose the recommended 5% of their initial body weight [11]. Furthermore, in the year following treatment, participants typically regain about 30–35% of the weight they lost during treatment. Although weight regain tends to slow down after the first year, by 5 years post-treatment, 50% or more patients are likely to have returned to their baseline weight [13].

With this in mind, the new generation of BT-OB generally involves a prolonged treatment period. For example, that studied in the Look AHEAD (Action for Health in Diabetes) trial was administered continuously over 4 years. Despite this, and although that treatment produced a clinically meaningful weight loss (≥5%) in 50% of patients with type 2 diabetes at year 8 [14], a large group of patients failed to reach its ultimate goal, namely, long-term maintenance of the weight lost.

1.1.3 Bariatric Surgery

In recent years, bariatric surgery treatment for obesity—also known as weight-loss surgery—has been growing in popularity and acclaim. Indeed, bariatric surgery can achieve drastic weight loss by limiting the capacity of the stomach (gastric banding) or removing a portion of the stomach (e.g. via sleeve gastrectomy), thereby reducing the amount of food that is necessary to feel full. Alternatively, physiological malabsorption can be achieved by resecting and re-routing the small intestine into a small stomach pouch (e.g. biliopancreatic diversion), or both techniques can be applied simultaneously (e.g. gastric bypass, sleeve gastrectomy with duodenal switch). The weight loss at 2–3 years following such surgical procedures in adults with obesity ranges from a mean of 20–35% of their initial body weight, while the mean weight loss at 10 years is approximately 16%, meaning that, on average, patients regain 7% of the weight they had lost through surgery in the long term [12].

In spite of the success of bariatric surgery, which is more effective in terms of weight loss and comorbidity reduction than all the other treatments for obesity, the 2013 AHA/ACC/TOS Guidelines for the Management of Overweight and Obesity in Adults recommend that it be considered only in a "small" number of patients with severe obesity, i.e. those with a body mass index (BMI) ≥40.0 or a BMI between 35.0 and 39.9 with obesity-related comorbid conditions, provided that they are motivated to lose weight but have not responded to weight-loss lifestyle modification interventions with or without pharmacotherapy [12]. This is because the complications of bariatric surgery may be severe, and long-term side effects—such as the need for reoperation, gallbladder disease and malabsorption—are common. Moreover, long-term randomised controlled trials have yet to confirm that bariatric surgery does indeed reduce mortality. Finally, a multidisciplinary team experienced in bariatric surgery, preferably in a centre dealing with a high volume of such cases, is required to handle the relatively few patients who qualify.

1.1.4 Summary of the Main Problems Associated with Current Treatments for Obesity

In summary, therefore, though bariatric surgery treatment for obesity is effective, it is only indicated for a small subgroup of patients with severe obesity. Of the remaining options, biomedical treatment is associated with relatively poor weight-loss outcomes, in addition to high rates of dropout and long-term failure, while BT-OB is plagued by poor long-term weight maintenance, even though it provides good and healthy weight loss in the short term. It is clear, then, that there is an urgent need for new approaches for managing obesity that will be effective in the majority of patients.

1.2 The Neglected Role of Cognitive Processes

There is a general consensus that the main driving forces behind weight gain are the biological pressure on individuals to overeat in order to restore their original weight, combined with exposure to an environment rich in highly palatable and hypercaloric food, not to mention the availability of labour-saving devices, which exacerbate the human predisposition to conserve energy. Nonetheless, data from the National Weight Control Registry (NWCR) clearly shows that many individuals are able to overcome these pressures in the long term and to maintain significant weight loss by adopting specific lifestyle modification behaviours [15]. The NWCR compared the behavioural strategies adopted by successful individuals in this regard (i.e. an average weight loss of 37 lb maintained for over 7 years) with those who regained weight, and weight-stable controls [15]. In addition to reporting higher levels of strenuous physical activity and a greater frequency of self-weighing, those who managed to keep the weight off reported the continued use of many more behavioural strategies to control their dietary intake. Unfortunately, however, this report was not designed to answer the central question that this finding raises, namely, why some individuals do manage to continue to practice weight-control behaviours—and therefore maintain weight-loss in long term—while others do not.

That being said, since the "complex behaviours" involved in losing and maintaining weight via lifestyle modification are influenced by conscious cognitive processes, it is plausible that these may play an influential role in an individual's success or failure to maintain weight loss [10]. Cognitive factors have largely been overlooked in traditional weight-loss lifestyle modification programmes, but this hypothesis is supported by basic scientific findings that clearly demonstrate the role of cognitive processes in maintaining unhealthy eating habits and making healthier eating difficult [16]. It is also supported by the results of several clinical studies that have, respectively, shown associations between specific cognitive factors and treatment discontinuation, as well as the amount of weight lost and long-term weight-loss maintenance [17].

Over the past 10 years, attempts have been made to investigate the role of several cognitive factors associated with attrition, weight loss and weight maintenance in more depth. For example, the data provided by the QUOVADIS study (QUality of life in Obesity: eVAluation and DIsease Surveillance) has proved invaluable in this regard. QUOVADIS was a purely observational study designed to investigate quality of life in 1944 treatment-seeking patients with obesity in a "real-world" setting—specifically 25 medical centres (including our own) authorised to treat obesity by the Italian National Health Service [18]. All centres were expected to treat patients according to their own specific programmes, which included dieting and/or BT-OB, weight-loss drugs and/or bariatric surgery (<2% of patients). Patients were evaluated at baseline—approximately 1 week before beginning the treatment in question—and again 6 and 12 months after treatment. Eighteen of the participating centres also conducted telephone interview follow-up, on average 36 months after enrolment. This, along with other datasets derived from real-world settings, enables us to shed considerable light on the role of cognitive factors in several processes serving to hinder weight loss and weight-loss maintenance.

1.2.1 Cognitive Factors and Attrition

Attrition is undoubtedly the greatest obstacle to treatment success. In the QUOVADIS study, 51.7% of participants had interrupted their treatment by 12 months [19], and the strongest predictors of attrition were lower age and higher expectations; attrition was also high in subjects with a primary goal for weight loss based on their appearance. At baseline, the group as a whole reported a mean "dream" BMI that would entail an overall weight loss of 32%, and a maximum BMI perceived as acceptable corresponding to a weight loss of 23%. Neither of these targets is achievable by non-surgical treatments for obesity. Interestingly, the risk of dropout, which was particularly high in the first 6 months, increased systematically per unit increase in expected BMI loss at 12 months [19]. After 36 months, only 15.7% of the patients in the 15 medical centres that provided a continuous care programme remained in active treatment, and, again, the strongest predictors of adherence were lower expected 1-year BMI loss and older age [6]. This study also supports the notion that continuous care is a therapeutic option that is only useful in a minority of patients.

The association between weight-loss expectation and attrition was confirmed by the QUOVADIS 2 study, another observational study of 634 women with obesity consecutively seeking treatment for obesity at eight Italian medical centres [20]. This study too revealed "acceptable" weight-loss goals that were highly unrealistic. On average, participants said that they would be happy with any weight reduction over 20%, which is more than twice the mean amount usually achieved by lifestyle modification programmes. This may explain why the dropout rate from this study was about 32% at 12 months. Indeed, the data showed that adherence was mainly influenced by more realistic but challenging weight goals (i.e. acceptable or disappointing weight) rather than largely unrealistic expectations (i.e. dream or desirable weight) [21].

Lending weight to the hypothesis that realistic treatment goals could be a highly influential factor in terms of attrition is our observation that dissatisfaction with weight-loss outcomes was reported as a major cause of attrition by 25% of dropouts [22]. This is further supported by other research linking higher initial weight-loss expectations with a higher dropout rate [23].

That being said, some studies have failed to find any association between initial expectations and attendance in BT-OB programmes [24, 25]. However, it is likely that this is related to the treatment being delivered in a research setting. Indeed, the BT-OB trials that found no association between higher weight loss expectations and attrition featured a frequent recall system, which could feasibly blunt the effect of expectations on attrition. Moreover, in such trials participants receive treatment free of charge, which creates a powerful incentive for them to complete the programme, even if they are not achieving their own weight-loss goals. In many real-world settings—such as those observed in QUOVADIS—patients are responsible for funding their own treatment, which generates a powerful disincentive to continue treatment if they are not achieving their expected weight-loss and/or other specific goals (i.e. improving appearance).

In summary, the available data raises some key issues that need to be addressed in order to improve the long-term outcomes of obesity treatment, specifically, (1) patients who seek treatment have unrealistic weight loss expectations; (2) the greater the expected BMI loss (especially among the more realistic expectations), the earlier the dropout—probably due to early dissatisfaction with the weight loss achieved; and (3) attrition is associated with a younger age and goals other than weight loss, such an overriding motivation to improve appearance.

1.2.2 Cognitive Factors and Weight Loss

The QUOVADIS team also analysed several cognitive factors associated with weight loss at a 12-month follow-up after the various treatments in 500 participants [26]. After 12 months, a substantial reduction in BMI, general psychopathology, binge eating and body image dissatisfaction was accompanied by reduced scores for dietary disinhibition and hunger and a considerable increase in dietary restraint in both females and males. After controlling for age, sex and baseline BMI, the most influential factors associated with a reduction in BMI at 12 months were an increase in dietary restraint and a reduction in disinhibition. 63.7% of cases exhibited a 5% weight loss at 1 year, and the probability of achieving this target increased significantly for every point increase in dietary restraint and point decrease in disinhibition. A weight loss exceeding 10% was observed in 34.4% of participants and was also predicted by changes in dietary restraint and disinhibition. This suggests that a treatment that can promote an increase in dietary restraint and a reduction in disinhibition may lead to weight loss via decreased calorie intake [26].

However, in a randomised controlled trial comparing two types of energy-restricted diets (high protein vs. high carbohydrate) combined with CBT-OB, we found that higher expected weight loss (in kilograms) was associated with greater weight loss [27]. In light of the association between higher expected weight loss and with treatment discontinuation, this observation raises some issues regarding the management of obesity, which CBT-OB addresses with the strategies described in Sect. 2.2.2.

1.2.3 Cognitive Factors and Weight-Loss Maintenance

Although many types of treatment show some degree of success, a very large subset of patients is unable to keep the weight off in the long term. Hence, the QUOVADIS study also sets out to analyse the effect of cognitive factors on weight-loss maintenance at 36 months in 15 medical centres (those offering patients a continuous care programme) [6]. After an average of 36 months, 157 (15.7%) of the initial 1000 patients were still in ongoing treatment (continuers). These were generally older, with lower BMI loss expectations, and the percentage of subjects who achieved a weight loss of 5% was considerably higher in continuers (40.8%) than in dropouts (22.7%), confirming that continuous care may improve weight-loss maintenance [28], at least in the subgroup that adhere to long-term treatment. Dropouts, on the other hand, cited many different reasons for abandoning treatment, including family problems, problems at work, living too far from the medical centre and health problems other than obesity. That being said, not all dropouts can be considered failures, as some—7.0% of the entire sample—were in fact satisfied with the results of treatment in terms of the body weight achieved. In fact, this subset of patients, alongside those who were confident in their ability to lose additional weight without professional help (11.7%), not only lost significantly more weight than other dropouts but also achieved a greater mean weight loss than continuers.

Therefore, it is feasible that, while achievement of results perceived as less than satisfactory may lead to loss of motivation, a substantial weight loss in the initial phases of treatment may strengthen adherence. This bolsters the idea that satisfaction with the results of treatment might be a cognitive factor that can help promote weight-loss maintenance in the long term, even without continuous care. This is further supported by data from another study in which we found that both the amount of weight loss and weight-loss satisfaction were independent predictors of weight maintenance at 1-year follow-up [27].

Indeed, in further study we assessed the association between weight maintenance and session-by-session diet adherence, weight loss and weight-loss satisfaction in 58 patients who participated in a randomised controlled trial and who lost at least the 10% of their baseline BMI. We grouped these participants into weight-loss "maintainers" (i.e. those who maintained a weight loss of ≥10% of baseline body weight at 6 months after the weight-loss phase) and "regainers" (i.e. those who did not maintain >10% weight loss at 6 months after the weight-loss phase) [29]. In support of the above, regainers displayed lower adherence to dietary restriction after the initial 11 weeks, accompanied by a progressive decline in weight loss and weight-loss satisfaction from week 15 or 19 of the weight-loss phase. We also found that a cut-off score of 7 or less on a Likert weight-satisfaction scale (0–10) 3–4 months after the beginning of treatment appeared to identify those patients who would not go on to maintain weight loss. It is therefore possible that the declining rate of weight loss produced by a reduced adherence to diet may trigger a reduction in weight-loss satisfaction, which in turn decreases adherence to calorie control—a vicious cycle that eventually results in patients regaining the weight they have lost.

1.2.4 Summary of Findings

The findings from the above studies clearly indicate that some cognitive processes may have an important role in the management of obesity. As shown in Table 1.1, there are clear and significant associations between certain cognitive factors and treatment discontinuation, as well as the amount of weight lost and/or long-term weight-loss maintenance. Furthermore, results show that attrition is associated with younger age [6, 19] and weight regain with both a lower adherence to diet and decline in weight loss 3–4 months after the beginning of treatment. With this in mind, treatments should directly target these factors where possible in order to facilitate adherence and foster successful outcomes in terms of long-term weight loss and satisfaction.

Table 1.1 Cognitive factors associated with attrition, weight loss and weight maintenance

Factors associated with attrition:
• Higher expected 1-year BMI loss [6, 19]
• Primary goal for weight loss based on appearance [19]
• Acceptable or disappointing weight with respect to personal expectations [21]
• Dissatisfaction with weight loss obtained through treatment [22]
Factors associated with weight loss:
• Increase in dietary restraint and reduction in disinhibition [26]
• Higher expected weight loss at baseline [27]
Cognitive factors associated with weight maintenance:
• Satisfaction with the results achieved [6]
• Weight-loss satisfaction [27]
• Confidence in the ability to lose additional weight without professional help [6]
• Declining weight-loss satisfaction from week 15 or 19 of the weight-loss phase (associated with weight regain) [29]

1.3 From BT-OB to CBT-OB

There are many ways in which behavioural treatments and cognitive behavioural treatments overlap [10]. In particular, both use a short-term problem-solving approach focused on the present, rather than on the past. They also both adopt a specific model of how the disorders they are designed to treat are maintained and a collaborative therapeutic style that actively involves the patients. Moreover, practitioners of both are committed to assessing the empirical evidence of treatment efficacy and to improving the treatment in response to clinical and research findings.

Nevertheless, there is a major difference between the two types of treatment; while behavioural programmes are mainly aimed at producing changes in behaviour, the ultimate goal of cognitive behavioural treatment is to help patients to achieve *cognitive* change, which should in turn influence their behaviour. Although BT-OB, for example, makes use of some generic cognitive procedures for tackling obstacles to losing weight, its major focus is changing eating habits rather than producing cognitive change.

Cognitive behavioural treatments, on the other hand, are generally based on a "cognitive conceptualisation" of both the core psychopathology and the main psychosocial mechanisms maintaining the disorder in question. For example, in eating disorders the target core psychopathology is the "overvaluation of shape or weight" (i.e. judging self-worth predominantly in terms of body shape or weight), as most other features of these disorders appear to be secondary to this underlying trait and its repercussions (e.g. undereating leading to being underweight; rigid and extreme dietary restraint leading to binge eating) [30].

The theory behind maintenance of the disorder is then used as a basis for "specific" cognitive behavioural treatments that are designed to address and change the mechanisms involved, as disruption of these mechanisms will be required to obtain lasting change [10]. So, in eating disorders (in which CBT approaches have been particularly successful and well-studied), for example, the treatment is designed to address [30] (1) dietary restraint and restriction, excessive exercising, low weight and/or binge eating and purging episodes—the main behavioural expressions of the disorder in question; (2) the main mechanisms that are maintaining the individual patient's eating disorder; and (3) any potential setbacks, with a view to preventing relapse.

In CBT, the postulated maintenance mechanisms behind the disorder are tackled using a combination of procedures that includes: (1) the collaborative development of a Personal Formulation, which highlights the main cognitive and behavioural expressions of the disorder and the mechanisms that maintain them; (2) the use of behavioural "experiments", which give patients the opportunity to "trial" different behaviours and to test their expectations regarding the consequences of such behavioural change; and (3) the identification and restructuring of dysfunctional thoughts and assumptions.

In the early 2000s, Cooper et al. were the first to integrate specific cognitive behavioural strategies into an alternative treatment for obesity [31]. Their treatment was designed to address the disappointing long-term results of BT-OB through cognitive behavioural analysis of the processes responsible for weight regain. It explicitly distinguishes weight loss from weight maintenance and addresses two interrelated factors postulated to underlie a patient's failure to engage in effective weight-maintenance strategies, namely, unrealistic weight goals and a lack of training in weight maintenance.

Preliminary data showed that adding cognitive procedures to weight-loss lifestyle modification is associated with better maintenance of weight loss [32] and less weight regain [33]. Moreover, a recent randomised controlled trial has found that participants allocated to a BT-OB intervention featuring integrated cognitive procedures (derived from acceptance and commitment therapy), in addition to dialectical behaviour therapy and relapse prevention for substance abuse, achieved significantly greater weight loss at 12 months than those assigned to standard BT-OB [34]. Although this finding contrasts with results from a controlled clinical trial that failed to find a positive effect of the treatment proposed by Cooper et al. in terms of long-term weight-loss maintenance [35], it is possible that this conclusion was at least in part determined by the time-limited duration of the treatment in question. As noted by the authors themselves, it is also possible that the treatment was insufficiently effective in changing the cognitive processes thought to be involved in weight regain, despite this being the main aim. It is also plausible that it failed to target other key cognitive processes responsible for weight regain.

Since then, more data on the important role of cognitive factors and procedures in influencing obesity-treatment outcomes, as well as the significant limitations of BT-OB, has emerged and made it obvious that innovative treatments based on cognitive change are urgently required. Moreover, the research suggests that patients with severe obesity often need more intensive interventions that can address their individual requirements. In the light of this need, and based on our consolidated clinical experience, we developed CBT-OB, a new, personalised multistep approach to obesity. Described in the following chapters, CBT-OB integrates specific procedures designed to address the cognitive processes that our previous research has found to be associated with attrition, weight loss and weight maintenance with several of the traditional procedures of BT-OB. The treatment is designed to treat patients with obesity of varying severity at a level of care and in a treatment setting that is most appropriate to their recovery and long-term health.

References

1. Banting W. Letter on corpulence, addressed to the public. 3rd ed. London: Harrison; 1864.
2. Foster GD, Wyatt HR, Hill JO, McGuckin BG, Brill C, Mohammed BS, et al. A randomized trial of a low-carbohydrate diet for obesity. N Engl J Med. 2003;348(21):2082–90. https://doi.org/10.1056/NEJMoa022207.
3. Pagoto SL, Appelhans BM. A call for an end to the diet debates. JAMA. 2013;310(7):687–8. https://doi.org/10.1001/jama.2013.8601.
4. Rodgers RJ, Tschop MH, Wilding JP. Anti-obesity drugs: past, present and future. Dis Model Mech. 2012;5(5):621–6. https://doi.org/10.1242/dmm.009621.
5. Rodgers RJ, Holch P, Tallett AJ. Behavioural satiety sequence (BSS): separating wheat from chaff in the behavioural pharmacology of appetite. Pharmacol Biochem Behav. 2010;97(1):3–14. https://doi.org/10.1016/j.pbb.2010.03.001.
6. Dalle Grave R, Melchionda N, Calugi S, Centis E, Tufano A, Fatati G, et al. Continuous care in the treatment of obesity: an observational multicentre study. J Intern Med. 2005;258(3):265–73. https://doi.org/10.1111/j.1365-2796.2005.01524.x.
7. Carels RA, Cacciapaglia HM, Douglass OM, Rydin S, O'Brien WH. The early identification of poor treatment outcome in a women's weight loss program. Eat Behav. 2003;4(3):265–82. https://doi.org/10.1016/s1471-0153(03)00029-1.
8. Stuart RB. Behavioral control of overeating. 1967. Obes Res. 1996;4(4):411–7.
9. Wadden TA, Butryn ML, Wilson C. Lifestyle modification for the management of obesity. Gastroenterology. 2007;132(6):2226–38. https://doi.org/10.1053/j.gastro.2007.03.051.
10. Cooper Z, Fairburn CG, Hawker DM. Cognitive-behavioral treatment of obesity: a clinician's guide. New York: Guilford Press; 2003.
11. Butryn ML, Wadden TA. Behavioral treatment of obesity. In: Brownell KD, Walsh BT, editors. Eating disorders and obesity: a comprehensive handbook. 3rd ed. New York: Guilford Press; 2017. p. 512–8.
12. Jensen MD, Ryan DH, Apovian CM, Ard JD, Comuzzie AG, Donato KA, et al. AHA/ACC/TOS guideline for the management of overweight and obesity in adults: a report of the American College of Cardiology/American Heart Association Task Force on Practice Guidelines and The Obesity Society. J Am Coll Cardiol. 2014;63(25 Pt B):2985–3023. https://doi.org/10.1016/j.jacc.2013.11.004.
13. Wadden TA, Sternberg JA, Letizia KA, Stunkard AJ, Foster GD. Treatment of obesity by very low calorie diet, behavior therapy, and their combination: a five-year perspective. Int J Obes. 1989;13(Suppl 2):39–46.
14. Look AHEAD Research Group. Eight-year weight losses with an intensive lifestyle intervention: the look AHEAD study. Obesity (Silver Spring). 2014;22(1):5–13. https://doi.org/10.1002/oby.20662.
15. McGuire MT, Wing RR, Klem ML, Hill JO. Behavioral strategies of individuals who have maintained long-term weight losses. Obes Res. 1999;7(4):334–41.
16. Jansen A, Houben K, Roefs A. A cognitive profile of obesity and its translation into new interventions. Front Psychol. 2015;6:1807. https://doi.org/10.3389/fpsyg.2015.01807.
17. Dalle Grave R, Calugi S, Marchesini G. The influence of cognitive factors in the treatment of obesity: lessons from the QUOVADIS study. Behav Res Ther. 2014;63:157–61. https://doi.org/10.1016/j.brat.2014.10.004.

18. Melchionda N, Marchesini G, Apolone G, Cuzzolaro M, Mannucci E, Grossi E. The QUOVADIS study: features of obese Italian patients seeking treatment at specialist centers. Diabetes Nutr Metab. 2003;16(2):115–24.
19. Dalle Grave R, Calugi S, Molinari E, Petroni ML, Bondi M, Compare A, et al. Weight loss expectations in obese patients and treatment attrition: an observational multicenter study. Obes Res. 2005;13(11):1961–9. https://doi.org/10.1038/oby.2005.241.
20. Dalle Grave R, Calugi S, Marchesini G, Beck-Peccoz P, Bosello O, Compare A, et al. Personality features of obese women in relation to binge eating and night eating. Psychiatry Res. 2013;207(1–2):86–91. https://doi.org/10.1016/j.psychres.2012.09.001.
21. Dalle Grave R, Calugi S, Compare A, El Ghoch M, Petroni ML, Tomasi F, et al. Weight loss expectations and attrition in treatment-seeking obese women. Obes Facts. 2015;8(5):311–8. https://doi.org/10.1159/000441366.
22. Grossi E, Dalle Grave R, Mannucci E, Molinari E, Compare A, Cuzzolaro M, et al. Complexity of attrition in the treatment of obesity: clues from a structured telephone interview. Int J Obes. 2006;30(7):1132–7. https://doi.org/10.1038/sj.ijo.0803244.
23. Teixeira PJ, Going SB, Sardinha LB, Lohman TG. A review of psychosocial pre-treatment predictors of weight control. Obes Rev. 2005;6(1):43–65. https://doi.org/10.1111/j.1467-789X.2005.00166.x.
24. Fabricatore AN, Wadden TA, Womble LG, Sarwer DB, Berkowitz RI, Foster GD, et al. The role of patients' expectations and goals in the behavioral and pharmacological treatment of obesity. Int J Obes. 2007;31(11):1739–45. https://doi.org/10.1038/sj.ijo.0803649.
25. Lent MR, Vander Veur SS, Peters JC, Herring SJ, Wyatt HR, Tewksbury C, et al. Initial weight loss goals: have they changed and do they matter? Obes Sci Pract. 2016;2(2):154–61. https://doi.org/10.1002/osp4.45.
26. Dalle Grave R, Calugi S, Corica F, Di Domizio S, Marchesini G. Psychological variables associated with weight loss in obese patients seeking treatment at medical centers. J Am Diet Assoc. 2009;109(12):2010–6. https://doi.org/10.1016/j.jada.2009.09.011.
27. Calugi S, Marchesini G, El Ghoch M, Gavasso I, Dalle Grave R. The influence of weight-loss expectations on weight loss and of weight-loss satisfaction on weight maintenance in severe obesity. J Acad Nutr Diet. 2016;117:32–8. https://doi.org/10.1016/j.jand.2016.09.001.
28. Perri MG, Sears SF Jr, Clark JE. Strategies for improving maintenance of weight loss: toward a continuous care model of obesity management. Diabetes Care. 1993;16(1):200–9.
29. Calugi S, Marchesini G, El Ghoch M, Gavasso I, Dalle Grave R. The association between weight maintenance and session-by-session diet adherence, weight loss and weight-loss satisfaction. Eat Weight Disord. 2018. https://doi.org/10.1007/s40519-018-0528-8.
30. Fairburn CG. Cognitive behavior therapy and eating disorders. New York: Guilford Press; 2008.
31. Cooper Z, Fairburn CG. A new cognitive behavioural approach to the treatment of obesity. Behav Res Ther. 2001;39(5):499–511.
32. Stahre L, Tarnell B, Hakanson CE, Hallstrom T. A randomized controlled trial of two weight-reducing short-term group treatment programs for obesity with an 18-month follow-up. Int J Behav Med. 2007;14(1):48–55. https://doi.org/10.1080/10705500701317070.
33. Werrij MQ, Jansen A, Mulkens S, Elgersma HJ, Ament AJ, Hospers HJ. Adding cognitive therapy to dietetic treatment is associated with less relapse in obesity. J Psychosom Res. 2009;67(4):315–24. https://doi.org/10.1016/j.jpsychores.2008.12.011.
34. Forman EM, Butryn ML, Manasse SM, Crosby RD, Goldstein SP, Wyckoff EP, et al. Acceptance-based versus standard behavioral treatment for obesity: results from the mind your health randomized controlled trial. Obesity (Silver Spring). 2016;24(10):2050–6. https://doi.org/10.1002/oby.21601.
35. Cooper Z, Doll HA, Hawker DM, Byrne S, Bonner G, Eeley E, et al. Testing a new cognitive behavioural treatment for obesity: a randomized controlled trial with three-year follow-up. Behav Res Ther. 2010;48(8):706–13. https://doi.org/10.1016/j.brat.2010.03.008.

2 Treatment Overview

In this chapter, we provide an overview of CBT-OB, describing its goals, main strategies and procedures and how it has been adapted for different settings. We then go on to discuss the respective roles of patient and therapist and how to optimise the environments in which the treatment is delivered. Finally, we report upon our experience of administering CBT-OB in the real world, presenting the data we have obtained thus far on its effectiveness.

2.1 Goals

The primary goals of CBT-OB are to help patients to (1) reach, accept and maintain a healthy weight loss; (2) adopt a lifestyle conducive to weight control; and (3) develop a stable "weight-control mindset".

Being able to reach, accept and maintain a healthy—but not necessarily "normal"—weight is a vital goal, as no available treatment (including bariatric surgery) has demonstrated efficacy in terms of helping the majority of patients with obesity to achieve and maintain a "normal" weight (i.e. a BMI of between 18.5 and 24.9). Several studies have, however, shown that a more achievable weight reduction target, of 5–10%, is able to reduce the main health risks associated with obesity and produce numerous psychological benefits [1].

As for the goal of making weight control a central part of life, this distinguishes CBT-OB from traditional dietary treatment in at least three fundamental ways. Firstly, it underscores the long-term change that will be required if patients are to lose weight and keep it off. Secondly, it shifts the emphasis from physical appearance (which, as we have already seen, is a motivation associated with treatment failure) to physical health; patients are taught the importance of developing a healthy lifestyle with a view to obtaining the significant health benefits it is associated with, irrespective of the total amount of weight lost. Last but not least, it directs patients' attention away from the unpredictable nature of weight modification in favour of more controllable—and therefore achievable—changes in lifestyle. As discussed

R. Dalle Grave et al., *Treating Obesity with Personalized Cognitive Behavioral Therapy*, https://doi.org/10.1007/978-3-319-91497-8_2

above, satisfaction with outcomes is a strong incentive for continuing treatment, and moving the onus away from a single, ultimate goal (i.e. losing an unachievable amount of weight) may promote adherence.

Similarly, the "weight-control mindset" goal sets apart CBT-OB from BT-OB. Indeed, the latter pays scant attention to the cognitive processes influencing the control of weight, as its primary aim is to change eating and physical activity habits. CBT-OB, on the other hand, is designed to foster cognitive change, enabling patients to take control of their own mindset and therefore their obesity, with a view to promoting long-term change.

2.2 Strategies and Procedures

2.2.1 General Strategies and Procedures

CBT-OB uses a therapeutic style similar to that of generic cognitive behavioural therapy. In other words, it is based on the development of a collaborative working relationship in which the therapist and patients work together as team. Like other treatments, it involves providing specific physical activity and dietary recommendations, in addition to some procedures adopted by standard BT-OB programmes (such as self-monitoring, goal setting, stimulus control, contingency management, behavioural substitution, skills for increasing social support, problem solving, and relapse prevention) [2]. However, CBT-OB also includes a battery of specific cognitive behavioural strategies and procedures. These enable the treatment to be individualised and to help patients to address the processes that previous research has found to be, respectively, associated with treatment discontinuation, the amount of weight lost and long-term weight-loss maintenance. Some of these procedures have been developed by our team, while others have been adapted from of Cooper et al.'s cognitive behavioural therapy for obesity [3], enhanced cognitive behavioural therapy (CBT-E) [4] and multistep CBT-E for eating disorders [5], as well as dialectical behavioural therapy (DBT) [6] and relapse prevention for substance abuse (RPSA) [7].

CBT-OB places great emphasis on engaging patients in their own treatment; they are encouraged to make the treatment a priority and to play an active role in changing their own habits. As in generic cognitive behavioural therapy, self-monitoring in real time and doing the strategically planned "homework" tasks are of fundamental importance. Unlike generic cognitive behavioural therapy, however (but like CBT-E [4]), CBT-OB does not require that patients keep a formal "thought record", although the last column of their Monitoring Record may be used for this purpose at certain stages of the treatment. For example, patients may be asked to record the events, thoughts and feelings that arise when they encounter an obstacle to weight loss or weight maintenance, with a view to heightening self-awareness and identifying any personal triggers. Moreover, in CBT-OB, no explicit reference is made to several concepts adopted by generic cognitive behavioural therapy, such as schema, assumptions and automatic thoughts. Although CBT-OB addresses some cognitive bias, such as dichotomous thinking and generalisation, it does not frequently use cognitive restructuring. Instead, it promotes cognitive change by encouraging patients to change the way that they behave and analysing the effects and implications of such behavioural changes [4]. Patients are encouraged to observe themselves and to identify their individual obstacles to adopting a lifestyle that will enable them to lose weight and keep off the weight that they have lost. The idea is to get them interested in the effects and implications of trying different ways of behaving.

Once they have developed new eating and physical activity habits and a persistent weight-control mindset, patients are helped to identify stimuli that are likely to reinstate their weight-gain mindset and to recognise the signs that this is occurring; they are then taught how to take action immediately, to "Do the right thing"—generally the opposite of the behaviour driven by the weight-gain mindset [4]. In this way, patients learn to manipulate not only their behaviour but also their frame of mind. The theory is that, with these skills, patients are able to deal more effectively with weight gain and to respond immediately and effectively to setbacks that might otherwise develop into full-scale relapse.

Since early weight-loss success is a good predictor of long-term weight loss [8], the frequency of sessions in initial stage of CBT-OB is higher to help patients "start well". As we have seen, early success makes patients satisfied with the weight loss achieved so far and reduces the risk of early dropout. With this in mind, some patients, i.e. those with disability, may benefit from the first part of CBT-OB being delivered in more intensive settings, such as day hospital or residential units (see Chap. 12) [9].

2.2.2 Strategies and Procedures for Minimising Attrition

As mentioned, attrition is one of the major causes of the failure of treatments for obesity, which occurs in about 50% of cases in real-world clinical settings [10]. Adherence to treatment is therefore a key factor for long-term weight-loss success [11, 12], and, with this in mind, therapists should do their best to help patients complete the treatment. As described in Chap. 1, we have already identified several baseline predictors of early treatment discontinuation which need to be taken into consideration, namely, younger age, higher weight-loss expectations and improving appearance as a primary goal for losing weight. Moreover, in another joint study, we asked patients with obesity their reasons for attrition [13]. More than half of dropouts reported practical difficulties—such as family problems, problems at work and logistics—as the leading causes of attrition. These were followed by perceived failure of treatment, lack of motivation, sense of abandonment and a poor interaction with their therapists. CBT-OB therefore includes specific strategies designed to address many of these factors with a view to minimising patient attrition.

To address a patient's practical difficulties, and thereby promote adherence, CBT-OB recommends that therapists routinely ask whether they are experiencing any difficulties as regards attending the sessions (e.g. the time of day for appointments, the time it takes to get to and from sessions, etc.). If such a barrier is identified, the therapists should devote time to understanding and/or overcoming it. Needless to say, sessions should always be scheduled at times compatible with a patient's work commitments.

Indeed, it is firmly recommended that CBT-OB therapists do their best to show that they are interested in each patient as a person, irrespective of their weight and/or other issues. It is crucial to avoid any attitude that might be perceived as stigmatising by the patients. In fact, "abandonment syndrome" is reported by several patients with obesity and cited as one of the major reasons for treatment discontinuation, and it appears that this is in part derived from the social stigma of obesity [14]. Persons with obesity are often reminded that their body frame deviates from social norms by everyday contacts with family members, peers, healthcare providers and casual acquaintances, and, accordingly, they experience a pattern of denigration and condemnation reported as "civilized oppression" [14]. This may be a major cause of attrition, and therapists must therefore take steps to ensure that they are not unwittingly contributing to this condition. Since the terminology and language used to describe body weight may be offensive and perceived as stigmatising to persons with obesity, as suggested by a document published by the Rudd Center for Food Policy and Obesity, The Obesity Society (TOS), Obesity Action Coalition (OAC), Obesity Medicine Association (OMA) and American Society for Metabolic and Bariatric Surgery (ASMBS) [15], CBT-OB therapists should avoid any use of potentially pejorative adjectives or adverbs or any language that implies moral judgements or highlights patients' "character flaws". For instance, the descriptive terms used by CBT-OB therapists to refer to body weight should be confined to clinical terms such as "obesity", "BMI", "weight" and "excess weight", rather than the stigmatising "fat", "weight problem" and "morbidly obese". Moreover, CBT-OB adopts the OAC's "People-First" policy—putting individuals before the disability or disease when describing persons affected by obesity [16], incorporating the appropriate Language for Obesity (e.g. stating "people with obesity have an increased risk of diabetes" instead of "obese people have an increased risk of diabetes").

Another key factor to bear in mind is the paradoxical problem associated with high weight-loss expectations (i.e. higher expectations are associated with treatment discontinuation but greater weight loss). CBT-OB does not attempt to tackle unrealistic expectations directly at the beginning of treatment, except for encouraging patients to pursue and be satisfied with achievable short-term weight-loss goals (i.e. a weight loss of between 0.5 kg and 1.0 kg/week). Unrealistic goals may be addressed later on, when patients have achieved some success in reaching intermediate goals, and have developed a trusting and collaborative relationship with the therapist, but manifest dissatisfaction with the weight loss achieved.

CBT-OB also places great emphasis on establishing and maintaining *therapeutic momentum* [4]. To this end the therapist encourages patients to identify the best time for them to embark on the CBT-OB programme, stressing the importance of avoiding any interruptions in treatment. In particular, patients need to be able to commit to not going away during the first 8 weeks. If, however, an unforeseen interruption is unavoidable, the therapist should try to arrange a weekly web chat or telephone session following the usual session structure (bar the in-session weighing). Likewise, therapists should do their best to be consistently available to the patient. In the event of any necessary absence, the CBT-OB therapist should explain to the patient in advance that they will have to be away but that another therapist will take their place so that the treatment can continue virtually uninterrupted. Interestingly, it is our experience that patients always agree to this arrangement, seeming to prefer it to missing sessions.

In a similar vein, CBT-OB has developed a protocol for dealing with late attendance or non-attendance. The therapist should try to prevent this problem by encouraging patients to arrive a little early for session (e.g. 10–15 min) in order to relax and mentally prepare themselves. Patients are asked to let the therapist know as soon as possible if they are unable to attend a specific appointment, so that this can be rescheduled and the slot offered to another patient. If patients are running late for an appointment, it is important that the therapist call them after 15 min and express concern about their absence. It may be that patients have decided to drop out, and this is an ideal opportunity for therapist to determine why (perhaps they feel they are not losing enough weight and the programme is not working). Once the cause of the absence has been ascertained, the therapist should try to reschedule the appointment as soon as possible and make addressing these issues a priority.

Encouragingly, by adopting the strategies described above, our clinic has registered a progressive decline in dropout rate from 30% to 15–20%.

2.2.3 Strategies and Procedures for Enhancing Weight Loss

To increase dietary restraint and decrease dietary disinhibition—two cognitive factors that, as we have seen, predict the amount of weight loss—CBT-OB incorporates several specific strategies designed to help patients improve their adherence to the meal plan.

Firstly, since it has been found that adherence to diet may be enhanced by increasing diet structure and limiting food choices—thereby reducing temptation and potential mistakes in the calculation of energy intake [17]—CBT-OB suggests to patients that they plan meals in advance on a specific Monitoring Record. They should record when, what and where they are going to eat and make reference to the structured meal plans recommended to them by the therapist [18]. These serve both to provide a structural framework to the diet (promoting adherence) and, indirectly, to increase dietary restraint and reduce dietary disinhibition. As part of the CBT-OB programme, patients are also supplied with grocery lists, menus and recipes.

It is important for patients to adopt a regular eating procedure, and they are encouraged to eat three meals per day, plus two planned snacks (which they should plan in advance on their Monitoring Record), and to refrain from eating in the intervals between. Indeed, data from CBT-E for eating disorders has consistently shown that this procedure significantly reduces the frequency of overeating and binge-eating episodes [4].

As well as for meal planning, CBT-OB suggests that patients use their Monitoring Record in real time, to check off or amend their meal plan in the precise moment at which food and drink is consumed. This strategy provides an accurate picture of a patient's eating habits and brings to their attention any obstacles to weight loss; it serves to increase patients' awareness of what they are doing while they are eating and thereby helps to interrupt dysfunctional and automatic eating habits that previously seemed uncontrollable [4].

Indeed, CBT-OB trains patients to eat consciously (i.e. "think while you are eating") following the planned meals and snacks without being influenced by external (e.g. the sight of food, events) or internal eating cues (e.g. cravings, the need for gratification, hunger, thoughts of food, changes in mood). This is an integral part of developing a mindset focused on weight loss and needs to be applied until the new way of eating (facilitated by the real-time monitoring of food intake) becomes an automatic habit that does not require continuous cognitive effort. To overcome short-term aversive experiences (e.g. hunger and craving for highly palatable foods) and loss of pleasure (e.g. not eating dessert) that may accompany such dietary restraint, patients are asked to "ride it out" and to see that these impulses are transitory states that they can tolerate. Patients are encouraged to consider this effort as a necessary condition of their reaching a healthy weight, which would allow them to benefit from the physical and psychological advantages that this would bring.

Another procedure that is fundamental for patients developing a weight-loss mindset is their identification of any personal obstacles to weight loss. Hence, CBT-OB actively involves patients in a collaborative review of their Monitoring Records, and they are asked to complete the "Weight-Loss Obstacles Questionnaire" (see Appendix D) on a weekly basis. Thus identified, these obstacles will be included in the patients' cognitive behavioural formulation—a visual representation (a flow chart) of the cognitive behavioural processes that are acting to obstruct their adhesion to the lifestyle changes needed to lose weight. This procedure helps to personalise CBT-OB and ensures that only procedures aimed at addressing the specific obstacles encountered by each patient are incorporated into the treatment.

Last but not least, CBT-OB takes into account the influence that a person's social environment may have on their ability to lose weight. As such, and with the consent of the patient, their significant other(s) (i.e. partner or parental figures) are involved in the treatment through joint sessions. By educating and involving significant others, they can be recruited to aid in the creation of the optimal environment for facilitating a patient's attempt to change their eating habits [4].

2.2.4 Strategies and Procedures for Improving Weight-Loss Maintenance

As reported above, increased dietary restraint and reduced dietary disinhibition help patients to adhere to the diet, lose more weight and be satisfied with the weight loss they have achieved. These three factors are interlinked and associated with long-term weight maintenance, which is why they are a focus of the treatment from the very beginning. However, CBT-OB also includes several other strategies that are designed to help patients to maintain the weight they have lost.

First, during the weight-loss phase, CBT-OB therapists assess dietary adherence, weight-loss rate and weight-loss satisfaction session by session, by means of the "Weight-Loss Obstacles Questionnaire" (see Appendix D). If a patient reports a reduction in one or more of the three factors that our research has found to be associated with weight regain, namely, dietary adherence, a decline in weight loss rate and/or a reduction weight-loss satisfaction (7 or less on the Likert (0–10) scale), the therapist should implement the procedures designed to address weight-loss dissatisfaction (described in Module 5).

The CBT-OB weight-maintenance phase follows the recommendations in the AHA/ACC/TOS Guidelines for the Management of Overweight and Obesity in Adults [1] in that it has a duration of 48 weeks. Patients are, however, invited to attend post-treatment review sessions at 3-month intervals after the end of treatment for at least 1 year. This maintenance phase of about 12 months has been included due to the data emerging from some studies that patients who attend continuous care of similar duration after the weight-loss phase tend to better maintain the weight they have lost in comparison to those who are not followed up on [19].

Before commencing the weight-maintenance phase, one or two CBT-OB sessions should be dedicated to preparing patients for weight maintenance. This will entail patients agreeing to stop any attempts to lose weight and instead dedicate themselves to learning and practicing the skills required to maintain weight for a long period of time. This needs to be reiterated during the weight-maintenance phase itself, which includes several procedures designed to hone their weight-control mindset and maintain a healthy lifestyle to ensure that they do not regain weight in the long term. Specifically, patients are encouraged to:

- Establish weekly self-weighing, a procedure found to be associated with better weight maintenance [20], and ensure they maintain weight within a specific range of 4 kg.
- Adopt specific eating and physical activity habits that research has found to be associated with better weight maintenance, such as a high-protein, low-glycaemic-index diet with moderate fat content [21] and burning on average about 2600 kcal/week through physical activity (i.e. ~60–75 min/day of moderate-intensity physical activity such as brisk walking) [22].
- Build a mindset centred around weight maintenance by creating a list of personal reasons to maintain weight to refer to, persisting in adhering to the newly acquired eating and exercise habits and keeping a constant but flexible focus on weight control and self-awareness regarding their diet and physical activity.
- Identify and address the eraly sign of weight regain in order to prevent a lapse becoming a relapse and to deal with any weight regain in a timely and effective fashion.

Towards the end of the weight-maintenance phase, patients are encouraged to discontinue real-time self-monitoring of food intake, to discuss and prepare for possible future weight-loss attempts and to collaboratively create a written weight-maintenance plan with the therapist.

2.3 The Versions of CBT-OB

CBT-OB is delivered within a *stepped-care* approach, i.e. one that can be applied, with appropriate adaptation, at three levels of care (outpatient, day hospital and residential) to treat all classes of obesity. For this reason, the treatment is referred to as "multistep CBT-OB" [9].

Outpatient CBT-OB can be delivered individually or in group sessions, led, respectively, by a single therapist or two therapists. It includes the following phases (Fig. 2.1):

- Preparatory Phase. This comprises one or two sessions aimed at assessing the nature and the severity of a patient's obesity, as well as any associated medical and psychosocial comorbidities, and engaging patients in the treatment.

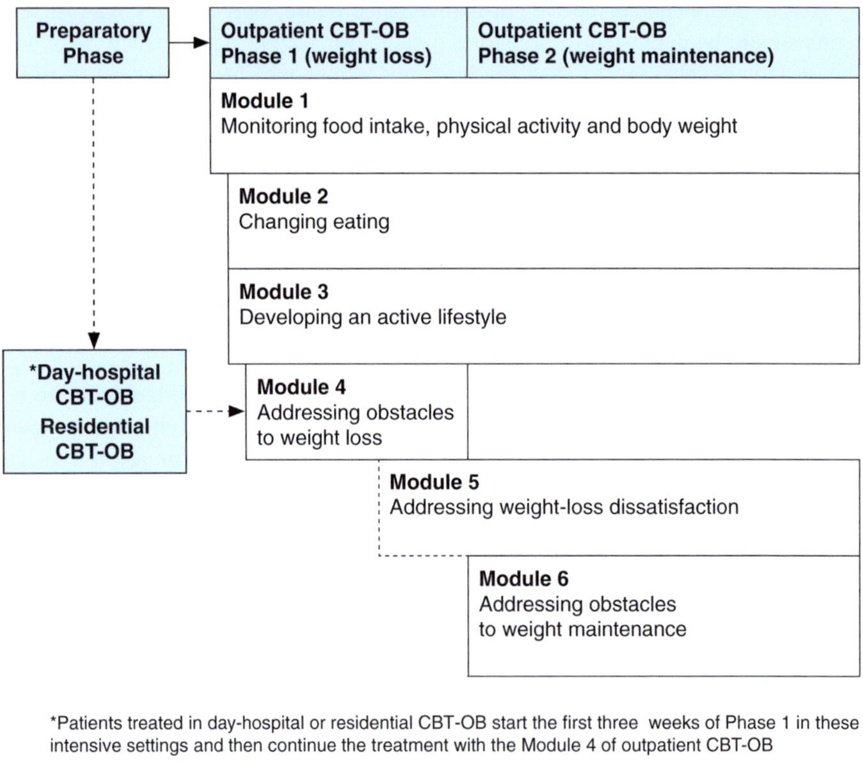

Fig. 2.1 The map of personalised cognitive behavioural therapy for obesity (CBT-OB)

- Phase 1. This is the weight-loss phase, which is aimed at helping patients to achieve a healthy weight loss (e.g. a weight loss of at least 10%) and to be satisfied with this weight. It usually lasts about 24 weeks and is delivered in 16 sessions, the first 8 of which are held once a week and the remainder every 2 weeks.
- Phase 2. This is the weight-maintenance phase, designed to help patients to develop a lifestyle and mindset conducive to keeping the weight off in the long term. It usually lasts 48 weeks and is delivered in 12 sessions held at 4-week intervals.

The strategies and procedures involved in CBT-OB are delivered across the following six modules:

- Module 1—Monitoring food intake, physical activity and body weight
- Module 2—Changing eating
- Module 3—Developing an active lifestyle
- Module 4—Addressing weight-loss obstacles
- Module 5—Addressing weight-loss dissatisfaction
- Module 6—Addressing weight-maintenance obstacles

In general, Module 1 is introduced in the first session, Modules 2 and 3 in the second session, Module 4 in the third session and Module 6 at the beginning of Phase 2, with Module 5 being integrated when patients report weight-loss dissatisfaction unrelated to poor adherence to the recommended diet and physical activity. However, modules should be introduced in a flexible and individualised way, according to the patient's needs. Similarly, the strategies and procedures involved in each module should be adapted to each patient's individual progress and barriers.

That being said, 45 min (90 min when the treatment is delivered in group) should be set aside for each session, which will be divided into the following five parts:

1. In-session collaborative weighing (up to 5 min).
2. Reviewing the Monitoring Record and other homework (up to 10 min).
3. Collaboratively setting the agenda for the session (about 2 min). This should include issues that need to be addressed (identified during the homework review), items relevant to the treatment that patients want to discuss and new topics introduced by the therapist based on the particular stage in treatment.
4. Working through the agenda and agreeing on the homework task(s) (up to 30 min).
5. Concluding the session (about 3 min). This part of the session includes summarising what has been addressed in the session, reiterating the homework assignment(s) and arranging the next appointment.

Sessions are cumulative, meaning that the third session, for example, will include the topics, strategies and procedures introduced in Modules 1–4.

The treatment has also been adapted for delivery in more intensive settings—namely, day hospital and residential rehabilitation units—to benefit those who are more unwell (as assessed by the Comprehensive Appropriateness Scale for the Care of Obesity in Rehabilitation (CASCO-R); see Sect. 3.6). Intensive CBT-OB is a highly personalized approach (see Chap. 12) which adopts the same theory and procedures as the outpatient version, with the only difference being the intensity of treatment. In particular, intensive CBT-OB enables the management of patients with severe comorbidities and disability associated with obesity, who, incidentally, are not usually included in traditional weight-loss lifestyle-modification trials.

The day hospital and residential CBT-OB "steps" both last 21 days and are delivered by a non-eclectic multidisciplinary team composed of physicians, dieticians, psychologists, physiotherapists and nurses who have all been trained in CBT-OB. Each patient is given an individualised rehabilitation programme that includes the following principal procedures: (1) a low-energy diet (LED), (2) a motor/functional rehabilitation program and (3) a daily group CBT-OB session in which patients are actively trained to use the procedures in Modules 1–3 of outpatient CBT-OB. Once patients have completed this intensive phase, they are advised to "step down" and continue their CBT-OB treatment in an outpatient setting. Since such patients have already implemented the procedures in Modules 1–3 (generally delivered during the first two sessions of outpatient CBT-OB; see Fig. 2.1) during the intensive CBT-OB phase, post-intensive outpatient treatment does not include these.

It is also important to note that CBT-OB is not a barrier to weight-loss drugs and/or bariatric surgery, which may be seamlessly integrated in selected cases (see Chap. 14).

2.4 The Role of the Patient

Patients are advised that CBT-OB distinguishes itself from most treatments for obesity because it does not adopt a "prescriptive" approach, but rather collaborative procedures designed to empower patients, enabling them to take control of their own behaviour. In other words, patients will never be asked to do things that they do not agree to. Instead, they will be led through the following four steps:

1. Education on specific issues that need to be addressed (e.g. an individual obstacle to meal plan adherence) and the mechanisms that are keeping them in place (e.g. a lack of tolerance of food "cravings")
2. Discussion of the pros and cons of addressing these obstacles and maintenance mechanisms, with a view to achieving consensus on the benefits of change
3. Collaborative planning of the procedures that will be required to address the patient's individual obstacles and maintenance mechanisms and agreement on the necessary maximum commitment to these procedures
4. Review of the outcomes of the procedures applied

It is clear that CBT-OB requires patients to play an active role during and between sessions if they are to change their habits, and the treatment has little possibility of success if patients are not wholeheartedly committed. Hence, CBT-OB suggests that patients consider treatment a priority and "start well", since, as previously mentioned, the amount of weight lost in the first 2 months is predictive of long-term weight loss [8]. The motto we advise patients to adopt is the following: "It'll be hard, but it'll be worth it".

Patients are told that they will have to work collaboratively with the therapist as a team and that together they will agree on specific homework tasks that will have to be done between sessions. It should be emphasised that the homework is of fundamental importance for the success of treatment, and it should therefore be given absolute priority. Indeed, it is what the patients do between sessions that will determine the outcome of the treatment.

To foster commitment, patients are also told that it is important for every session to begin and end on time. As previously stated, they are encouraged to arrive 10–15 min in advance, which will give them the opportunity to relax and prepare the topics that will be addressed in the session.

Finally, patients are advised to avoid any interruption in treatment, as this will obstruct the therapeutic momentum needed for the creation of the new habits and weight-control mindset that will enable them to overcome their obesity.

2.5 The Role of the Therapist

Therapists who desire to practice personalised CBT-OB must be familiar with obesity and its medical and psychosocial complications, the cognitive behavioural perspective of the processes hindering weight loss and weight maintenance, the details of the treatment and the CBT-OB formulation (i.e. conceptualisation of the case). Ideally, the therapist should have completed specific training in CBT-OB (please contact us for further information), have experience working with patients with obesity and be able to recognise and address the medical complications of obesity, or have access to other specialists that are able to do it. Clinical expertise is the most important factor, but please bear in mind that therapists with current overweight or obesity may be disadvantaged in terms of engaging the patients in the treatment. That being said, personal experience may help a therapist to set a personal example in terms of accepting a moderate but healthy weight loss within the condition of obesity. Finally, the therapist should be active and empathetic, but also firm when needed. They should dedicate their efforts to working collaboratively with the patient, keeping them engaged in the treatment and lifestyle change, taking care to avoid any interruptions in the treatment.

2.6 The Office Environment

An appropriate office environment is essential for effectively managing patients with obesity. Patients with obesity should be made comfortable, and embarrassment should be avoided at all costs. Attention to patients' practical needs demonstrates understanding and sensitivity. Some suggestions for establishing an appropriate treatment setting for these patients are the following:

- The office should be free of architectural barriers (e.g. steep steps), easily accessible by public transport and near to a car park.
- Chairs in the waiting room should be strong, capacious and without armrests.
- Weighing scales should be suitable for heavier patients, with a wide, sturdy base.
- Sphygmomanometers used to measure blood pressure should have an ample cuff.
- All of the office staff (doctors, psychologists, dieticians, interns and secretaries, etc.) should be empathetic, respectful and devoid of prejudice against patients with obesity.
- Educational material and manuals for the management of obesity should be easily accessible to patients.

2.7 The Effectiveness of CBT-OB

The effectiveness of CBT-OB, as described above and below, has been assessed in 88 patients with severe obesity, allocated either to a high-protein diet (HPD) or a high-carbohydrate diet (HCD), as part of a randomised control trial [23]. The specific version of treatment studied in this trial included 3 weeks of residential CBT-OB followed by a course of outpatient CBT-OB. Encouragingly, the attrition rate observed in both the HPD (25.6%) and HCD (17.8%) groups was far lower than the 50% attrition rate commonly reported for standard weight-loss treatments delivered in a community setting [13]. Among completers ($n = 69$), weight loss at 43 weeks was 15% for HPD and 13.3% for HCD, with no significant difference in this regard being noted between the two arms throughout the study period. It should be stressed that the percentage weight loss achieved by both of these arms was much higher than the mean 8%–10% typically reported in conventional BT-OB-based lifestyle-modification programmes. Equally importantly, both diets produced a similar improvement in cardiovascular risk factors and psychological profiles, and no tendency to regain weight was observed at either 6 or 12 months after CBT-OB.

In fact, in another study, comparing the long-term effects of residential CBT-OB in 54 patients with severe obesity and with or without binge-eating disorder (BED), 51.5% of the former group no longer met the diagnostic criteria for BED at 5 years of follow-up [24]. There was no difference between the two groups of patients in terms of mean weight loss (6.3 kg in BED vs. 7.4 kg in non-BED), despite the fact that patients in this study received no outpatient CBT-OB after discharge.

With a view to building on these promising findings, two observational studies conducted in a real-world clinical setting are currently underway. One is designed to assess outpatient CBT-OB delivered to individuals, and one to evaluate the same treatment administered in group sessions.

References

1. Jensen MD, Ryan DH, Apovian CM, Ard JD, Comuzzie AG, Donato KA, et al. AHA/ACC/TOS guideline for the management of overweight and obesity in adults: a report of the American College of Cardiology/American Heart Association Task Force on Practice Guidelines and The

Obesity Society. J Am Coll Cardiol. 2014;63(25 Pt B):2985–3023. https://doi.org/10.1016/j.jacc.2013.11.004.

2. Butryn ML, Wadden TA. Behavioral treatment of obesity. In: Brownell KD, Walsh BT, editors. Eating disorders and obesity: a comprehensive handbook. 3rd ed. New York: Guilford Press; 2017. p. 512–8.
3. Cooper Z, Fairburn CG, Hawker DM. Cognitive-behavioral treatment of obesity: a clinician's guide. New York: Guilford Press; 2003.
4. Fairburn CG. Cognitive behavior therapy and eating disorders. New York: Guilford Press; 2008.
5. Dalle Grave R. Multistep cognitive behavioral therapy for eating disorders: theory, practice, and clinical cases. New York: Jason Aronson; 2013.
6. Linehan MM. Cognitive behavioral treatment of borderline personality disorder. New York: Guilford Press; 1993.
7. Marlatt GA, George WH. Relapse prevention: introduction and overview of the model. Br J Addict. 1984;79(3):261–73.
8. Unick JL, Neiberg RH, Hogan PE, Cheskin LJ, Dutton GR, Jeffery R, et al. Weight change in the first 2 months of a lifestyle intervention predicts weight changes 8 years later. Obesity (Silver Spring). 2015;23(7):1353–6. https://doi.org/10.1002/oby.21112.
9. Dalle Grave R, Sartirana M, El Ghoch M, Calugi S. Personalized multistep cognitive behavioral therapy for obesity. Diabetes Metab Syndr Obes. 2017;10:195–206. https://doi.org/10.2147/DMSO.S139496.
10. Dalle Grave R, Calugi S, Compare A, El Ghoch M, Petroni ML, Tomasi F, et al. Weight loss expectations and attrition in treatment-seeking obese women. Obes Facts. 2015;8(5):311–8. https://doi.org/10.1159/000441366.
11. Dalle Grave R, Melchionda N, Calugi S, Centis E, Tufano A, Fatati G, et al. Continuous care in the treatment of obesity: an observational multicentre study. J Intern Med. 2005;258(3):265–73. https://doi.org/10.1111/j.1365-2796.2005.01524.x.
12. Perri MG, Sears SF Jr, Clark JE. Strategies for improving maintenance of weight loss: toward a continuous care model of obesity management. Diabetes Care. 1993;16(1):200–9.
13. Grossi E, Dalle Grave R, Mannucci E, Molinari E, Compare A, Cuzzolaro M, et al. Complexity of attrition in the treatment of obesity: clues from a structured telephone interview. Int J Obes. 2006;30(7):1132–7. https://doi.org/10.1038/sj.ijo.0803244.
14. Rogge MM, Greenwald M, Golden A. Obesity, stigma, and civilized oppression. ANS Adv Nurs Sci. 2004;27(4):301–15.
15. Rudd Center for Food Policy and Obesity. Guidelines for media portrayals of individuals affected by obesity http://www.uconnruddcenter.org/files/Pdfs/Media_Guidelines.pdf.
16. Obesity Action Coalition (OAC). People-first language for obesity. Tampa, Florida; 2017. http://www.obesityaction.org/weight-bias-and-stigma/people-first-language-for-obesity.
17. Fabricatore AN. Behavior therapy and cognitive-behavioral therapy of obesity: is there a difference? J Am Diet Assoc. 2007;107(1):92–9. https://doi.org/10.1016/j.jada.2006.10.005.
18. Wing RR, Jeffery RW, Burton LR, Thorson C, Nissinoff KS, Baxter JE. Food provision vs structured meal plans in the behavioral treatment of obesity. Int J Obes Relat Metab Disord. 1996;20(1):56–62.
19. Middleton KM, Patidar SM, Perri MG. The impact of extended care on the long-term maintenance of weight loss: a systematic review and meta-analysis. Obes Rev. 2012;13(6):509–17. https://doi.org/10.1111/j.1467-789X.2011.00972.x.
20. Shieh C, Knisely MR, Clark D, Carpenter JS. Self-weighing in weight management interventions: a systematic review of literature. Obes Res Clin Pract. 2016;10(5):493–519. https://doi.org/10.1016/j.orcp.2016.01.004.
21. Larsen TM, Dalskov SM, van Baak M, Jebb SA, Papadaki A, Pfeiffer AF, et al. Diets with high or low protein content and glycemic index for weight-loss maintenance. N Engl J Med. 2010;363(22):2102–13. https://doi.org/10.1056/NEJMoa1007137.
22. Catenacci VA, Ogden LG, Stuht J, Phelan S, Wing RR, Hill JO, et al. Physical activity patterns in the National Weight Control Registry. Obesity (Silver Spring). 2008;16(1):153–61. https://doi.org/10.1038/oby.2007.6.

23. Dalle Grave R, Calugi S, Gavasso I, El Ghoch M, Marchesini G. A randomized trial of energy-restricted high-protein versus high-carbohydrate, low-fat diet in morbid obesity. Obesity (Silver Spring). 2013;21(9):1774–81. https://doi.org/10.1002/oby.20320.
24. Calugi S, Ruocco A, El Ghoch M, Andrea C, Geccherle E, Sartori F, et al. Residential cognitive-behavioral weight-loss intervention for obesity with and without binge-eating disorder: a prospective case-control study with five-year follow-up. Int J Eat Disord. 2016;49(7):723–30. https://doi.org/10.1002/eat.22549.

3 Preparatory Phase

It is important that patients are adequately prepared to participate actively in the treatment, and for this reason, CBT-OB includes a dedicated Preparatory Phase. This generally lasts one or two sessions and has three main goals: (1) to assess the nature and severity of obesity using an obesity-focused history; (2) to engage patients in the treatment by adopting an engaging style, providing education on obesity and CBT-OB and involving them actively in the decision to change; and (3) deciding how best to proceed.

3.1 Developing a Collaborative and Trusting Relationship

A key strategy of CBT-OB is developing a collaborative and trusting relationship between the therapist and patient(s). This collaborative approach should be established at the first contact with the patients in the Preparatory Phase and continue throughout the entire duration of the treatment.

First the therapist should greet the patient warmly and make them feel at ease. A good "ice-breaker" question to start with is asking them whether the decision to come to the assessment interview was their own or whether they were advised to attend by others (e.g. family doctor, specialist, significant other). This question aids in the creation of an empathetic bond and may foster a patient's willingness to share information about their problems. To this end, the patient should be given all the time they need to describe their problems, without overloading them with questions and questionnaires. It is also worthwhile remembering to set aside time to answer any questions they may have.

R. Dalle Grave et al., *Treating Obesity with Personalized Cognitive Behavioral Therapy*, https://doi.org/10.1007/978-3-319-91497-8_3

3.2 Assessing the Nature and Severity of Obesity

After having put the patients at ease, the therapist should take an obesity-focused history. Table 3.1 shows a list of points that are usually addressed. They include asking first about general personal information and then about social circumstances that may have a bearing on treatment. Once this general information has been gathered, therapists should take a detailed history of the specifics of the patient's obesity, investigating its development (i.e. how the problem began), age of obesity onset

Table 3.1 List of points to address when assessing the nature and severity of obesity

Personal information:
• Age • Race • Marital status and attitude of spouse or significant other(s) towards the treatment • Education • Living situation (who is at home) • Children • Occupation and working hours • Interests
Weight history:
• Weight at different periods of life (birth, menarche or puberty, 20 years, before and after pregnancy, menopause) • Minimum and maximum weight • Age of obesity onset • Weight change in the last year • Events associated with weight gain
Previous treatments for obesity:
• Nature and duration • General compliance • Maximum weight loss and degree of satisfaction • Duration of weight-loss maintenance • Possible reasons for weight regain • Number of cycles of weight loss and regain
Current status:
• Current weight and height (measured) and calculation of body mass index (BMI)[a] • Waist circumference[b] • Menstrual status (in females) • Eating behaviour (e.g. portion size, food choice and frequency of food intake) • Binge-eating episodes: Frequency and triggers • Physical activity (nature and frequency of lifestyle activities and formal exercising) • Extreme weight control behaviours (e.g. self-induced vomiting, laxative and/or diuretic misuse): Frequency and triggers • Alcohol and/or substance misuse: Frequency and triggers • Body checking and body avoidance: Frequency and triggers

(continued)

- Overall view of shape and body parts and the importance of shape and weight in personal self-evaluation
- Effects of obesity on physical health, psychological wellbeing, social functioning and school and/or work-related performance

Weight goals and reasons for wanting to lose weight:

- Dream weight, desirable weight and maximum acceptable weight
- Reasons for wanting to lose weight (e.g. improving health, physical fitness, appearance, interpersonal relationships, self-confidence, etc.)

Barriers to weight loss:

- Personal (e.g. poor motivation, low self-efficacy, low mood, using food to modulate mood)
- External (e.g. difficulties in the family, stress at work, exposure to food during work)

Personal and family medical history:

- Current and past medical and psychiatric comorbidities
- Current medications
- Medical and psychiatric family history (including family history of obesity or eating problems)

[a]BMI < 18.5 (underweight), BMI 18.5 < 25.0 (normal weight), BMI 25.0 < 30.0 (overweight), BMI 30.0 < 35.0 (class I obesity), BMI 35.0 < 40.0 (class II obesity), BMI $\geq$40.0 (class III obesity [extreme obesity]). BMI $\geq$30.0 identifies adults who may be at increased risk of cardiovascular diseases (CVD) and other obesity-related conditions. BMI $\geq$30.0 identifies adults who may be at elevated risk of mortality from all causes [5]

[b]A waist circumference >88 cm in women and > 102 cm in men is associated with central fat distribution [6], and the greater the waist circumference, the greater is the risk of CVD, type 2 diabetes, and all-cause mortality [5]

(when it began) and what was happening in their life at the time. For many patients, the onset of obesity is associated with smoking cessation, change in life events (e.g. marriage, employment and illness), stressful events, initiation of medication, pregnancy and menopause (in women) [1].

The next step is to ask the patients about the nature of any previous attempts to treat their condition, taking particular care to note the extent of their compliance, the maximum weight lost, the degree of satisfaction with the weight loss achieved, the duration of weight-loss maintenance, possible reasons for weight regain and the number of cycles of weight loss and regain. Since it is common for patients to repeat the same behavioural patterns, this type of information may help both the therapist and patient to focus attention on specific, potentially recurring issues.

At this stage, the patient's current status should be thoroughly assessed. An exhaustive assessment will include the measurement of weight and height to calculate the BMI; waist circumference should also be measured (at the level of the iliac crest of the pelvis), as this is associated with an increased risk of cardiovascular disease. It is also clinically useful to collect the patient's short-term dietary history at this point, asking them to recall what they have eaten over the previous 24 h, how often they ate and how they judge their portion sizes and the type of food they eat. As part of this procedure, the therapist should also take the opportunity to enquire about any binge-eating episodes, extreme weight-control behaviours (e.g. self-induced vomiting, laxative and/or diuretic misuse) and/or alcohol and substance misuse. Their physical activity history should also be obtained, asking patients about their current engagement in lifestyle activities and formal exercising. It may be useful (if possible) to assess physical fitness at this stage, as described in Module 3, so that personalised physical recommendations can be suggested to the patient. They should also be asked about their attitude towards their appearance, assessing the frequency and nature of some behavioural expressions of negative body image, such as body checking and body avoidance, as well as their view on their overall shape and body parts, and the importance of shape and weight in personal self-evaluation. Patients should also be asked how obesity is affecting their health, psychological wellbeing, social functioning and school and/or work-related performance.

Without commenting, the therapist should also investigate the patient's personal weight goals and reasons for losing weight. Although these factors should not be addressed at this stage, as described in Chap. 1, our research indicates that weight-loss expectations can have a bearing on weight loss [2]. Once again, it is also important to bear in mind that higher weight-loss expectations are, like seeking weight loss to change appearance, associated with a higher rate of dropout [3, 4].

When assessing weight-loss expectations and reasons for losing weight, it is also helpful to analyse the patient's perceived general barriers to weight loss. These may be internal, like poor motivation, low self-efficacy, low mood and using food to modulate mood, or external, such as difficulties within the family, stress at work and exposure to food during work, and will be addressed later on (see Chap. 7).

The final step of a thorough evaluation is to obtain an accurate assessment of the physical, psychological and psychiatric history of the patient [1]. In particular, the therapist should ask about past or present mood disorders, as these are common among treatment-seeking patients with obesity and may be an obstacle to weight loss if not adequately addressed. It is also important to assess whether or not patients are taking any medications that may contribute to weight gain, and in particular if there was a change in the trajectory of body weight associated with starting a new drug [1]. Common drugs that may promote weight gain are antidiabetics (sulfonylureas, insulin), antidepressants (mirtazapine, amitriptyline, paroxetine), neuroleptics (olanzapine, clozapine), mood stabilisers (valproate, lithium), corticosteroids and beta-blockers (atenolol). Substitution with a medication that is not associated with weight gain should be considered (if possible). Finally, it is also important to assess the patient's family history of medical and psychiatric conditions, in particular a family history of obesity or eating problems [1].

In brief, recording a patient's obesity-focused history will enable the therapist to:

- Establish a collaborative and effective therapeutic relationship.
- Assess the severity of obesity.
- Assess the presence of any weight-associated risk factors and complications.
- Assess the indications and contraindications to weight loss (see Sect. 3.3).
- Identify the patient's weight goals and reasons for wanting to lose weight.
- Begin to relate the cognitive behavioural model to the individual obstacles to weight loss that will be included in the patient's Personal Formulation (Module 4; see Chap. 7).
- Modulate the intervention on the basis of the patient's specific issues.

The initial assessment can be improved by asking patients to fill in some self-report questionnaires, which can also be used as a "baseline" against which to evaluate the effects of CBT-OB. In our clinical practice, for example, we rely the following tools:

- *The Eating Disorder Questionnaire* (EDE-Q) [7, 8]. The EDE-Q is a self-report measure of relevant attitudes and behaviours of eating disorder over the previous 28 days. The items are rated on a 7-point forced-choice format (0–6), with higher scores reflecting greater severity of eating-disorder psychopathology or frequency of eating-disorder behaviours. Items are grouped into subscales (restraint, eating concern, weight concern and shape concern), and the global score is taken as the mean score of the four subscales. A number of behavioural measures (objective and subjective binge eating, vomiting, laxative and diuretic misuse, driven exercising) are also recorded to assess the behaviours and attitudes of eating disorder in the previous 28 days.
- *The Brief Symptom Inventory* (BSI) [9]. The BSI is a 53-item self-report tool that assesses psychological distress and psychiatric disorders over the previous 7 days. The Global Severity Index (GSI) is calculated from scores assigned to participants' responses.
- *The ORWELL-97* [10]. The ORWELL-97 is an 18-item questionnaire measuring obesity-related quality of life. For each item on the scale, patients are asked to score the intensity of the symptoms and the subjective relevance of these symptoms to their own lives. Scoring is based on a 4-point Likert scale, and the final score reflects the intensity and subjective relevance of physical and psychological distress generated by excess weight. Higher scores indicate higher levels of distress.

These tools should be administered at baseline, at the end of the weight-loss and weight-maintenance phases and at 12 months from the end of treatment. If we suspect the presence of an eating disorder (e.g. BED or bulimia nervosa), we use the *Eating Disorder Examination Interview* (EDE 17.0D) [11, 12] to confirm the diagnosis and to assess the core eating disorder psychopathology (i.e. the overvaluation of shape and weight) and behavioural symptoms (i.e. binge eating, self-induced vomiting, laxative misuse, diuretic misuse, excessive exercising and dietary restraint) over the preceding 28 days and over the previous 3 months; this enables us to make an accurate diagnosis of eating disorder according to the DSM-5.

3.3 Assessing the Indications and Contraindications to Weight Loss

According to the 2013 AHA/ACC/TOS Guideline for the Management of Overweight and Obesity in Adults [5], weight-loss treatment is indicated for (1) individuals with obesity and (2) individuals with overweight and one or more indicators of increased CVD risk (e.g. diabetes, pre-diabetes, hypertension, dyslipidaemia, elevated waist circumference) or other obesity-related comorbidities.

Weight loss is not indicated if individuals have a BMI <25 or are overweight but without indicators of increased CVD risk or other obesity-related comorbidities [5].

We also do not recommend weight loss via CBT-OB during pregnancy or breastfeeding or in individuals with bulimia nervosa, major depressive disorders and/or other severe diseases in which caloric restriction is contraindicated.

However, BED, an eating disorder characterised by recurrent episodes of binge eating (i.e. episodes of uncontrolled overeating) in the absence of recurrent inappropriate compensatory behaviours [13], is not a contraindication of CBT-OB. Nonetheless, as described in Chap. 13, the treatment should be adapted to such patients by including an initial preparatory stage of 5 weeks. We recommend using CBT-E for eating disorders for this purpose [14]. CBT-E aims to help patients regulate their eating and reduce the frequency of binge-eating episodes; any attempt to lose weight should be discouraged during this period.

3.4 Engaging the Patient in the Treatment

CBT-OB does not generally involve a long period of preparatory motivational work to engage patients in the treatment, because the treatment itself is inherently motivating. Patients generally readily engage once they feel that they are being listened to and understood. Hence, the therapist that successfully adopts an engaging style (see below) has a good chance of achieving early change. Patients should therefore be asked to share with the therapist their personal reasons and motives for losing weight, any previous history of weight-loss attempts, their attitude towards physical activity and if they feel ready to change. The aims, duration, organisation, procedures and potential outcomes of the treatment are also discussed with patients in the initial stages, which represent an opportunity to educate them about obesity and the benefits of weight loss—which in itself is likely to promote engagement.

3.4.1 Adopting an Engaging Style

The adoption of an engaging style is of vital importance for motivating the patient to change and establishing a trusting therapeutic relationship. The approach for engaging the patient varies on the basis of their individual degree of motivation to change, but in all cases it includes transmitting empathy, understanding and competence, instilling hope and providing a clear picture of what the treatment will involve.

Although there is no simple formula to becoming an engaging therapist, we include a list of general guidelines, which our clinical experience indicates may help to achieve this goal [15, 16]:

- *Conceptualisation of motivation*. Motivation is a dynamic entity that waxes and wanes as a function of shifting personal, cognitive, behavioural and environmental determinants. This means that CBT-OB therapists should pay continuous attention to a patient's motivation, not only during the engagement process but also throughout the course of treatment.

- *Collaborative therapeutic style*. CBT-OB therapists should adopt a collaborative therapeutic style as opposed to a confrontational approach [17]. The collaborative style of CBT is considered one of the main reasons for its greater success in engaging resistant patients with respect to other interventions [18].
- *Showing empathy*. Patients in general, and especially those with obesity—who tend to often receive criticism regarding their excess weight—appreciate a friendly therapist who shows interest in them as people.
- *Acceptance and change*. CBT-OB therapists should validate a patient's experiences within a balanced framework of acceptance and change, firmness and empathy [19].
- *Functional analysis*. CBT-OB therapists should involve each patient in a functional analysis of the pros and cons of lifestyle change, because change is facilitated by communicating in a way that elicits a person's own reasons for and advantages of change [15].
- *Rolling with resistance*. CBT-OB therapists should not address resistance with confrontation, but with a collaborative evaluation of the variables involved in maintaining their unhealthy lifestyle [15].
- *Supporting self-efficacy*. Self-efficacy refers to a person's belief that they are capable of adhering to a specific behaviour [20], and it plays an important role in achieving healthy behavioural change [21]. In the initial assessment interview, clinicians should already begin to promote self-efficacy by raising the hope that lifestyle changes are achievable. Later, during the programme itself, self-efficacy should be promoted by co-designing an individualised eating and physical activity plan that patients are confident they will be able to stick to.
- *Being sensitive to stigma against individuals with obesity*. Stigma influences a patient's decision to start treatment for obesity [22]. To avoid displaying any signs that could be interpreted as stigmatisation, clinicians should recognise that obesity is derived from a complex interaction of genetic, epigenetic, environmental, emotional, cognitive and behavioural factors that is only partially understood [23]; it is not simply the product of a lack of willpower, and patients should be never judged for their excess of weight; they should instead receive all the respect and support that they need [24].
- *Inviting questions*. CBT-OB therapists should ask patients if they have any doubts or questions. This will encourage engagement, commitment and the development of an open and empathetic therapeutic relationship.

3.4.2 Educating the Patient on Obesity and CBT-OB

A strategy that we find helpful in engaging patients is to ask them if they are interested in having some information about obesity and CBT-OB. If they respond yes, as always occurs, we provide them with the following general information:

- The causes of obesity are not fully known, but it appears to derive from a complex interaction of genetic and environmental factors, and some learned habits.

- Obesity is a chronic condition, like diabetes, and its management requires the adoption of a persistent lifestyle change and the development of a long-term weight-control mindset.
- The currently available treatments for obesity rarely allow people with obesity to reach and maintain a condition of normal weight.
- Fortunately, even a moderate weight loss of 5–10%, if maintained over time, reduces most of the physical complications associated with obesity and often produces significant psychosocial benefits.
- Most obesity treatments are able to produce this short-term weight loss in a large subgroup of patients but tend to fail in terms of helping patients to maintain the weight lost.
- CBT-OB has been designed to help patients to achieve and maintain a healthy weight.
- The treatment includes several strategies and procedures designed to help patients to develop specific skills and a mindset that will enable them to control their weight in the long term.
- The treatment is tailor-made to address their specific obesity issues and individual needs, and it will enable them to become an expert on their own condition and the processes that maintain it.
- The treatment is therefore divided into two phases: Phase 1, which lasts about 24 weeks and has the aim of helping patients to achieve and be satisfied with a healthy weight loss, and Phase 2, which lasts 48 weeks and has the aim of helping patients to develop a mindset and habits that will enable them to maintain the weight lost in the long term. In the first 8 weeks of Phase 1, sessions will take place once a week and thereafter every 2 weeks. Phase 2 sessions will take place every 4 weeks.
- During Phase 1, patients can expect to achieve a weight loss of between 0.5 and 1 kg/week. The amount of weight loss achievable does, however, vary considerably from person to person and week-by-week, as it is influenced by individual physical characteristics (e.g. age, gender, body weight) and by the degree of adherence to dietary and physical activity changes. There is also variation in how long people maintain the weight they have lost. However, CBT-OB has been specifically designed to reduce the risk of weight regain, and patients will learn and practice long-term weight-maintenance skills in Phase 2, in which they will be asked to interrupt any further weight-loss efforts and focus their endeavours solely on weight maintenance.
- After the end of the therapy, four review sessions will be scheduled at 3-month intervals to assess a patient's progress and how they are handling the almost inevitable setbacks.
- It is crucial not to have breaks in the treatment so as not to interrupt the "therapeutic momentum", in which patient and therapist work together to develop new eating and exercise habits and a long-term weight-control mindset.
- Each session will last 45 min, and it is important that it starts and finishes on time. It is also advisable to arrive 15 min before the appointment to have time to prepare the topics to address in the session. Likewise, the therapist will do their best to always be on time.

- The style of treatment is collaborative in nature, and patients must expect to play an "active" role in determining the content of the sessions. They will work together with the therapist to address their own obstacles to weight loss and maintenance, and from time to time agree on specific homework tasks that should be done between sessions. These tasks are of paramount importance, since it is what patients do between sessions that will determine the outcome of their treatment.
- The treatment should be seen as a priority that requires commitment and a radical change in lifestyle. The more effort is put into the treatment, the greater the rewards that can be attained.
- It is fundamental to "start well", because the amount of weight lost in the first and second months is a powerful predictor of weight loss in the long term.
- The treatment should be considered as a special opportunity to start a new, healthier life. As with every change, there are risks, but the benefits that the patient can get are enormous and include better health, improved physical fitness and self-confidence.
- Losing weight and keeping it off is hard, but will be worth it!

3.4.3 Involving the Patient Actively in the Decision to Change

Although logic would dictate that most of the adult patients seeking weight-loss treatment are motivated to lose weight, it is nonetheless advisable to discuss with them their reasons for and against losing weight and initiating lifestyle change. This can be achieved by collaboratively producing a list of pros and cons of lifestyle modification. It is best to start by asking patients to list their reasons against change—e.g. whether they are afraid or whether their current lifestyle provides them with perceived advantages that they would be unwilling to give up. Subsequently, patients should be asked to evaluate the benefits of change; the CBT-OB therapist should encourage patients to reflect on both the short- and long-term effects of changing their eating and exercise habits on body-weight control, and on their physical and psychosocial quality of life. This list of pros and cons, and the conclusions resulting thereof, should be written down in table form for future reference (see Table 3.2).

This table should then be analysed in detail together with the patient. During this discussion, the CBT-OB therapist should focus the patient's attention on their long-term goals, not just on the immediate future. Every reason for change should be positively reinforced. That being said, it is also important to deal with the cons of change, in order to help patients to reach the conclusion themselves that changing eating and exercise in a lasting way will be necessary for them to control body weight in the long term and to reduce the medical and psychosocial complications associated with obesity.

In practice, this often occurs naturally, when a patient begins to make statements such as "If lose weight I will be able to…"—a sign that they see their present lifestyle as problematic. Should this occur, clinicians should not forget to make a

Table 3.2 Example table showing individual pros and cons of losing weight

Reasons for not losing weight	Reasons for losing weight
I will have to resist feelings of hunger	*I will be in better shape*
I will have to give up snacks and dinners with friends	*I will improve my health*
I will have to cope with my emotions without	*I will reduce my risk of diabetes and cardiovascular disease*
Resorting to comfort eating	*I will meet new people*
I will have to exercise, even when I don't feel like it	*I will be happier*
	I will be more attractive
	I will increase my self-confidence

Conclusions: *I want lose weight to improve my physical fitness and health, to reduce my risk of diabetes and cardiovascular disease and to improve my interpersonal relationships and psychological wellbeing*

confirmatory statement such as "I see that you have decided to try and change your lifestyle and to lose weight. That's great". At this point clinicians should also suggest that patients actively try to change. In reluctant patients, clinicians could recommend that they "take the plunge" and make a fresh start (e.g. "I encourage you to take the plunge, and to start changing your eating and exercise habits. The sooner you try, the sooner you will see the benefits"), even if only on a trial basis.

The importance of discussing the pros and cons of lifestyle changes with patients has been confirmed by the results of a study that added motivational interviewing (i.e. a brief intervention eliciting the patients' own reasons and arguments for change) to a BT-OB programme. This combined approach improved body weight-loss outcomes and glycaemic control in specific groups of overweight women with type 2 diabetes [25].

3.4.4 Assessing the Patient's Readiness to Change

One vital aspect to consider before starting CBT-OB proper is to assess whether or not a patient is ready to begin. In general, it is better not to start a weight-loss treatment until the odds of success are at their best. Hence, if patients are moving house, changing job or school, getting married, expecting a child, going away or have some other major obstacle, it would be wise to suggest that they postpone treatment until they are able to fully devote themselves to it. As weight change in the first 2 months of a lifestyle intervention predicts long-term weight changes [26], patients will need the first 8 weeks free of important commitments in order to start well and therefore increase their likelihood of a good outcome.

3.4.5 Assessing Whether a Patient Will Make the Programme a Priority

Changing habits and losing weight require persistent commitment, and a fundamental condition for weight loss is therefore to consider the programme a priority. To ensure that this is indeed the case, the CBT-OB therapist should ask the patients if they are willing and able to put the programme first among their day-to-day commitments. They should remind the patient that planning meals, buying food, cooking and compiling the Monitoring Records take time—on average 45–60 min a day. If this time does not immediately appear to be available, the therapist should help the patient make a list of daily activities, putting those that are not a priority on one side. In our experience, even the busiest people can find 45–60 min a day to devote to the weight-loss programme if they so desire. However, if a patient claims that they cannot find the time, the therapist should nevertheless discuss with them the pros and cons of starting treatment, thereby giving them an opportunity to reassess their priorities. At the same time, the therapist should also try to help in any practical way that they can, rescheduling appointment times so that they are compatible with the patient's other commitments.

Vignette

The patient, a 40-year-old divorced dentist, mother of an 8-year-old-child, was very reluctant to start the treatment, because she did not feel that she had enough time to dedicate to it. She was working about 7 h a day and spent the rest of the day doing housework and looking after her son. The therapist reviewed with the patient her daily schedule, and together they realised that she might delegate some housework to the nanny and that in reality she spent much of the day doing things that she could postpone or delegate to others. In addition, the therapist set the sessions 45 min after the end of the patient's working day to facilitate her attendance. In light of this review, the patient decided that she would, in fact, start CBT-OB. She later expressed appreciation not only for the improvement in her eating and physical activity habits, and the weight loss she achieved on the programme, but also the improvement in her lifestyle in general and the time that she was finally able to dedicate to herself.

3.4.6 "To Lose Weight or Not to Lose Weight" Questionnaire

The "To Lose Weight or not to Lose Weight" questionnaire (Fig. 3.1) is designed to assess a patient's degree of motivation not only to lose weight but also to change their eating habits and commit to exercise. It assesses whether a patient is willing to consider the treatment a priority, ready to change and agrees with the goal of the programme. The questionnaire comprises six questions, measured on a Likert scale (0–10); responses for each item are added together and then divided by six. The higher the resulting score (from 0 to 10), the stronger the patient's motivation to change. However, it should be noted that a "perfect" score is not necessary for a patient to start the programme—a score greater than 6 is more than sufficient. Indeed, the motivation of the patients to change is likely to increase with the benefits they get from CBT-OB.

How motivated am I to lose weight?

0 1 2 3 4 5 6 7 8 9 10

Not at all **Completely**

How motivated am I to change my eating habits?

0 1 2 3 4 5 6 7 8 9 10

Not at all **Completely**

How motivated am I to exercise?

0 1 2 3 4 5 6 7 8 9 10

Not at all **Completely**

How motivated am I to consider the programme as a priority?

0 1 2 3 4 5 6 7 8 9 10

Not at all **Completely**

How ready am I to start the programme?

0 1 2 3 4 5 6 7 8 9 10

Not at all **Completely**

How much do I agree with goals of the programme?

0 1 2 3 4 5 6 7 8 9 10

Not at all **Completely**

Total score: sum of scores divided by 6 ....

Fig. 3.1 The "To lose weight or not to lose weight" questionnaire

3.4.7 Assessing the Involvement of Significant Others

Some research has found that interpersonal relationships can exert a social influence on obesity [27]. Significant others may transfer dietary habits that can promote a change of weight in adults [28]. For this reason, the therapist should assess with the patient the possibility of involving their partner (or anyone that may influence their eating and physical activity habits) in the treatment. If the patient feels that this would be a good idea, what type of participation they will be asked to contribute should be discussed. It is important to underline, however, that in CBT-OB significant others are involved only with the consent of the patient, and if both the patient and therapist agree that their involvement might be useful to facilitate change in the patient's eating and exercise habits. How significant others may be involved in CBT-OB is described in detail in Chap. 10.

3.5 Addressing Concerns and Questions About the Treatment

The therapist should always ask the patient to raise any questions and concerns they may have about the treatment. Some examples are listed below, together with appropriate responses by the therapist.

- *Patient*: "How much weight will I lose on the programme?"
- *Therapist*: "The goal of the treatment is to lose between 0.5 and 1 kg a week. The weight loss you achieve will depend on the degree of your adherence to the diet and physical activity plans. I suggest you focus on a weekly weight loss rather than your long-term weight goal, because it is more rewarding and easier to achieve".
- *Patient*: "Can I continue to lose weight after the 24 weeks of Phase 1?"
- *Therapist*: "Yes, you can, although a distinctive characteristic of this treatment is to help you to develop and practice skills for maintaining weight. It is for that reason that the programme suggests you stop any attempt at weight loss after about 24 weeks and instead put all your efforts into weight maintenance. However, for now, I advise you to focus your attention only on the changes in your lifestyle that will help you to lose weight. We will discuss when to start the weight-maintenance phase later in the treatment".
- *Patient*: "You are right. It would be better for me to concentrate on weight loss for now. However, I like the fact that the programme places so much importance on the maintenance of weight. Keeping the weight off was a problem with my previous treatments".
- *Patient*: "The weekly goals of this programme seem too modest. My orthopaedic specialist says I need to lose a lot of weight rapidly so I can have knee replacement surgery".
- *Therapist*: "I understand, but losing weight too quickly is associated with a significant loss of muscle mass—this may be counterproductive to recovery from knee surgery. In contrast, a weight loss of between 0.5 and 1 kg a week produces an optimal change in body composition percentages, especially if you include regular physical activity to build muscle. In any case, if you agree, I will call your orthopaedic surgeon to discuss this issue".
- *Patient*: "Thank you. I really appreciate it. Here is the phone number".
- *Patient*: "I am afraid of not being able to follow the diet. I am always so hungry".
- *Therapist*: "I understand your concerns. However, the programme includes specific procedures that will help you to tolerate hunger and change your eating habits. Set aside your fears, and concentrate your efforts on implementing the treatment procedures; if you are having difficulty we can discuss it then".
- *Patient*: "I do not have enough willpower to lose weight. I cannot stop eating sweets".
- *Therapist*: "Taking control over eating is not a question of willpower. In our treatment, willpower is the commitment you put into the programme, which will teach you specific skills that will enable you to control your eating".

- *Patient*: "I don't understand".
- *Therapist*: "Here's an example: you can try to prevent boiling water from escaping a pot; you can press down on the lid, but in the end the water pressure will be too strong and you will not be able to stop it escaping. This is the approach based on willpower. Alternatively, you can lower the flame and reduce the intensity of the boil. This is the approach based on skills acquisition".
- *Patient*: "Now it is clear. Thank you".
- *Patient*: "Is it possible for me to take weight-loss drugs?"
- *Therapist*: "Yes, it is. However, I suggest that you start the treatment without any drugs, so you can decide whether or not you really do need them. I am quite sure that if you apply the procedures of the programme, you will not need any drugs to control your eating and weight loss".

3.6 Assessment Outcomes

At the end of the evaluation, the therapist should decide, together with the patient, on one of the following treatment options:

- *Individual outpatient CBT-OB*. This is appropriate for patients with obesity who are willing to actively engage in treatment and prefer an individual, rather than a group, approach.
- *Group outpatient CBT-OB*. This is appropriate for patients with obesity who are willing to actively engage in treatment and prefer a group, rather than an individual, approach. It is also preferred by some patients because is less expensive than individual treatment.
- *Day hospital or residential CBT-OB*. These intensive treatments are reserved solely for the subgroup of patients with disabling obesity. The appropriateness of these treatments is assessed by the Comprehensive Appropriateness Scale for the Care of Obesity in Rehabilitation (CASCO-R) [29], as described in Chap. 12. Day hospital CBT-OB is appropriate when the CASCO-R score is between 20 and 25 and residential CBT-OB when the score is >25.
- *Additional assessment sessions*. With ambivalent patients, the therapist should set one additional assessment interview to engage them in the decision to start the treatment.
- *CBT-OB after a preliminary intervention*. If the patient has comorbid clinical depression, it is not appropriate to start CBT-OB immediately, as clinical depression interferes with treatment in various ways. Depressive thoughts prevent the patient having any hope of making a change and hinder their ability to engage in treatment—an effect that is intensified by their apathy. Moreover, clinical depression is associated with impaired concentration, which will interfere with the reception and retention of information. Hence, it is best for the clinical depression to be addressed first, with drugs that do not adversely affect eating control (e.g. fluoxetine). Once the patient has displayed a full response to this treatment,

CBT-OB can be commenced. Likewise, if a patient has coexisting BED, we suggest that patients embark on an initial preparatory stage of 5 weeks derived from CBT-E for eating disorders [20], as discussed above. This should help the patient regulate their eating and reduce the frequency of binge-eating episodes, as such behaviour is counterproductive to any attempt to lose weight.

- *CBT-OB with other forms of treatment.* In patients who are not convinced about the possibility of losing weight through lifestyle modification because several such treatments have already failed in their case, the therapist should discuss the option of integrating CBT-OB with a weight-loss drug or bariatric surgery (if they have severe obesity, e.g. BMI $\geq$ 40 or between 35 and 39.9 with obesity-related comorbidity) (see Chap. 14).
- *Advice on avoiding weight gain.* If patients do not feel ready to commit to any of the above options at this stage, the therapist should advise them to weigh themselves on a weekly basis, to avoid weight gain and to get treatment for any risk factor and comorbidity associated with their obesity. If the patient chooses this option, the therapist should remind the patient that their door will be open when they decide they are ready to start CBT-OB.

Vignette

The patient, a 55-year-old married lawyer with two children, was referred to us by his family doctor. The patient had a BMI of 34 and a waist circumference of 115 cm; he was being prescribed an ACE inhibitor for hypertension and was also with prediabetes and high triglyceride levels. According to his wife, his snoring had recently intensified, and he was probably experiencing episodes of sleep apnoea. He had previously attempted to lose weight at the ages of 40, 45 and 48, but in all cases, after a weight loss of 5–7% in about 4–5 months, he gradually regained all the weight lost in about 1 year. In the year preceding the consultation, he had gained approximately 5 kg, which he attributed to a sedentary lifestyle and a disordered and excessive food intake, especially at dinner when he often overate and drank too much wine. However, he reported no objective binge-eating episodes or severely negative body image, although he was dissatisfied with his body weight and the shape of his stomach. He had a weight loss goal of 20 kg, and his primary reason for losing weight was to improve his health and physical fitness so that he would not end up like his father, who suffered from diabetes and died of myocardial infarction at the age of 65. The patient was enthusiastic about the nature and goals of CBT-OB, in particular the collaborative approach and its focus on developing a long-term weight-control mindset, and agreed to start individual CBT-OB.

3.7 Medical Management

The following sections provide some general information for non-medical CBT-OB practitioners on the medical management of patients with obesity.

3.7.1 Points for Non-medical Therapists to Keep in Mind

- The health and safety of patients with obesity are paramount and must never be neglected or underestimated.
- Obesity can be associated with several physical complications, and therapists must be aware of them.
- Non-medical therapists conducting the Preparatory Phase of CBT-OB should always send the patients to a physician for the assessment and management of physical complications associated with obesity.
- Non-medical therapists who deliver CBT-OB should make sure that patients have a medical doctor who will take responsibility for their medical management. The therapists should also exchange contact information with this physician so that they can liaise if necessary.
- The majority of risk factors and complications associated with obesity improve with a 5–10% reduction in weight, the normalisation of eating habits and the adoption of an active lifestyle. However, in some cases the medical doctor may prescribe pharmacological treatment for some specific risk factors (e.g. hypertension, high fasting blood glucose, hypercholesterolemia, hypertriglyceridaemia) to potentiate the effects of lifestyle modification and weight loss.
- There is no need for specific laboratory or clinical tests to make the diagnosis of obesity; it is sufficient to measure weight and height (to calculate BMI) and waist circumference. However, some in vivo and in vitro diagnostic tests are recommended to assess the presence of risk factors and complications associated with obesity.

3.7.2 Recommended Medical Tests

A list of laboratory and clinical tests that should be administered to patients with obesity before starting CBT-OB is the following (N.B. non-medical therapists should not attempt to interpret the results of these tests and instead defer to the medical doctor who is treating the patient):

- Haemachrome with formula (to identify the possible presence of anaemia, leukopenia and thrombocytopenia)
- Alanine aminotransferase (ALT), aspartate aminotransferase (AST), gamma-glutamyl transferase (GGT) (to assess hepatic function)
- Creatinine (to assess renal function)
- Potassium, sodium, calcium, magnesium and phosphorus (to assess electrolyte status)
- Glucose, insulin, LDL and HDL cholesterol and triglycerides (to assess cardiovascular risk factors)
- C-reactive protein and fibrinogen (to assess for any an inflammatory condition)
- Thyroid-stimulating hormone (TSH) (to assess thyroid function)
- Vitamin D [25(OH)D] (to assess vitamin D status)

- Urine analysis (to assess hydration status and detect urinary infections or other complications)
- Electrocardiogram (to assess any changes in heart rhythm)
- Systolic and diastolic blood pressure (to detect any hypertension)
- Abdominal ultrasound (in case of suspected non-alcoholic fatty liver disease)
- Pelvic ultrasound (in case of suspected polycystic ovary syndrome)
- Epworth Sleepiness Scale and polysomnography (in case of suspected obstructive sleep apnoea syndrome)
- Indirect calorimetry (to measure basal metabolic rate)
- Bioelectrical impedance analysis or Dual Energy X-ray Absorptiometry (DEXA) (to measure body composition)

References

1. Kushner RF. Clinical assessment of patients with obesity. In: Brownell KD, Walsh BT, editors. Eating disorders and obesity: a comprhensive handbook. 3rd ed. New York: Guilford Press; 2017. p. 473–9.
2. Calugi S, Marchesini G, El Ghoch M, Gavasso I, Dalle Grave R. The influence of weight-loss expectations on weight loss and of weight-loss satisfaction on weight maintenance in severe obesity. J Acad Nutr Diet. 2016;117:32–8. https://doi.org/10.1016/j.jand.2016.09.001.
3. Dalle Grave R, Calugi S, Compare A, El Ghoch M, Petroni ML, Tomasi F, et al. Weight loss expectations and attrition in treatment-seeking obese women. Obes Facts. 2015;8(5):311–8. https://doi.org/10.1159/000441366.
4. Dalle Grave R, Calugi S, Molinari E, Petroni ML, Bondi M, Compare A, et al. Weight loss expectations in obese patients and treatment attrition: an observational multicenter study. Obes Res. 2005;13(11):1961–9. https://doi.org/10.1038/oby.2005.241.
5. Jensen MD, Ryan DH, Apovian CM, Ard JD, Comuzzie AG, Donato KA, et al. AHA/ACC/TOS guideline for the management of overweight and obesity in adults: a report of the American College of Cardiology/American Heart Association Task Force on Practice Guidelines and The Obesity Society. J Am Coll Cardiol. 2014;63(25 Pt B):2985–3023. https://doi.org/10.1016/j.jacc.2013.11.004.
6. Lean ME, Han TS, Morrison CE. Waist circumference as a measure for indicating need for weight management. BMJ. 1995;311(6998):158–61.
7. Calugi S, Milanese C, Sartirana M, El Ghoch M, Sartori F, Geccherle E, et al. The Eating Disorder Examination Questionnaire: reliability and validity of the Italian version. Eat Weight Disord. 2016;22:509–14. https://doi.org/10.1007/s40519-016-0276-6.
8. Fairburn CG, Beglin SJ. Eating Disorder Examination Questionnaire (EDE-Q 6.0). In: Fairburn CG, editor. Cognitive behavior therapy and eating disorders. New York: Guiford Press; 2008. p. 309–13.
9. Derogatis LR, Spencer PM. The Brief Symptom Inventory: administration, scoring and procedures manual. Baltimore: Clinical Psychometric Research; 1982.
10. Mannucci E, Ricca V, Barciulli E, Di Bernardo M, Travaglini R, Cabras PL, et al. Quality of life and overweight: the obesity related well-being (Orwell 97) questionnaire. Addict Behav. 1999;24(3):345–57.
11. Calugi S, Ricca V, Castellini G, Lo Sauro C, Ruocco A, Chignola E, et al. The Eating Disorder Examination: reliability and validity of the Italian version. Eat Weight Disord. 2015;20(4):505–11. https://doi.org/10.1007/s40519-015-0191-2.
12. Fairburn CG, Cooper Z, O'Connor M. Eating Disorder Examination (EDE 16.0D). In: Fairburn CG, editor. Cognitive behavior therapy and eating disorders. New York: Guilford Press; 2008. p. 265–308.

13. American Psychiatric Association. Diagnostic and statistical manual of mental disorders, fifth edition (DSM-5). Washington, DC: American Psychiatric Association; 2013.
14. Cooper Z, Fairburn CG, Hawker DM. Cognitive-behavioral treatment of obesity: a clinician's guide. New York: Guilford Press; 2003.
15. Miller WR, Rollnick S. Motivational interviewing. 2nd ed. New York: Guilford Press; 2002.
16. Wilson GT, Schlam TR. The transtheoretical model and motivational interviewing in the treatment of eating and weight disorders. Clin Psychol Rev. 2004;24(3):361–78. https://doi.org/10.1016/j.cpr.2004.03.003.
17. Meichenbaum D, Gilmore J. Resistance: from a cognitive–behavioral perspective. In: Wachtel P, editor. Resistance: psychodynamic and behavioral approaches. New York: Plenum; 1982. p. 133–56.
18. Guidano VF, Liotti G. Cognitive processes and emotional disorders: a structural approach to psychotherapy. New York: Guilford Press; 1983.
19. Linehan MM. Cognitive behavioral treatment of borderline personality disorder. New York: Guilford Press; 1993.
20. Bandura A. Social foundations of thought and action: a social cognitive theory. Englewood Cliffs, NJ: Prentice-Hall; 1986.
21. Strecher VJ, DeVellis BM, Becker MH, Rosenstock IM. The role of self-efficacy in achieving health behavior change. Health Educ Q. 1986;13(1):73–92. https://doi.org/10.1177/109019818601300108.
22. Ciao AC, Latner JD, Durso LE. Treatment seeking and barriers to weight loss treatments of different intensity levels among obese and overweight individuals. Eat Weight Disord. 2012;17(1):e9–16.
23. Reddon H, Gueant JL, Meyre D. The importance of gene-environment interactions in human obesity. Clin Sci (Lond). 2016;130(18):1571–97. https://doi.org/10.1042/cs20160221.
24. Kushner R. Roadmaps for clinician practice: case studies in disease prevention and health promotion—assessment and management of adult obesity: a primer for physicians. Chicago, IL: American Medical Association; 2003.
25. West DS, DiLillo V, Bursac Z, Gore SA, Greene PG. Motivational interviewing improves weight loss in women with type 2 diabetes. Diabetes Care. 2007;30(5):1081–7. https://doi.org/10.2337/dc06-1966.
26. Unick JL, Neiberg RH, Hogan PE, Cheskin LJ, Dutton GR, Jeffery R, et al. Weight change in the first 2 months of a lifestyle intervention predicts weight changes 8 years later. Obesity (Silver Spring). 2015;23(7):1353–6. https://doi.org/10.1002/oby.21112.
27. Christakis NA, Fowler JH. The spread of obesity in a large social network over 32 years. N Engl J Med. 2007;357(4):370–9. https://doi.org/10.1056/NEJMsa066082.
28. Rossini R, Moscatiello S, Tarrini G, Di Domizio S, Soverini V, Romano A, et al. Effects of cognitive-behavioral treatment for weight loss in family members. J Am Diet Assoc. 2011;111(11):1712–9. https://doi.org/10.1016/j.jada.2011.08.001.
29. Donini LM, Dalle Grave R, Di Flaviano E, Gentile MG, Mezzani B, Pandolfo Mayme M, et al. Assessing the appropriateness of the level of care for morbidly obese subjects: validation of the CASCO-R scale. Ann Ig. 2014;26(3):195–204. https://doi.org/10.7416/ai.2014.1977.

Module 1: Monitoring Food Intake, Physical Activity and Body Weight

4

Module 1 starts in the first session after the Preparatory Phase and features the following components:

1. Explaining what the treatment will involve
2. Educating on energy balance
3. Establishing real-time monitoring of food intake and physical activity
4. Initiating weekly weighing
5. Concluding the session

Exceptionally, the first session is longer than the others and will usually last about 90 min.

4.1 Explaining What the Treatment Will Involve

The therapist should start the first session in Module 1 by welcoming the patients and reviewing the nature and general organisation of the treatment. Although many of these issues should have already been addressed in the Preparatory Phase, it is important to explain again to the patient what the treatment will involve, given the differences between CBT-OB and the traditional obesity treatments that they may already be familiar with. Specifically, the therapist should explain that the treatment has two main goals, the first losing weight and the second maintaining the weight lost. As the first goal is reached by a large subset of patients and many programmes, but the second goal is more difficult, CBT-OB is designed to tackle these goals in two distinct phases. In Phase 1 (which will last about 24 weeks), patients should focus on the goal of achieving a healthy weight loss, while in Phase 2 (about 48 weeks) their goal will be to maintain the weight lost (even if they have not yet reached their desired weight). As suggested by Cooper et al. [1], it is important for patients to commit to maintaining the weight lost in Phase 1 without attempting to lose weight in Phase 2 so that they have the opportunity to learn and practise the

R. Dalle Grave et al., *Treating Obesity with Personalized Cognitive Behavioral Therapy*, https://doi.org/10.1007/978-3-319-91497-8_4

skills and mindset for maintaining weight in the long term—the most challenging and much desired ultimate goal of obesity treatments. In other words, CBT-OB is designed to enable and assist patients both to lose and maintain weight, empowering them to take control of their own health and BMI.

With this in mind, the therapist should point out that, unlike traditional treatments for obesity—which rely heavily on willpower—CBT-OB will expose them to specific strategies and procedures that will help them to improve their adherence to the lifestyle habits needed first to lose and then maintain the weight (i.e. diet and exercise). This will involve them not only making changes to their behaviour but also adjusting their way of thinking. The aim is to develop a "weight-control mindset" that will give them greater control over their eating, exercising and weight.

As described in Chap. 1, patients' unrealistic weight-loss goals are not discussed or directly addressed at the beginning of CBT-OB, because our research has found that higher weight-loss expectations are associated with greater weight loss [2]. However, to prevent the early dropout often associated with higher weight-loss expectations [3], the therapist agrees with the patients on short-term weight-loss goals, such as a weekly weight-loss rate from 0.5 to 1 kg. Unrealistic weight-loss expectations are addressed later on in the programme, in Module 5, but only if patients report a decrease in weight-loss satisfaction. Indeed, this is associated with poor weight maintenance [2, 4], and it is fundamental that patients start Phase 2 of the treatment satisfied with the weight loss achieved at the end of Phase 1.

The therapist should also describe to patients how the sessions will be run, saying that they will start with in-session weighing and homework review, discussing the progress and the obstacles encountered over the past week. Then the patient and the therapist will set and work collaboratively through the agenda. Finally, the session will be concluded by agreeing on the homework to be done for the next session, summarising collaboratively what has been addressed in the session and setting the next appointment.

As mentioned, the therapist should always emphasise to patients the importance of giving priority to the treatment and playing an active role in the attempt to change. The benefits of "starting well" and not having any breaks should be pointed out—namely, that the amount of weight loss in the first 4–8 weeks is a powerful predictor of long-term weight-loss outcomes [5]. The fundamental importance of doing the agreed homework between sessions should also be stressed at this stage.

The therapist should make sure that the patient is free to ask any questions they may have and should do so if they do not understand or disagree with anything that is said. In patients who express the feeling that they will never be able to lose weight, the therapist should instil the hope that by working together, it will be possible to identify and overcome their personal obstacles to weight loss and thereby reach a reasonable, healthy weight for them.

Finally, the therapist should take time to address the practical aspects of the programme with the patient, such as whether there are any difficulties getting to the office and whether the session times are compatible with their other commitments. In general, therapists should do their best to address any such obstacle reported by patients and exchange (work) phone numbers and e-mail addresses in case there is any need to reschedule, etc.

4.2 Educating on Energy Balance

A key strategy of CBT-OB is educating patients on energy balance, describing, with the aid of handouts, the following points:

- The *energy balance* is the balance between the amount of calories (kcal) burned and the amount of calories consumed.
- From a physical point of view, the "calorie" is a unit of energy measurement equivalent to the amount of heat needed to raise the temperature of a litre of distilled water at sea level from 14.5 to 15.5 °C.
- The *daily energy intake* corresponds to the energy (i.e. the caloric) value of the foods and liquids that we introduce every day.
- The calorie content of the food depends on its composition in *macronutrients*. The calorie values for the macronutrients are:
  - Protein: 4 kcal/g
  - Carbohydrate: 4 kcal/g
  - Fat: 9 kcal/g
  - Alcohol: 7 kcal/g
- The *daily energy expenditure* is determined by three major components [6]: (1) basal metabolic rate, (2) diet-induced thermogenesis and (3) energy expenditure through physical activity.
- The *basal metabolic rate* is the amount of energy, expressed in kcal, that a person needs to keep the body functioning at rest. It accounts for about 60–75% of the daily calorie expenditure and may be measured using a test called indirect calorimetry or estimated using the Harris–Benedict equation (see below). It represents the calories expended by the body to maintain the body's normal functions (e.g. breathing, blood and nerve activity, metabolic and glandular activity and maintaining body temperature). The basal metabolic rate is influenced by body temperature, food intake, body weight (the higher the weight, the greater the expenditure), gender (it is lower in women) and age (it declines by 1–2% per decade after age 20, mostly due to loss of fat-free mass over the years).
- *Diet-induced thermogenesis* (DIT) is the energy required to digest, absorb, transport and deposit food, and in healthy subjects with a balanced diet, it represents about 10% of the total amount of energy ingested over 24 h [7] (e.g. if an individual introduces 2000 kcal, the DIT corresponds to about 200 kcal).
- The *energy expenditure through physical activity* accounts for about 20–30% of the total daily energy expenditure. It is useful to distinguish between two types of physical activity: (1) active lifestyle (i.e. the physical activity that is part of everyday life, such as walking around, standing, climbing, cleaning the house, gardening, etc.) and (2) formal exercise (i.e. physical activity that involves effort and increases heart and respiratory rate, such as swimming, tennis, running, etc.).
- A *neutral energy balance* occurs when the calories taken in through food are equal to the calories expended. A neutral energy balance is required to *maintain* weight.

- A *positive energy balance* arises when more calories are taken in with food than those expended. A positive energy balance leads to weight *gain* and increased fat deposition.
- A *negative energy balance* is caused by fewer calories being taken in than those that are expended. A negative energy balance is necessary to achieve weight *loss*.
- To lose about 1 kg of body weight, it is necessary to create a negative energy balance of about 7000 kcal. In other words, if you wish to lose 1 kg/week, you will have to expend 7000 more calories than you take in.

We find that Fig. 4.1 is an effective means of illustrating to patients how the various components of the energy balance described above serve to maintain, increase or reduce weight.

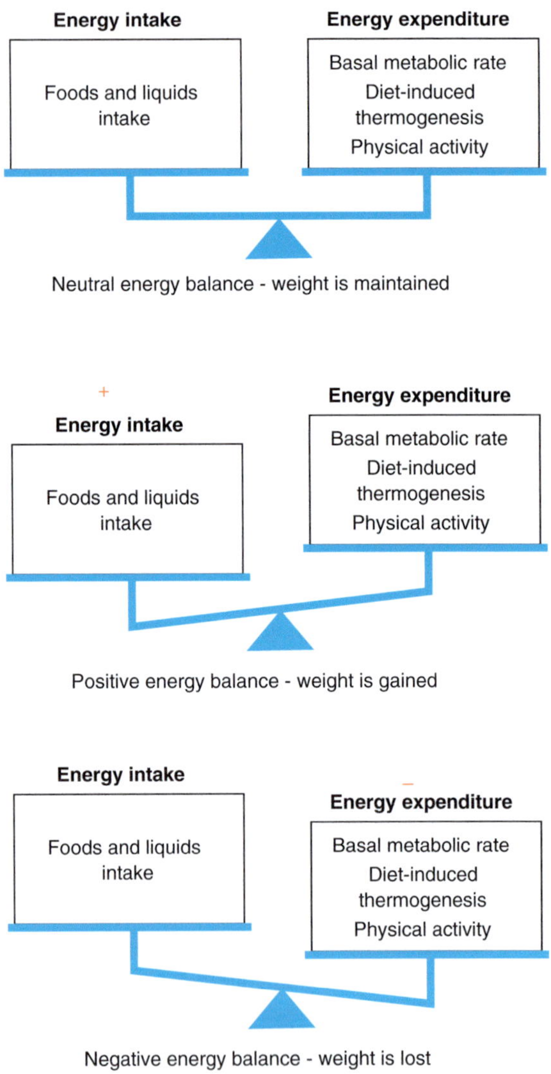

Fig. 4.1 The energy balance

4.3 Initiating Real-Time Monitoring of Food Intake and Physical Activity

Self-monitoring of food intake and physical activity is a core procedure of CBT-OB, because the greater the use of self-monitoring, the greater the amount of weight lost [8, 9]. However, the Monitoring Record adopted as part of CBT-OB (see Appendix A) differs from a traditional "food diary", as it is used to record mealtimes and the food, drink and calories that the patients are consuming both in advance and in "real time" (i.e. in the precise moment at which the food is consumed). In Module 1, the Monitoring Record is used by patients to record their eating in real time, noting *where* the food or drink is consumed; they are also asked to place asterisks in the fourth column adjacent to any episodes of eating or drinking that they felt were excessive and to use the last column to record any events, thoughts, emotions and/or physical sensations that influenced their eating at that time. In Module 2 the Monitoring Record is also used for planning meals in advance (see Chap. 5).

The therapist should carefully explain to patients how to use the Monitoring Record in Session 1, after they have been educated on energy balance. Patients should be informed that numerous studies have shown the importance of using self-monitoring in the treatment of overweight and obesity and that people who consistently compile the Monitoring Record lose more weight than those who do not [8]. Greater weight loss seems to derive from a more accurate control of portion sizes and increased adherence to the diet and physical activity. The therapist should also tell the patient that, by providing a detailed picture of their eating habits in real time, this procedure is designed to bring to their attention their individual obstacles to weight loss (e.g. comfort eating). Moreover, by making them aware of what they are doing while they are eating, monitoring helps them to eat consciously and interrupt dysfunctional and automatic eating habits that may seem uncontrollable. This way of eating should continue until new habits conducive to weight control have become automatic.

Naturally, for successful monitoring, the therapist should provide the patients with detailed information on how to calculate the calorie content of foods in kcal. To this end, we give the patients a calorie guide [10] and suggest some websites and apps that show how many calories are in the foods they are eating. The calorie guide is deliberately simple, with foodstuffs listed in alphabetical order and grouped in food groups according to classical divisions; it reports only the amount of calories and fat in 100 g of food or the average amount calorie per serving (e.g. an average apple). Since people tend to underestimate their food intake [11], the therapist should suggest that patients adjust their estimate upward when they are uncertain about how much they have eaten. To reinforce this skill, we also do in-session calorie counting exercises with patients until they learn to rapidly calculate the calorie content of foods. Patients are also encouraged to use known-capacity measuring tools, such as cups, spoons and food scales, and taught how to read nutritional information labels. Practical in-session exercises are dedicated to these activities.

The therapist must also train patients how to calculate a rough estimate of their energy expenditure. Although this is complex and can only be accurately performed with the aid of costly and sophisticated instruments that are generally only available in research settings, patients can be taught a simple formula that will provide a rough estimate of their daily energy expenditure. In spite of an inevitably high margin of error, this task helps patients to understand how calories are burned and enables them to relate these amounts to those they are introducing through food and drink. Patients are taught, by means of practical in-session exercises, to estimate their daily energy expenditure by adding together the kcals they burn through the following components:

- *Basal metabolic rate.* Measured by indirect calorimetry (if available) or estimated by means of the Harris–Benedict formula [12]
- *Diet-induced thermogenesis.* Estimated as 10% of the total amount of energy ingested over 24 h [7]
- *Lifestyle activities* (in terms of daily step count). Estimated with a pedometer or a digital wristband step counter, which will preferably be supplied by the therapist
- *Formal exercise.* Estimated using the metabolic equivalent of task (MET) table, which is provided to the patients [13] (see Table 4.1; a more detailed list of activities and MET intensities can be found on the Compendium of Physical Activity website [14]). MET is the ratio of the rate of energy expended during an

Table 4.1 Examples of physical activity and metabolic equivalent of task (MET) [13]

Physical activity	MET
Low-intensity activities	**<3**
Sleeping	0.9
Watching television	1.0
Writing, desk work, typing	1.5
Walking 2.7 km/h, level ground, strolling, very slow	2.3
Walking, 4 km/h	2.9
Moderate-intensity activities	**3–6**
Cycling, stationary, 50 W, very light effort	3.0
Doing yoga	3.0
Walking, 4.8 km/h	3.3
Calisthenics, home exercise, light or moderate effort, general	3.5
Walking, 5.5 km/h	3.6
Cycling <16 km/h, leisure, to work or for pleasure	4.0
Playing ping-pong	4.0
Dancing	4.5
Golfing	4.8
Cycling, stationary, 100 W, light effort	5.5
Playing volleyball	5.5
Vigorous-intensity activities	**≥6**
Swimming	6.0
Playing tennis, doubles	6.0
Jogging, general	7.0
Playing football	7.0
Playing tennis, single	7.0
Playing basketball	8.0
Calisthenics (e.g. push-ups, sit-ups, pull-ups, jumping jacks), vigorous effort	8.0
Playing rugby	8.3

activity to the rate of energy expended at rest. For example, 1 MET is the rate of energy expenditure while at rest. A 4-MET activity expends 4 times the energy used by the body when it is at rest.

This procedure enables the patient to make a rough estimation of their daily energy balance by subtracting their daily energy expenditure from their daily energy intake. In our clinical experience, understanding the energy balance motivates patients to increase their daily energy expenditure through exercise and reduce their energy intake via their diet.

A blank CBT-OB Monitoring Record is provided in Appendix A, while Fig. 4.2 shows an example of one that has been filled in with a neutral energy balance; we use this to illustrate to patients how to use self-monitoring. The therapist should provide the patients with 20 blank copies of the Monitoring Record, accompanied by written instructions on how to use it (see Table 4.2). Patients are recommended to keep their Monitoring Records private but to take them with them wherever they go so that they can record their intake in real time, whatever the occasion. Patients are also advised to file their Monitoring Records in sequential order in a large ring-binder. This will make it easy to review earlier records and compare changes in their eating and exercising habits over the course of treatment.

4.3.1 Addressing Concerns and Questions About Self-Monitoring

The therapist should always ask the patients to raise any questions and concerns they may have about the prospect of self-monitoring. Some examples are listed below, together with appropriate responses by the therapist:

- *Patient*: "I can control what I eat using willpower. I don't need to use the Monitoring Record".
- *Therapist*: "Maybe this is true. However, we often eat automatically without paying attention to what we eat. It is a habit. Recording in real time will help you to eat in a conscious way, to interrupt automatic and apparently uncontrollable dysfunctional eating behaviours, and to increase your capacity to decide when, what, and how much to eat. Why don't you give it a try?"
- *Patient*: "This sounds too hard".
- *Therapits*: "Yes, at first it can be challenging, but in a few days it will become easier and very useful, because it will help you to improve control over your eating behaviours".
- *Patients*: "I used a food diary in the past, but I did not lose any weight".
- *Therapist*: "The Monitoring Record that I have suggested is very different from the traditional food diary, in which you report the food eaten several hours afterwards. The purpose of monitoring in CBT-OB is to help you to interrupt automatic eating behaviours and to understand which factors influence your behaviour, and this requires real-time recording of your behaviours, thoughts and feelings".

Day Monday, February 4th Daily calorie goal 1,500 kcal

A. ENERGY INTAKE

Time	Food and drink consumed	Calories	*	Place	Comments and contexts
8:00	coffee with 5 g of sugar	20		Kitchen	101 kg. This is my weight at the start of the treatment
	low fat milk (1.8%) 20 g	10			
	1 small slice of fruit tart	180			
10:30	3 apricots 125 g	35		Office	
13:00	rise 90 g	300		Kitchen	
	sauce with mushrooms 40 g	30			
	parmesan cheese 10 g	40			
	frozen spinach	45			
	olive oil 10 g	90			
	1 pear 250 g	65			
16:30	1 yogurt cream 150 g	150		Office	
17:30	2 cookies 15 g	80	*	Office	They were on my table and I could not resist
20:00	soft cheese 100 g	300		Kitchen	
	potatoes 225 g	190			
	boiled zucchini 300 g	35			
	olive oil 20 g	180			
	1 apple 190 g	80			
	coffee with 5 g of sugar	20			
	Daily energy intake	1,850			

B. ENERGY EXPENDITURE

			Calories
Steps	Number 4,351		140
Formal exercise	Type exercise bike	minutes 10	76
Forma exercise	Type	minutes	
Basal metabolic rate			1,449
Diet induced thermogenesis (about 10% of the total calories consumed)			185
		Daily energy expenditure	1,850

C. ENERGY BALANCE

1,850	–	1,850	=	0
Daily energy intake		**Daily energy expenditure**		**Energy balance**

Fig. 4.2 Example of a completed CBT-OB Monitoring Record

Table 4.2 Patient's handout explaining how to use the Monitoring Record

Self-monitoring is one of most important procedures of CBT-OB and has four main aims:

1. To help you lose more weight
2. To provide an accurate record of what you are eating, drinking and doing in terms of physical activity and to help you understand the factors that influence your behaviour. If we understand this, we can find solutions for the things that are making it difficult for you to lose weight
3. To help you change some automatic eating behaviours. You will realise that by becoming aware of what you are doing, thinking and feeling in the precise moment that you are eating, you will learn that you have the choice to decide what to eat. This will help you interrupt some behaviours that now seem automatic and uncontrollable. However, remember that you can achieve this control only by doing accurate real-time monitoring. Reporting in the Monitoring Record after the fact does not work
4. To enable you to choose the foods that are best for you to eat and introduce a wide variety of foods that are normally excluded from traditional low-calorie diets

At the beginning, you may find writing down everything that you eat, etc. irritating and boring, but after a few days, it will become natural and useful

Here are instructions on how to complete your Monitoring Record:

- Date and day of the week:
  - Here you should write the date and the day of the week
- Daily calorie goal:
  - Here you should indicate the daily calorie goal, as agreed with your therapist
- A—Energy intake:
  - *Time*. In this column you should report the time when you eat and drink
  - *Foods and drinks consumed*. In this column you should report in real time all solids and liquids that you consume immediately after their ingestion, not at the end of the meal
  - *Calorie*. In this column you should report the calorie content of the foods and drinks that you consume. To calculate the calorie content of the food you eat, you should look at your calorie guide and use the following formula:

    kcal content of the food = (kcal in 100 g × g of food to consume)/100
  - *Place*. In this column you should record the place where you consumed the food. If you are eating at home, you should describe where and how you are eating (e.g. in the kitchen, at the breakfast bar or in the living room, with the family, etc.)
  - *. In this column, you should put an asterisk when you think that you have eaten an excessive amount of food and/or eaten without control. In this way, the column of asterisks will highlight any episode of overeating or binge eating/drinking
  - *Comments*. You should use this column as a diary to record the events, thoughts, emotions and/or physical states that might have influenced your eating/drinking. For example, if an event triggered an uncontrolled episode of overeating, you should report the nature of the episode in this column
  - *Daily energy intake*. At the end of day, you should calculate the sum of all the calories you consumed through food and drink and report it in this column
- B—Energy expenditure:
  - *Steps*. In this box you should report the number of steps you took throughout the day. The number of steps can be measured with a pedometer, which you should wear all day and reset in the morning, or with a digital wristband step counter. You should calculate the calories you expend through steps using the following formula:

    kcal consumed = weight (kg) × 0.0005 × number of steps

(continued)

Table 4.2 (continued)

- *Formal exercise*. Here you should report the type of formal exercise you did during the day and how long (in minutes) that you did it for. Formal exercise is any activity that involves effort and an increase in heart rate and respiratory rate (e.g. swimming, tennis, running, etc.). You should include a line for each type of formal exercise you performed during the day. Remember to remove your step counter during formal exercising. To calculate the amount of energy consumed during formal exercise, you should use the metabolic equivalent task (MET) table to identify the MET corresponding to the physical activity that you did. The following formula should be used to calculate the energy you expended during each type of exercise you performed:
  kcal consumed = MET × weight (kg) × minutes of physical activity/60
- *Basal metabolic rate*. In this column you should report the value of your basal metabolic rate, that is, the amount of energy required at rest with no additional activity. If your basal metabolic rate has not been measured through indirect calorimetry, you can estimate the basal metabolic rate using the Harris–Benedict equation (if you do not want to do the calculation yourself, you can use the following Internet address: http://www.bmi-calculator.net/bmr-calculator/metric-bmr-calculator.php):
  BMR (men) = 66.47 + (13.75 × weight in kg) + (5.003 × height in cm) – (6.755 × age in years)
  BMR (women) = 655.1 + (9.563 × weight in kg) + (1.850 × height in cm) – (4.676 × age in years)
- *Diet-induced thermogenesis*. In this box you should report the value of diet-induced thermogenesis (i.e. the energy consumption that occurs after ingestion of a meal), which represents about 10% of the total amount of energy ingested over 24 h (e.g. if your daily energy intake was 1800 kcal, your diet-induced thermogenesis was 180 kcal)
- *Daily energy expenditure*. Here you should report your daily energy expenditure, adding together the calories that you burned through your step count, formal exercise, basal metabolic rate and diet-induced thermogenesis

• **C—Energy balance**
  - In this box you should report your daily energy balance, which you should calculate from your daily energy intake (A) minus your total energy expenditure (B). Remember that to lose about 0.5 kg/week, you need to create a negative energy balance of approximately −3500 kcal

- *Patient*: "I am afraid of becoming obsessed with food".
- *Therapist*: "It is possible that at the beginning you will be more preoccupied with food, but in the long term this will help you to become more aware of the events, thoughts, emotions, and physical states influencing your eating, and to find solutions for improving your eating control. In any case, the increase of preoccupations with food is transitory and will disappear within a few weeks".
- *Patient*: "Do I also have to record in real-time when I eat out?"
- *Therapist*: "Yes you do. If you are embarrassed to get your Monitoring Record out in a restaurant, for example, you can jot down what you are eating on your smartphone or a slip of paper and fill in the Monitoring Record later. Alternatively, you could go to the bathroom at intervals to fill in your Monitoring Record".

- *Patient*: "Can I use my smartphone or a laptop instead of these forms?"
- *Therapist*: "That is not a good idea. This Monitoring Record has been specially designed to allow you to record not only what you eat but also events, thoughts, feelings and physical states that influence your eating. If you use another means of recording what you eat, you risk missing information that you will need to deal effectively with these influences".
- *Patient*: "Do I have to record all the food I eat? That would be very embarrassing".
- *Therapist*: "Try to record everything. I am here to help you to improve your control over eating, and I will never judge your behaviour. However, I suggest that you do not show your records to other people, as this might affect what you write down".

Vignette
The patient, a 60-year-old retired woman, manifested some doubts about her ability to use the Monitoring Record and disputed its usefulness for losing weight. However, after completing the in-session exercises of calorie counting food intake and energy expenditure, she realised that the task was not as difficult as she had believed. She agreed to use the Monitoring Record in real time for 1 week to test its utility. In the next session, she reported that self-monitoring had helped her to become aware that she eats far more calories than what she had thought and that writing down the food she was eating in real time helped her to reduce the episodes of overeating during meals. She also reported that using a pedometer prompted her to increase her number of daily steps, because when, in the late afternoon, she realised that she had only taken 2000–3000 steps, she would take a walk for about half an hour.

4.4 Establishing Weekly Weighing

Regular self-weighing is one of most important behaviours associated with weight loss and weight maintenance [15], but people with obesity often shift from avoiding weighing (when their diet is uncontrolled) to an excessive frequency of weighing (when they are on a diet). Needless to say, both of these behaviours are problematic [1, 16]. Avoiding weighing does not enable collection of information about weight variations and, particularly in individuals predisposed to obesity, is often associated with a progressive weight gain. Frequent weighing (e.g. every day or several times each day), on the other hand, may create concerns about irrelevant fluctuations in weight due to changes in hydration. These, if misinterpreted, may promote a temporary abandonment of food control, often determined by an all or nothing mode of thinking (e.g. "My efforts are useless because my weight hasn't changed. It is not worth continuing this diet"). Checking weight regularly—generally once a week—is the best approach, as it enables examination of the relationship between eating and weight variations and establishing lifestyle changes necessary to lose or maintain weight.

Collaborative weighing is a core procedure of CBT-OB that has been designed to educate patients to check their weight at the right frequency, i.e. once a week, and to interpret variations in body weight correctly. The procedure involves the patient being weighed in their indoor clothing and no shoes on a scale with 0.5 kg intervals, to avoid too minute reading of the weight. The number shown on the scale is then plotted on a "weight-loss graph" (see the example in Fig. 4.3) and interpreted by the patients with the aid of the therapist. Patients are educated in the correct form of interpreting changes in their weight—that is, to consider the trend over a period of 4 weeks. In other words, they are advised to look at five weight measurements (the current weight and the four previous ones) on the weight-loss graph, using a transparent ruler to link the current weight with that of 4 weeks before. The therapist should say to the patients that this is the only way to really understand whether the weight is fluctuating or has in fact decreased or increased.

The two dotted lines on the weight-loss graph represent the recommended weekly weight loss of between 0.5 and 1 kg/week. This illustrates to patients whether their rate of weight loss is in line with the goals of the treatment. Patients are asked also to check their weight at home, if possible the same day as the session,

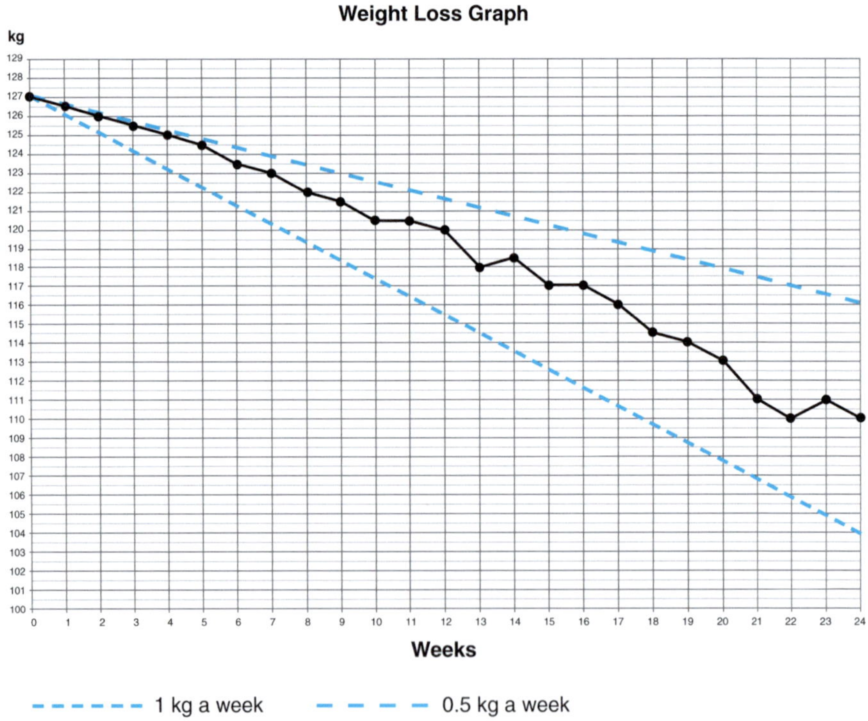

Fig. 4.3 An example weight-loss graph

and to write this "unofficial" weight and their interpretation on it in the "Comments" column of the Monitoring Record. However, it is important for the therapist to underline that the "official" weight in the first 8 weeks will be that measured in the office. It is not important if there is any difference between the two figures, but this difference should remain constant throughout the course of the treatment. In the event of any discrepancy, the therapist should suggest that the patient recalibrate their personal scale.

Vignette

The patient, a 22-year-old woman who had suffered from obesity since childhood, had not weighed herself for 5 years, during which she experienced a weight gain of about 30 kg. After listening to the therapist's explanation of the weekly weighing procedure, she admitted that she had avoided weighing herself because she was very concerned about her body weight and wanted to block out the fear of weight gain. However, she agreed that avoiding weighing was counterproductive, because she had put on a large amount of weight without being fully aware of what was happening, and, paradoxically, her concerns about weight had increased in the long term. She agreed on the importance of starting the weekly weighing, but she reiterated her anxiety regarding this task. The therapist empathetically told the patient that he understood her concerns but that weekly weighing was a necessary first step on the way to taking back control of her body weight. He explained to her that although there was a possibility of her worries about her weight getting worse in the short term, they would fade in a few weeks as she gained control over her weight. The patient started weekly weighing and in the following weeks realised that this procedure helped her to increase her adherence to the meal plan. She also realised that her fear of weighing gradually diminished and was in fact replaced by curiosity—checking the effect of the changes she had made to her eating and physical activity habits became an interesting and encouraging, rather than frightening, experience.

4.5 Bringing the Session to a Close

In the last part of the session, the therapist should agree with the patients on the homework they will do before the next session. At this stage, this will be to start real-time monitoring from the beginning of the next day and weekly weighing. The therapist should remind the patient that homework is integral to CBT-OB and fundamental to change. Patients should also be informed that suggestions on changing eating and physical activity will be discussed in the subsequent session—at this stage the focus is on raising awareness of current behaviour. To close the session, the therapist should collaboratively summarise the material covered to help patients to remember the major points and then book the next appointment.

References

1. Cooper Z, Fairburn CG, Hawker DM. Cognitive-behavioral treatment of obesity: a clinician's guide. New York: Guilford Press; 2003.
2. Calugi S, Marchesini G, El Ghoch M, Gavasso I, Dalle Grave R. The influence of weight-loss expectations on weight loss and of weight-loss satisfaction on weight maintenance in severe obesity. J Acad Nutr Diet. 2016;117:32. https://doi.org/10.1016/j.jand.2016.09.001.
3. Dalle Grave R, Calugi S, Compare A, El Ghoch M, Petroni ML, Tomasi F, et al. Weight loss expectations and attrition in treatment-seeking obese women. Obes Facts. 2015;8(5):311–8. https://doi.org/10.1159/000441366.
4. Calugi S, Marchesini G, El Ghoch M, Gavasso I, Dalle Grave R. The association between weight maintenance and session-by-session diet adherence, weight loss and weight-loss satisfaction. Eat Weight Disord. 2018. https://doi.org/10.1007/s40519-018-0528-8.
5. Lent MR, Vander Veur SS, Peters JC, Herring SJ, Wyatt HR, Tewksbury C, et al. Initial weight loss goals: have they changed and do they matter? Obes Sci Pract. 2016;2(2):154–61. https://doi.org/10.1002/osp4.45.
6. IOM. Institute of Medicine and Food & Nutrition Board. Dietary reference intakes—energy, carbohydrate, fiber, fat, fatty acids, cholesterol, protein, and amino acids (macronutrients). Washington, DC: National Academy Press; 2002.
7. Westerterp KR. Diet induced thermogenesis. Nutr Metab (Lond). 2004;1(1):5. https://doi.org/10.1186/1743-7075-1-5.
8. Burke LE, Wang J, Sevick MA. Self-monitoring in weight loss: a systematic review of the literature. J Am Diet Assoc. 2011;111(1):92–102. https://doi.org/10.1016/j.jada.2010.10.008.
9. Boutelle KN, Kirschenbaum DS. Further support for consistent self-monitoring as a vital component of successful weight control. Obes Res. 1998;6(3):219–24.
10. Dalle Grave R, Pasqualoni E, De Kolitscher L, Ginetti S. Il contacalorie AIDAP. Verona: Positive Press; 2007.
11. Lichtman SW, Pisarska K, Berman ER, Pestone M, Dowling H, Offenbacher E, et al. Discrepancy between self-reported and actual caloric intake and exercise in obese subjects. N Engl J Med. 1992;327(27):1893–8. https://doi.org/10.1056/nejm199212313272701.
12. Harris JA, Benedict FG. A biometric study of human basal metabolism. Proc Natl Acad Sci U S A. 1918;4(12):370–3.
13. Ainsworth BE, Haskell WL, Herrmann SD, Meckes N, Bassett DR Jr, Tudor-Locke C, et al. 2011 compendium of physical activities: a second update of codes and MET values. Med Sci Sports Exerc. 2011;43(8):1575–81. https://doi.org/10.1249/MSS.0b013e31821ece12.
14. Ainsworth BE, Haskell WL, Herrmann SD, Meckes N, Bassett Jr DR, Tudor-Locke C, et al. The compendium of physical activities tracking guide. Healthy Lifestyles Research Center, College of Nursing & Health Innovation, Arizona State University. Retrieved [2017] from the World Wide https://sites.google.com/site/compendiumofphysicalactivities/.
15. Zheng Y, Klem ML, Sereika SM, Danford CA, Ewing LJ, Burke LE. Self-weighing in weight management: a systematic literature review. Obesity (Silver Spring). 2015;23(2):256–65. https://doi.org/10.1002/oby.20946.
16. Pacanowski CR, Linde JA, Neumark-Sztainer D. Self-weighing: helpful or harmful for psychological Well-being? A review of the literature. Curr Obes Rep. 2015;4(1):65–72. https://doi.org/10.1007/s13679-015-0142-2.

Module 2: Changing Eating

5

This chapter concerns the core strategies and procedures that will need to be implemented in the weight-loss phase of CBT-OB. It is essential that the patient be given ample education and chance to practise each, underlining the importance of consistency in these practices to successful weight-loss outcomes.

5.1 In-Session Weighing

The therapist starts CBT-OB Session 2 by weighing the patients. Although in the first week of treatment the patients did not receive any recommendations regarding losing weight, they will likely have lost some weight as the consequence of the real-time recording, which often provides an incentive to reduce food intake. In any case, as described in Chap. 4, the therapist should remind the patients that, due to variations in their hydration status, it will be impossible to perform an accurate evaluation of their changes in weight until 4 weeks have passed—it is not possible to interpret a single reading [1].

In the following sessions, after recording the patient's weight, the therapist should ask them about their progress. Any amount of weight loss should be praised, being careful always to stress the importance of looking at the trend that has emerged over the last 4 weeks. The therapist should also express concerns if there is no change in weight over this period and help the patients to identify and address anything that may be preventing weight loss (see Chap. 7 for obstacles to weight loss), emphasising that the key factor to losing weight is adherence to calorie restriction.

5.2 Reviewing Records and Other Homework

In Session 2, the therapist should dedicate about 10 min to reviewing collaboratively the patient's Monitoring Record in detail. This review should assess two specific aspects of recording:

R. Dalle Grave et al., *Treating Obesity with Personalized Cognitive Behavioral Therapy*, https://doi.org/10.1007/978-3-319-91497-8_5

1. *The process of recording*. A review of the recording quality should be undertaken by asking patients about their attitude towards this procedure, how it has gone from their perspective and whether they encountered any difficulties in recording. Points to investigate are whether their self-monitoring was done in real time, whether all episodes of eating and drinking were reported and whether the asterisk and comment columns were used correctly.
2. *The content of recording*. A review of the recording content should be performed in order to assess whether a patient's calculations of the daily calorie intake, step count and formal exercise and diet-induced thermogenesis were accurate. They should also be asked whether each day was typical or atypical and what they have learned by recording their behaviour (see the *Vignette* below).

During the review, the therapist should also provide information and advice on how to improve reporting and calculation of the caloric intake and expenditure if problems are noted. That being said, patients should always be praised for their efforts to record, even if it was not done very well. In this case, they should be further educated and encouraged to use the Monitoring Record according to CBT-OB indications (see Chap. 4). Likewise, if a patient attends the session without their Monitoring Records, the therapist should take the blame but investigate the reasons why and reiterate the procedure and the rationale behind it (e.g. "Maybe I did not explain the importance of self-monitoring very well. Can we review together why it is fundamental for losing weight?").

From Session 3 onwards, the records review is mainly focused on the content of recording, using one or two relevant Monitoring Records to identify the patient's individual obstacles to weight loss (see Chap. 7).

Vignette

The patient, a 40-year-old woman who had made many attempts to lose weight via a traditional prescriptive biomedical approach, reported numerous episodes of "grazing" during the day. At the end of the first session, she stated that she was sceptical that using a Monitoring Record could help her lose weight. She was also a little annoyed that the session was brought to a close without her being prescribed a diet. However, she agreed to perform real-time self-monitoring for a week as an experiment that would enable her to figure out if it could help her to improve her control over food intake. By Session 2, the patient had lost 1 kg and (to the therapist's surprise) presented with accurate daily Monitoring Records compiled in real time. A review of the records clearly demonstrated that her weight loss was ascribable to the fact that she had eaten regularly, without grazing. When asked by the therapist about the mechanisms that had helped her to eat regularly, the patient confirmed that real-time self-monitoring had helped her to improve her control over eating. Moreover, counting calories had helped her to realise that she had been eating much more than she had thought and therefore encouraged her to limit her intake of high-energy foods. These positive effects of real-time self-monitoring on her eating convinced her of the usefulness of the Monitoring Records and the accurate use of this procedure.

5.3 Introducing the Change in Eating

As stated above, the CBT-OB dietary recommendations are designed to produce a 500–1000 kcal energy deficit per day in order to obtain a variable weight loss of about 0.5–1 kg a week. In our clinical practice, we calculate this energy deficit by subtracting 250–500 kcal from the patient's basal metabolic rate (BMR) measured through indirect calorimetry and then adjusting the calorie deficit for the individual's physical activity level. We also educate patients on how to follow a low-energy diet (LED) eating plan based on the Italian Mediterranean diet, adapted to both the characteristics and preferences of the individual and their metabolic targets. Although the Mediterranean diet appears not to produce greater short- or medium-term weight loss than diets of other macronutrient compositions [2], the choice to adopt this dietary model derives from the fact that it determines better long-term weight loss than a low-fat diet [3]. It is also well known for its positive health effects [4] and is preferred by the population we treat. However, CBT-OB can be easily adapted to different cultures, patient preference and health statuses, as suggested by the AHA/ACC/TOS Guideline, by adopting any of the following methods of reducing food and calorie intake [5]:

- 1200–1500 kcal/day for women and 1500–1800 kcal/day for men (kcal levels should be adjusted to the individual's body weight)
- Any of the evidence-based diets that restrict certain food types (such as high-carbohydrate foods, low-fibre foods or high-fat foods) in order to create an energy deficit through reduced food intake

Indeed, as described in Chap. 1, our studies in real-world settings have shown that the amount of weight loss is associated with an increase in cognitive dietary restraint and a reduction in cognitive dietary disinhibition [6], irrespective of the (healthy) diet type. For this reason, CBT-OB has introduced some specific procedures to help patients improve their adherence to their particular diet plan by increasing their dietary restraint and reducing their dietary disinhibition. These procedures are explained in the following paragraphs.

5.3.1 Planning Ahead When, What and Where to Eat

The therapist should explain to patients that one of the most effective strategies for improving adherence to the meal plan and taking control over eating is planning ahead. Indeed, planning in advance what they are going to eat and drink helps patients to increase diet structure and limits food choices, thereby reducing temptation and potential mistakes in calculating energy intake [7]. Moreover, it is one of the key procedures in changing eating habits that are automatic and apparently difficult to change, as illustrated in the *Vignette* above.

To help patients to improve the quality of their diet, we provide patients with a meal plan based on the food exchange lists for meal planning published by the American Diabetes Association and the American Dietetic Association [8], adapted for the Mediterranean diet [9] (see Appendix C). The main advantage of the food exchange system is that it provides patients with a system that includes a wide selection of foods, thereby offering variety and versatility to the person who is trying to limit their caloric intake. Furthermore, the list provides a framework, grouping foods with similar nutrient contents, which can help patients to make substitutions on the basis on their preferences without going over their calorie limit. In addition to using these lists, however, patients are encouraged to count the calories in the planned food, because this may help them to avoid the rigidity and monotony of a prescribed diet and to become aware of the caloric content of the food they are eating.

Patients are taught how to use the first three columns of the Monitoring Record to plan and write in advance when, what and where they are going to eat (see Fig. 5.1). The therapist also suggests that patients choose a specific moment of the day to do this task, when they have no other chores or distractions. They should associate this task with a written shopping list, which will ensure that the food they have planned to eat is available. Some patients prefer to plan their meals each morning before breakfast, others the day before and others every 2–3 days or once a week.

5.3.1.1 When to Eat

A key strategy for improving control over eating is adopting the procedure of *regular eating*. This procedure, initially developed for the treatment of bulimia nervosa [10], has also proven to be very effective in reducing the frequency of binge-eating episodes in patients with BED [11] (see Chap. 13).

The therapist should explain to the patient that there is no right or wrong time of day to eat and that there are no differences in food absorption at different times of the day. However, delaying eating as much as possible increases the risk of having an episode of overeating or binge eating. Furthermore, eating regularly at intervals not exceeding 4 h provides structure to eating habits (and to the day) and prevents any alteration in the planned dietary restriction (e.g. skipping meals) and/or overeating. The following two behaviours should be adopted in order to ensure regular eating [1]:

1. Eating three meals plus two snacks at planned, regular intervals (of not more than 4 h), for example:
   (a) 8:00 am—Breakfast
   (b) 10:30 am—Snack
   (c) 1:00 pm—Lunch
   (d) 4:00 pm—Snack
   (e) 8:00 pm—Dinner
2. Not eating between planned meals and snacks

The therapist should explain to the patient that regularisation of eating will resynchronise their feelings of hunger to specific times of the day, which it will then be gradually possible to rely on. Patients are advised that the new eating pattern

Day ......Monday, February 11th...... Daily calorie goal ......1,200 kcal......

A. ENERGY INTAKE

Time	Food and drink consumed	Calories	*	Place	Comments and contexts
7:00	skimmed milk 150 g	69		Kitchen	
	3 crispbreads 24 g	98			
10:30	1 orange 190 g	35		Office	
13:00	spaghetti 80 g	282		Kitchen	
	tomato sauce 50 g	9			
	parmesan cheese 10 g	40			
	lettuce 100 g	19			
	olive oil 10 g	90			
	1 apple 150 g	80			
16:30	1 fruit yogurt cream 125 g	62		Office	
20:00	tenderloin 150 g	190		Kitchen	
	fennel 200 g	18			
	olive oil 10 g	90			
	1 apple 150 g	80			
	Daily energy intake	1,162			

B. ENERGY EXPENDITURE

			Calories
Steps	Number		
Formal exercise	Type	minutes	
Forma exercise	Type	minutes	
Basal metabolic rate			
Diet induced thermogenesis (about 10% of the total calories consumed)			
		Daily energy expenditure	

C. ENERGY BALANCE

______ − ______ = ______

Daily energy intake	**Daily energy expenditure**	**Energy balance**

Fig. 5.1 An example of a Monitoring Record used for planning ahead (when, what and where to eat)

should take precedence over other activities and circumstances. That being said, in the event of sudden changes in day-to-day commitments, patients should be advised to adopt a flexible approach, adapting the time of eating but sticking to the 4-h interval guideline.

If the records show that patients are skipping meals or snacks, they should be educated on the potential negative consequences of this behaviour. In particular, skipping meals increases the risk of overeating or binge eating and becoming too preoccupied with food and therefore undermines dietary restriction. At the other end of the spectrum, if patients have difficulty not eating between planned meals and snacks, the therapist should suggest that they apply the "things to think and do" procedure described in Chap. 7 (Module 4).

5.3.1.2 What to Eat

To start, the therapist should inform the patient that the amount of weight loss is not dependent on the qualitative composition of the diet but rather the adherence to caloric restriction. A safe weight loss of about 0.5–1 kg/week can be achieved by creating an energy deficit of 500–1000 kcal/day. There are two main strategies for attaining this energy deficit: (1) following a diet that restricts certain types of food (e.g. high-carbohydrate foods, low-fibre foods or high-fat foods) and (2) counting the calories in food intake. The approach we use combines these two strategies, suggesting calorie counting and a meal plan based on the Mediterranean diet.

The first step in this approach is agreeing with the patient a daily calorie goal. This can be identified through indirect calorimetry (see above) or from the mean total energy expenditure estimated by patients in their Monitoring Records (if an indirect calorimeter is not available). The therapist should inform the patient as the programme progresses to maintain a weight loss of about 0.5–1 kg/week; it may be necessary to further reduce the calorie content of their diet in line with the progressive reduction in their basal metabolic rate. However, patents should be aware that it is not advisable for them to follow a very low-calorie diet (i.e. a diet with a calorie content below 800 kcal/day) because these often lack nutrients, are associated with a high risk of overeating and will not help them develop long-standing healthy eating habits [12]. Patients are also educated that in the first weeks of caloric restriction, it is common to lose a greater amount of weight due to glycogen breakdown and loss of water in their tissues (up to 2–3 L) [13] and because their basal metabolic rate will be higher [14].

The second step in our approach is to explain to the patient the rationale behind restricting certain types of foods. As previously described, in our unit, we suggest that patients follow a meal plan based on the Mediterranean diet because it determines better long-term weight loss than a low-fat diet [3], is preferred by the population we treat and has well-known positive health effects [4]. The therapist should explain that the Mediterranean diet contains a healthy nutrient balance, as it ensures the daily intake of complex carbohydrates (i.e. pasta, bread, rice) and the correct ratio of animal and vegetable proteins (i.e. fish, meat, pulses), as well as healthy fat (i.e. olive oil), vitamins, mineral salts and soluble and insoluble vegetable fibre. Furthermore, olive oil and fish are rich in monounsaturated and polyunsaturated fatty acids—such as oleic, linoleic and linolenic acids—which are essential for the maintenance of cell membrane integrity and the containment of cholesterol levels within normal limits. The Mediterranean diet is also rich in antioxidants—like vitamin E—that prevent damage caused by free radicals in aging, inflammatory processes, tumours and atherosclerosis. Moreover, the high content of unrefined complex carbohydrates, as well as vegetable protein and dietary fibre, contributes to the reduction of blood fats and therefore reduces the risk of cardiovascular disease—as demonstrated by several epidemiological nutritional studies [4] and a randomised controlled trial [15]. Research also shows that the Mediterranean diet improves surrogates of cardiovascular disease such as waist-to-hip ratio, lipids and markers of inflammation and reduces the burden—or even prevents the development—of breast cancer, depression, colorectal cancer, diabetes, obesity, asthma, erectile dysfunction and cognitive decline [16].

The third step in helping the patient decide what to eat is suggesting some general dietary guidelines for enhancing the pleasure of eating, the feeling of satiety and the quality of the diet, which will protect against common diseases (e.g. heart disease, stroke, type 2 diabetes, several common cancers, cataracts, osteoporosis, dementia and other age-related diseases). The main informed instruction the therapist should provide in this regard is the following:

- *Reduce the intake of certain saturated fats* (i.e. butter, fat meat, processed meats, whole milk and yoghurt, cheese and many biscuits, cakes, pastries, pies, fast food, fried foods, potato chips, crisps and other savoury snacks and tropical oils) *and avoid trans fats*. This may help to decrease the "bad" low-density lipoprotein (LDL) cholesterol and reduce the risk of cardiovascular diseases by about 30%, in particular if they are replaced by polyunsaturated and monounsaturated fats, such as those found in vegetable oils (i.e. corn, soybean, safflower and cottonseed oils) [17] and the omega-3 fatty acids found in fish fat, seeds and wholegrains [18].
- *Reduce the intake of processed meat and red meat, in favour of protein from healthy sources such as beans, nuts, seeds, fish, poultry and eggs*. Processed meat, and probably red meat, is carcinogenic to humans. The association is mainly with colon cancer, but it also seems to be a factor in pancreatic and prostate cancers [19]. Moreover, getting more protein from plants, poultry and fish is linked to a lower risk of heart disease and diabetes. Finally, an adequate daily intake of proteins (e.g. 25%) improves weight loss and maintenance, because high-protein foods slow the movement of nutrients from the stomach to the small intestine; this increases the sensation of fullness and avoids the rapid, steep rises and falls in blood sugar caused by refined carbohydrates like those found in white bread and potatoes, for example [20].
- *Swap refined carbohydrates for wholegrains* (e.g. bread, pasta, brown rice, quinoa, whole oats and bulgur). This may help to reduce body weight via several mechanisms [21], through the lower energy density of wholegrain-based products and the increased feeling of satiety through the fermentation of non-digestible carbohydrates. Moreover, the rich fibre content of complex carbohydrates

improves intestinal transit, modulates gut bacteria and slows the absorption of carbohydrates and the stimulation of insulin secretion, which may otherwise increase the sensation of hunger. If whole carbohydrates are consumed without an excess of condiments, they may also help to reduce the calorie intake from fat, not to mention expand the range of tastes, textures and colours that are pleasing to the palate [20]. What is more, observational studies show that eating high-fibre cereals and foods with a low-glycaemic index helps reduce the respective risks of an individual developing diabetes and having a heart attack. In contrast, consuming soft drinks, white bread, white rice, French fries and cooked potatoes are all associated with an increased risk of diabetes, heart attack, stroke and heart-related deaths [20]. Finally, foods rich in fibre keep the stool soft and bulky and thereby help to prevent constipation—a common side effect of low-calorie diets—as well as diverticulosis and diverticulitis [20].

- *Increase the intake of water-rich foods such as fruits and vegetables.* Reducing the energy density of the diet is associated with substantial weight loss [22]. Moreover, water-rich foods contain large amounts of vitamins, minerals, antioxidants and fibre, whose intake is associated with a reduced risk of hypertension, cardiovascular disease, cancer and all-cause mortality [23]. For this reason, it is highly recommended that fruit and vegetables are always included in main meals and snacks, varying by variety and colour (e.g. dark green, leafy vegetables, yellow or orange fruits and vegetables, red or purple fruits and vegetables, pulses and peas, citrus fruits) [20]. Potatoes and corn, although vegetables, should be considered akin to starches like rice and pasta, since they deliver mostly easily digested starch, whose increased intake seems to be linked to weight gain [24].
- *Consume nuts (and fruit) as snacks.* Although nuts are energy-dense and high-calorie, they are excellent sources of proteins, vitamins, minerals and antioxidants. They also improve adherence to a low-calorie diet because they have a high satiety value, which leads to strong compensatory dietary responses. They are not associated with weight gain—due to the inefficiency of the body in absorbing the energy they contain—and evidence suggests that they may even increase resting energy expenditure and fat oxidation [25].
- *Drink at least 1.5–2.0 L of liquids every day.* This may help to prevent the development of dehydration associated with caloric restriction. The best drink is water, but other healthy alternatives are light tea, chamomile tea, herbal infusions and coffee in moderate amounts. It is advisable to limit or avoid altogether sugar-sweetened beverages, which contain on average 10% of simple sugars and have little nutritional value (i.e. they contain pure calories and are completely devoid of the healthy nutrients that may be present in real fruit juices, i.e. vitamins, minerals, other phytochemicals and maybe some fibre). Moreover, the simple sugars in fizzy drinks trigger rapid and intense rises in blood sugar, which causes the pancreas to produce more and more insulin; in the long term, this may increase the risk of developing type 2 diabetes [20]. Diet soda can be drunk in moderation—people who consume diet soda gain less weight than those who consume sugar-sweetened soda—but it should be noted that the sweet taste of artificially sweetened drinks may stimulate the brain to increase cravings for

more sweet food and drink, which can add up to extra calories. Fruit juice intake too should be moderate, because, although it contains water and healthy nutrients, it is easy to consume a large amount; this translates to a lot of sugar and thereby increases the daily intake of calories. It is equally important to limit the consumption of alcohol because, although in moderate doses (i.e. one drink a day) it could offer some protection against heart disease [20], its calorie content and its disinhibitory effect on control over eating may compromise weight loss.

- *Gradually reduce the amount of sugar* (e.g. from two teaspoons of sugar in a cup of tea or coffee to one and so on). This should obviate the need for artificial sweeteners, which, however, can be used in moderation.
- *Limit the use of salt.* This is particularly advisable in patients with high blood pressure. The taste buds can easily adapt to a gradual reduction of salt, so it is not very difficult to reduce the amount normally consumed at a time (provided, of course, that processed foods—often high in salt—are avoided altogether).
- *Remove all visible fat from meat and skin from chicken and turkey.* This helps to reduce the fat and therefore calorie content of these foods. Meat and fish should preferably be cooked without the addition of fat (e.g. grilled, boiled or steamed) and served with vegetables and spices rather than rich condiments and sauces. Fried foods should be avoided, but a dash of olive oil with vinegar or lemon is a good choice for seasoning vegetables. Accompaniments for pasta and rice should predominantly consist of vegetables, without adding fat, although small portions of lean meat or fish associated with pasta or rice can be healthy.
- *Adopt a consistent pattern of eating* (e.g. repeating a similar pattern of eating week by week). This helps to establish and consolidate new eating habits, which gradually become a lifestyle that does not require a continuous cognitive effort to control what to eat.
- *Follow a meal plan in a flexible way, introducing favourite foods on occasion.* This helps to improve control over eating, prevents the sense of deprivation and improves gratification. Adopting extreme and rigid dietary rules only increases risk of overeating and binge eating; if dietary rules are extreme (i.e. many dietary rules requiring constant vigilance), they will inevitably be broken, and the slightest deviation from rigid rules may be interpreted as a failure (dichotomous thinking) and lead to temporary abandonment of eating control [1].
- *Take a multivitamin and multimineral supplement every day.* This will prevent the onset of any deficiency associated with a low-calorie diet. It also provides a nutritional "safety net", as several ingredients in standard multivitamins (i.e. vitamins B6 and B12, folic acid, vitamin D and beta-carotene) are instrumental in preventing heart disease, cancer, osteoporosis, memory loss and other chronic diseases [20].

The fourth step in instilling healthy eating behaviour is to explain to patients the composition of the Mediterranean diet and how the food exchange system can be used to make substitutions on the basis on their preferences and the suggestions above (Appendix C reports some sample menus of 1200 and 1500 kcal, and the foods groups adapted for a Mediterranean-based meal plan). We also provide patients with a book containing menus and recipes if they like to cook tasty and low-calorie foods [26]. However, patients are informed that the menus should be used as a general guide, because calorie counting (a procedure that they learned through the Monitoring Record in the first week of treatment) can be used to create an individualised and flexible meal plan according to personal preferences and lifestyle. Indeed, it is not realistic to expect to follow a prescribed meal plan for life, and the goal of CBT-OB is that patients gradually became therapists of their own obesity. The importance of monitoring food intake and calorie counting has been demonstrated by several studies which show that the adoption of this procedure is associated with greater weight loss [27]. Moreover, in our clinical experience, we have observed that patients who count calories become more aware of the calorie content of foods and their effects on energy balance and that this awareness helps them to choose foods with lower energy density, become more flexible in their dietary planning and adhere better to dietary restriction.

The fifth and final step in planning what to eat is discussing how to reduce portion sizes, as making smaller portions of food is a key strategy for controlling weight [28]. In general, the therapist should give the patients the following advice:

- Weigh the food before cooking it (if possible).
- Adopt some easy-to-use reference measurements for estimating food portions (e.g. a cup for 80 g of rice, a glass for a portion of milk, a tablespoon for 10 g of olive oil, etc.).
- Only eat pre-packaged foods that report their calorie content.
- Go to restaurants that serve normal (i.e. small) portions of food.
- Use small dishes (a strategy that helps to reduce the portion size).
- Serve the food only once and in the right portion (no second helpings).

With patients who often eat out or have difficulty in calibrating the exact portions or controlling their food intake when they handle food, we discuss the possibility of using meal replacements. Indeed, some studies have shown that the use of meal replacements is associated with a greater weight loss and better weight maintenance [29]; meal replacements may in fact help to reduce food-related stimuli that promote excessive food intake, because there is less available "free" food at home, the portion is already quantified and there is no need to cook.

5.3.1.3 Where to Eat

In the first 4 weeks of CBT-OB, the therapist should suggest patients limit as much as possible social occasions in which there is a great exposure to food stimuli, and it is difficult to plan ahead what to eat. Indeed, one of the important initial goals of CBT-OB is to help patients to develop new eating habits, and this is facilitated if they only eat in an environment in which they have full control over what to eat and are exposed to as few food-related stimuli as possible (see Chap. 7). Ideally, patients should plan to consume as many meals at home as possible or in restaurants where they know the menu and calorie composition of the dishes they serve (which makes it possible to plan ahead what to eat). When eating at home, patients are encouraged to eat only at the table in the kitchen or dining room. Once the patients have developed new eating habits and are confident of having control over their eating, however, they are encouraged not to avoid high-risk social occasions and to accept sudden invitations to lunch or dinner—this will be the perfect opportunity for them to practise their ability to control what to eat without being influenced by the external environment.

Vignette

The patient, a 50-year-old business man with obesity, type 2 diabetes and hypertension, was very resistant to idea of planning when, what and where to eat in advance and to eating three meals and 2 snacks a day. When the therapist suggested this procedure, he immediately responded that it would be impossible for him to plan his meals in advance because he eats out regularly, often with clients, and that he doesn't eat snacks. The therapist therefore asked the patient to review his last seven Monitoring Records and to determine whether it would have been possible (even if difficult) to plan some of the meals in advance. From this review, the patient realised that in most cases, he ate in restaurants where he is familiar with the menu and collaboratively agreed to a meal plan for the following week. At the therapist's suggestion, he also undertook to include eating snacks as an experiment, to see if these procedures might assist him to lose weight. In subsequent sessions, the patient reported that meal planning and regular eating did in fact help him to improve control over eating and decrease food preoccupation. At the end of Phase 1 of the treatment, when the therapist asked the patient which procedures had helped him to lose a total of 18 kg, the patient stated that the most important procedure was regular eating and including snacks in his diet, which he declared he would never give up. He also stated that planning in advance had become more natural and not so difficult, even though he continued to eat in restaurants.

5.3.2 Continuing Real-Time Monitoring of Food Intake

Patients should be encouraged to continue real-time monitoring, as it helps to change some eating habits that are automatic and improves adherence to the meal planning [27]. The therapist should suggest that patients write in their Monitoring Record where they plan to eat the meals and snacks. They should then monitor their food intake in real time, by putting a tick (✓) next to the food planned and consumed, noting down any planned foods that were not eaten and any foods consumed that were not planned. In the event of any deviation from the meal plan, the patient is advised to recalculate their calorie intake and to put an asterisk in the "*" column, accompanied by a brief description of the associated events, thoughts and emotions in the "Comments" column (see Fig. 5.2).

Day Monday, February 11th Daily calorie goal 1,200 kcal

A. ENERGY INTAKE

Time	Food and drink consumed	Calories	*	Place	Comments and contexts
7:00	skimmed milk 150 g ✓	69		Kitchen	Weight 92 kg. I'm losing 0.5 kg a week and I'm achieving my weekly weight loss goal
	3 crispbreads 24 g ✓	98			
10:30	1 orange 190 g ✓	35		Office	
13:00	spaghetti 80 g ✓	282		Kitchen	
	tomato sauce 50 g ✓	9			
	parmesan cheese 10 g ✓	40			
	lettuce 100 g ✓	19			
	olive oil 10 g ✓	90			
	~~1 apple 150 g~~ slice of jam tart	198 ~~80~~	*		The tart was on the table, and I was tired. I felt the need to grafity myself
16:30	1 fruit yogurt cream 125 g	62		Office	
20:00	tenderloin 150 g	190		Kitchen	
	fennel 200 g	18			
	olive oil 10 g	90			
	1 apple 150 g	80			
22:00	Dark chocolate 10 g		*	Sitting room	Watching the television, I often eat automatically and without awareness
	Daily energy intake	~~1,162~~	1,335		

B. ENERGY EXPENDITURE

			Calories
Steps	Number 9,737		385
Formal exercise	Type	minutes	
Forma exercise	Type	minutes	
Basal metabolic rate			1,417
Diet induced thermogenesis (about 10% of the total calories consumed)			133
		Daily energy expenditure	1,935

C. ENERGY BALANCE

Daily energy intake		Daily energy expenditure		Energy balance
1,335	–	1,935	=	-600

Fig. 5.2 An example of a Monitoring Record used for planning ahead and real-time monitoring

5.3.3 Eating Consciously

Another key strategy that may help to improve adherence to caloric restriction and interrupt automatic dysfunctional eating habits is suggesting that patients eat consciously, observing their own behaviour during meals. Patients are educated to eat slowly, enjoying each mouthful and appreciating the smell, the textures, the colour and the taste of food, and adopt a mindset focused on weight control; this will entail following the meal plan without being influenced by external (e.g. seeing food, life events) or internal stimuli (e.g. craving, need for gratification, hunger, thoughts of food, changes in mood). This cognitive approach to eating—facilitated by the real-time self-monitoring of food intake— should be adopted by patients until they develop new healthy eating habits and can trust their internal hunger and satiety signals to regulate their food intake more naturally. The therapist should also inform patients that to reach this condition, it will be necessary for them to eat consciously for several weeks, until they realise that they have developed new eating habits that do not require a strong cognitive effort to maintain. Patients are also encouraged to adopt a mindset oriented towards the long-term goals of the treatment (e.g. reaching a healthy weight loss and its associated physical and psychological advantages)—a cognitive strategy that may help them tolerate the short-term aversive experiences (e.g. hunger and craving for high palatable foods) and loss of pleasure (e.g. not eating chocolate) that may occur when restricting energy intake [20].

5.3.4 Addressing Concerns and Questions About Meal Planning, Real-Time Monitoring and Eating Consciously

The therapist should always ask the patients if they have any concerns or questions about the procedures of meal planning, recording in real time and eating consciously. Here are some examples of typical concerns and appropriate responses:

- *Patient*: "I have no time to write in advance when, what and where to eat. Can't I just plan mentally?"
- *Therapist*: "I know that it may be a little time-consuming to write down in advance when, what and where to eat, but I suggest you try it out next week to see if it is useful or not in helping you improve your control over eating. Many reluctant patients of mine have found that meal planning enabled them to improve their adherence to the dietary recommendations and to lose more weight. When only planning mentally, it is common to forget when, what and where to eat, and you will be more susceptible to environmental and internal eating triggers".
- *Patient*: "I don't like the idea of planning in advance. I prefer to be more spontaneous and decide at the last moment when and what to eat".
- *Therapist*: "It is difficult to change eating habits without planning in advance. Indeed, eating habits like overeating or snacking are often automatic behaviours, and planning in advance may help to create a condition that facilitates adherence to the meal plan".

- *Patient*: "I have never eaten three meals and two snacks!"
- *Therapist*: "Try to use this pattern of eating as an experiment. It has been designed to help you to tolerate food restriction and reduce your preoccupation over eating and risk of overeating".
- *Patient*: "If I start the day eating breakfast, I will eat too much!"
- *Therapist*: "The weight you lose will depend on your total daily energy intake, not when the food is consumed. Try out this regular eating plan for a couple of weeks and see how you feel".
- *Patient*: "If I eat carbs, I will never lose weight!"
- *Therapist*: "It is a common belief that to lose weight one has to avoid carbs. However, data from several studies shows that there are no differences in long-term weight loss between a diet rich or poor in carbs. The key factor is adherence to the calorie restriction rather than the specific nutritional composition of the diet, and with this programme you will learn several strategies and procedures to improve your adherence to the meal plan" .
- *Patient*: "May I follow the menu without counting the calories?"
- *Therapist*: "Yes you can. However, I suggest that you count the calories because you will become more aware of the energy content of what you eat, and this will help you to create an individualised and flexible meal plan, according to your preference and lifestyle".
- *Patient*: "It is too hard to eat consciously all the time".
- *Therapist*: "Yes, it is hard, and a little unnatural. However, it is a procedure that you should apply for several weeks if you want to improve your control over eating. If you adopt this mindset, you will be better able to cope with sudden impulses to deviate from your meal plan and to decide consciously what to eat or not to eat. Once you have developed new eating habits that do not require a strong cognitive effort, you will eat more naturally".

5.4 Bringing the Session to a Close

As in Session 1, in the last part of this session, the therapist should agree on the homework for the next session, which at this stage will be planning in advance when, what and where to eat. This should be in line with the identified calorie goal (conducive to a weight loss of between 0.5 and 1 kg a week) and include real-time monitoring and eating consciously, as well as the homework set in Module 3 (see Chap. 6). Patients should also continue to check their weight once a week, both at home and in the therapist's office. Finally, and as always, the therapist should summarise the session collaboratively to help patients remember the main topics covered and confirm the date of the next appointment.

References

1. Fairburn CG. Cognitive behavior therapy and eating disorders. New York: Guilford Press; 2008.
2. Mancini JG, Filion KB, Atallah R, Eisenberg MJ. Systematic review of the Mediterranean diet for long-term weight loss. Am J Med. 2016;129(4):407–15.e4. https://doi.org/10.1016/j.amjmed.2015.11.028.
3. Schwarzfuchs D, Golan R, Shai I. Four-year follow-up after two-year dietary interventions. N Engl J Med. 2012;367(14):1373–4. https://doi.org/10.1056/NEJMc1204792.
4. Gotsis E, Anagnostis P, Mariolis A, Vlachou A, Katsiki N, Karagiannis A. Health benefits of the Mediterranean Diet: an update of research over the last 5 years. Angiology. 2015;66(4):304–18. https://doi.org/10.1177/0003319714532169.
5. Jensen MD, Ryan DH, Apovian CM, Ard JD, Comuzzie AG, Donato KA, et al. AHA/ACC/TOS guideline for the management of overweight and obesity in adults: a report of the American College of Cardiology/American Heart Association Task Force on Practice Guidelines and The Obesity Society. J Am Coll Cardiol. 2014;63(25 Pt B):2985–3023. https://doi.org/10.1016/j.jacc.2013.11.004.
6. Dalle Grave R, Calugi S, Corica F, Di Domizio S, Marchesini G, QUOVADIS Study Group. Psychological variables associated with weight loss in obese patients seeking treatment at medical centers. J Am Diet Assoc. 2009;109(12):2010–6. https://doi.org/10.1016/j.jada.2009.09.011.
7. Fabricatore AN. Behavior therapy and cognitive-behavioral therapy of obesity: is there a difference? J Am Diet Assoc. 2007;107(1):92–9. https://doi.org/10.1016/j.jada.2006.10.005.
8. Franz MJ, Barr P, Holler H, Powers MA, Wheeler ML, Wylie-Rosett J. Exchange lists: revised 1986. J Am Diet Assoc. 1987;87(1):28–34.
9. Dalle GR. Perdere e mantenere il peso. Verona: Positive Press; 2015.
10. Fairburn CG. Cognitive-behavioral treatment for bulimia. In: Garner DM, Garfinkel PE, editors. Handbook of psychotherapy for anorexia nervosa and bulimia. New York: Guilford Press; 1985. p. 160–92.
11. Grilo CM, White MA, Wilson GT, Gueorguieva R, Masheb RM. Rapid response predicts 12-month post-treatment outcomes in binge-eating disorder: theoretical and clinical implications. Psychol Med. 2012;42(4):807–17. https://doi.org/10.1017/s0033291711001875.
12. Astrup A, Brand-Miller J. Macronutrient composition and obesity treatment. In: Brownell KD, Walsh BT, editors. Eating disorders and obesity: a comprehensive handbook. 3rd ed. New York: Guilford Press; 2017. p. 480–7.
13. Muller MJ, Bosy-Westphal A. Reply to MG browning. Am J Clin Nutr. 2016;103(3):953–4. https://doi.org/10.3945/ajcn.115.127282.
14. Frey-Hewitt B, Vranizan KM, Dreon DM, Wood PD. The effect of weight loss by dieting or exercise on resting metabolic rate in overweight men. Int J Obes. 1990;14(4):327–34.
15. Estruch R. Ros E, Salas-Salvado J, Covas MI, Corella D, Aros F, et al. Primary Prevention of Cardiovascular Disease with a Mediterranean Diet Supplemented with Extra-Virgin Olive Oil or Nuts. N Engl J Med, 2018. 378(25):e34.
16. Widmer RJ, Flammer AJ, Lerman LO, Lerman A. The Mediterranean diet, its components, and cardiovascular disease. Am J Med. 2015;128(3):229–38. https://doi.org/10.1016/j.amjmed.2014.10.014.
17. Sacks FM, Lichtenstein AH, Wu JHY, Appel LJ, Creager MA, Kris-Etherton PM, et al. Dietary fats and cardiovascular disease: a presidential advisory from the American Heart Association. Circulation. 2017;136(3):e1–e23. https://doi.org/10.1161/cir.0000000000000510.

18. Briggs MA, Petersen KS, Kris-Etherton PM. Saturated fatty acids and cardiovascular disease: replacements for saturated fat to reduce cardiovascular risk. Healthcare (Basel). 2017;5(2):29. https://doi.org/10.3390/healthcare5020029.
19. Bouvard V, Loomis D, Guyton KZ, Grosse Y, Ghissassi FE, Benbrahim-Tallaa L, et al. Carcinogenicity of consumption of red and processed meat. Lancet Oncol. 2015;16(16):1599–600. https://doi.org/10.1016/s1470-2045(15)00444-1.
20. Willett WC, Skerrett PJ. Eat, drink, and be healthy: the Harvard medical school guide to healthy eating. New York: Free Press; 2017.
21. Giacco R, Della Pepa G, Luongo D, Riccardi G. Whole grain intake in relation to body weight: from epidemiological evidence to clinical trials. Nutr Metab Cardiovasc Dis. 2011;21(12):901–8. https://doi.org/10.1016/j.numecd.2011.07.003.
22. Rolls BJ. The relationship between dietary energy density and energy intake. Physiol Behav. 2009;97(5):609–15. https://doi.org/10.1016/j.physbeh.2009.03.011.
23. Aune D, Giovannucci E, Boffetta P, Fadnes LT, Keum N, Norat T, et al. Fruit and vegetable intake and the risk of cardiovascular disease, total cancer and all-cause mortality-a systematic review and dose-response meta-analysis of prospective studies. Int J Epidemiol. 2017;46:1029–56. https://doi.org/10.1093/ije/dyw319.
24. Bertoia ML, Mukamal KJ, Cahill LE, Hou T, Ludwig DS, Mozaffarian D, et al. Changes in intake of fruits and vegetables and weight change in United States men and women followed for up to 24 years: analysis from three prospective cohort studies. PLoS Med. 2015;12(9):e1001878. https://doi.org/10.1371/journal.pmed.1001878.
25. Tan SY, Dhillon J, Mattes RD. A review of the effects of nuts on appetite, food intake, metabolism, and body weight. Am J Clin Nutr. 2014;100(Suppl 1):412s–22s. https://doi.org/10.3945/ajcn.113.071456.
26. Dalle Grave R, Pasqualoni E. Perdere peso con gusto. 100 ricette AIDAP per perdere e mantenere il peso. Verona: Positive Press; 2017.
27. Burke LE, Wang J, Sevick MA. Self-monitoring in weight loss: a systematic review of the literature. J Am Diet Assoc. 2011;111(1):92–102. https://doi.org/10.1016/j.jada.2010.10.008.
28. Hollands GJ, Shemilt I, Marteau TM, Jebb SA, Lewis HB, Wei Y, et al. Portion, package or tableware size for changing selection and consumption of food, alcohol and tobacco. Cochrane Database Syst Rev. 2015;(9):Cd011045. https://doi.org/10.1002/14651858.CD011045.pub2.
29. Heymsfield SB, van Mierlo CA, van der Knaap HC, Heo M, Frier HI. Weight management using a meal replacement strategy: meta and pooling analysis from six studies. Int J Obes Relat Metab Disord. 2003;27(5):537–49. https://doi.org/10.1038/sj.ijo.0802258.

Module 3: Developing an Active Lifestyle

6

Exercise training plays a fundamental role in the management of obesity, and weight-loss programmes incorporating some form of physical activity are known to be more effective than those that rely on dietary prescription alone [1]. Moreover, exercise training limits the loss of fat-free (lean) tissue mass that tends to accompany calorie deficit and reduce abdominal fat [2]. Regular exercise is one of the most important factors associated with long-term body weight maintenance [3] and is known to produce significant health benefits independent of its effect on weight management. Indeed, regular exercise has been associated with significant reductions in the incidence of cardiovascular events [4], even in high-risk groups [5], and also has a protective effect against metabolic diseases (e.g. metabolic syndrome and type 2 diabetes); it reduces visceral adipose tissue accumulation, serum triglycerides and blood pressure, not to mention the risk of mortality [6].

6.1 Preparing the Patient for an Active Lifestyle

Although physical activity is of the utmost importance in obesity management, the majority of individuals with obesity find it difficult to get the amount of exercise necessary for weight loss and long-term control of body weight. This problem is compounded by the fact that many obesity therapists have not received adequate training in establishing effective communication with patients with a view to promoting radical change in terms of physical activity. However, patients with obesity can be encouraged to initiate and maintain regular exercise using simple cognitive behavioural techniques, the key principles of which are described in this chapter.

The aim of Module 3 is to help the patient to start and continue regular exercise. The relevant strategies are usually introduced in Session 2, after a review of the patient's Monitoring Record and an explanation of the main procedures of Module 2's "Changing Eating" (see Chap. 5).

R. Dalle Grave et al., *Treating Obesity with Personalized Cognitive Behavioral Therapy*, https://doi.org/10.1007/978-3-319-91497-8_6

6.1.1 Assessing a Patient's Eligibility for Exercise

The majority of sedentary patients with obesity with no signs of significant disease can start a moderate-intensity physical activity programme—such as walking slowly—with no contraindications [7]. However, non-medical therapists should refer patients to a medical doctor for a thorough medical examination before prescribing any type of exercise if they respond "Yes" to one or more questions in Table 6.1. If patients answer "No" to all questions, the therapist can be reasonably sure that it is safe for them to start becoming more physically active. Patients should begin slowly and build up gradually [8], taking note of their blood pressure—if the reading is over 144/94, they should see their doctor before becoming much more physically active [8]. The functional exercise capacity assessment described in the next session is also a good way of determining basic fitness.

6.1.2 Assessing the Patient's Functional Exercise Capacity

A patient's functional exercise capacity has traditionally been assessed by asking them how many flights of stairs they can climb or blocks they can walk. However, patients tend to overestimate or underestimate their actual functional capacity, and we therefore prefer to use objective measurements rather than self-reports. The tests that we use to determine functional exercise capacity are as follows:

1. *The 6-min walk test (6MWT).* This test, whose guidelines have been described in detail by the American Thoracic Society [9], measures the distance that a patient can quickly walk on a flat, hard surface in 6 min. It evaluates the global and integrated responses of all the systems involved during exercise, including the

Table 6.1 Questions to assess whether or not the patient requires a medical examination before starting to become more physically active[a]

	Yes	No
Have you ever had cardiovascular disease (e.g. cardiac infarction, angina pectoris, heart attack, cardiac arrhythmia, cardiac valve disease)?		
Have you had a stroke or any neurological problem?		
Do you suffer from high blood pressure?		
Do you suffer from type 1 or type 2 diabetes?		
Do you suffer from liver disease?		
Do you suffer from renal disease?		
Do you suffer from an endocrine metabolic disease?		
Do you suffer from severe orthopaedic or skeletal problems?		
Have you had any health problem that may prevent you doing physical activity?		
Do you think that exercise may be harmful of risky for you?		
Indication for medical examination		

[a]If the patient answers "Yes" to one or more question, a medical examination is indicated before any type of physical activity programme is begun

pulmonary and cardiovascular systems, systemic circulation, peripheral circulation, blood, neuromuscular units and muscle metabolism. Rather than the maximal exercise capacity, the 6MWT assesses the submaximal level of functional capacity—a more realistic reflection of the functional exercise level for daily physical activities, which are generally performed at submaximal levels of exertion. According to our data, a cut-off of 470 m can discriminate between patients with obesity and reduced lean body mass and those with obesity but no reduced lean body mass [10].

2. *The handgrip test.* The purpose of this test is to measure the maximum isometric strength of the hand and forearm muscles, as measured with a hand-grip dynamometer [11]. According to our data, 23.5 kg is a cut-off that can be used to distinguish between patients with obesity and reduced lean body mass and those with obesity but no reduced lean body mass [10].
3. *The five times sit-to-stand test.* This test measures the functional muscle strength of the lower limbs and the static and dynamic balance [12]. The test requires the patient to sit with their back against the chair and arms folded across their chest and then to stand up and sit back down five times as quickly as they can, without touching the back of the chair.
4. *The functional reach test.* The purpose of this test is to evaluate a patient's physical stability [13]. Patients are instructed to stand next to (but not touching) a wall with their dominant arm raised to shoulder height (90° of shoulder flexion) and their fist closed. They should then reach with this fist as far forward as they can without taking a step. Scores are determined by assessing the reach distance, i.e. the difference between the starting and ending positions.

Vignette

The patient, a 55-year-old businessman with central obesity (body weight 90.0 kg, BMI 35.0, waist circumference 155 cm) was assessed for physical activity eligibility before starting Module 3. The therapist helped him to complete Table 6.1, and the patient reported that in the past he had been seen by a cardiologist due to hypertension and that he was currently being prescribed pressure-lowering drugs. For this reason, the patient was referred to his cardiologist in order to determine his eligibility for exercise. The appropriate testing (EKG under stress), performed under medical supervision, revealed no contraindication to exercise, and the therapist was therefore able to administer the above physical fitness tests to the patient.

6.1.3 Strategies for Motivating Patients to Exercise

The adoption of an engaging style—by means of the strategies detailed described in Sect. 3.4.1—is vital for motivating patients to exercise. The CBT-OB therapist should always assess the motivation of the patients to exercise, proposing an achievable physical activity programme using a collaborative style and showing empathy for the patient's difficulties in exercising. The therapist should validate each patient's experience but within the framework of a balance between acceptance and change, firmness and empathy. It is advisable never to address resistance to exercise with confrontation but with a collaborative evaluation of the variables involved in maintaining a sedentary life. As in the Preparatory Phase, the therapist should make a functional analysis of the pros and cons of increasing physical activity, eliciting each person's own reasons for change and highlighting the advantages of regular exercise. The therapist should always foster self-efficacy in a patient by underlining that the physical activity programme has been designed to especially to be both suitable and achievable for them.

6.1.3.1 Educating on the Benefits of Regular Physical Activity

It may promote a patient's engagement in increasing their physical activity level to provide them with information about the general benefits of exercise and their specific need to increase their level of physical activity in order to achieve long-term body weight control. To this end, the topics described in Table 6.2 should be covered

Table 6.2 Main topics to cover when educating patients with obesity about exercise

Physical activity increases energy expenditure
• The amount of energy expended depends on the intensity and duration of activity, and the muscle groups involved, i.e. the more and the longer the patient exercises, and the more muscle groups they involve, the more calories they will burn off
Physical activity may help preserve fat-free mass during weight loss
• About 75% of body weight lost by dieting alone is composed of adipose tissue (which is good), with the remaining 25% being lean, or fat-free, mass (which is not) [15]. Exercise may, however, alter this ratio in favour of preserving fat-free mass
Physical activity alone results in minimal weight loss
• Although exercise does help lose weight, unless this is accompanied by a low-calorie diet, this will be minimal (an average of 2 kg less with respect to controls) [16]
Physical activity plays a fundamental role in the maintenance of weight loss
• Several studies have found that continued regular exercise is associated with successful long-term body weight loss [3] • However, considerable physical activity is necessary for weight-loss maintenance. The amount of physical activity required to reduce the rate of body weight regain is walking briskly 75 min/day (equivalent to burning about 2500 kcal/week) [17]
Exercising at home improves adherence to physical activity
• Long-term adherence to a walking programme was better in participants who were merely asked to walk in their own time rather than to participate in a supervised on-site programme [18]. Furthermore, home-based physical activity programmes seem to be associated with greater long-term weight loss than group-based programmes [18], in which barriers to exercising (e.g. cost, time constraints and embarrassment) may reduce attendance
Body weight maintenance can be achieved either with programmed activities or by changing lifestyle habits
• Increasing daily lifestyle activities is as effective as a structured endurance exercise programme in maintaining long-term weight loss [19]
Physical activity improves body image and psychological wellbeing
• Participants in exercise-intervention clinical trials report a more positive body image and psychological wellbeing post-intervention compared to non-exercising control participants [20]

interactively. Another effective strategy for promoting a patient's engagement in treatment is to give them detailed written information about the aims, duration, organisational procedures and expected results of lifestyle modification [14].

6.1.3.2 Assessing Individual Exercise Levels and Barriers to Change in a Non-judgmental Way

The CBT-OB therapist should empathetically enquire (rather than assume) how patients judge their current level of physical activity and whether they believe that it will be sufficient in their attempt to lose or maintain body weight. If, as is usually (but not necessarily) the case, patients report being sedentary, the therapist should ask them the reasons for their sedentary lifestyle and about any barriers to exercise they perceive that should be taken into consideration when designing their personalised physical activity programme.

In general, many barriers reported by our patients are shared with individuals without obesity and include low motivation and perceived self-efficacy, no history of learning to exercise, lack of coping skills and aversive environmental features—such as poor access to gyms or other facilities, high costs of training programmes, low social and cultural support and time constraints [21].

Other more specific barriers to individuals with obesity include low fitness, physical conditions (e.g. arthritis, obstructive sleep apnoea), boredom and lack of stimuli, laziness, negative comparisons with others, shame associated with exposing their body, weather constraints and fear of injury or death. Furthermore, it is important to bear in mind that women with obesity tend to report lower pleasure ratings during exercise of increasing intensity, and lower energy scores immediately after exercise, than women without obesity [22].

6.1.3.3 Involving the Patient Actively in the Decision to Change

The CBT-OB therapist should encourage patients to think about their personal reasons for and against exercising. It is best to start by asking patients to list the cons of changing—whether sedentary life provides them with perceived advantages that they are afraid or unwilling to lose. Subsequently, patients should be asked to evaluate the pros; at this stage, clinicians should encourage patients to reflect on both the short- and long-term effects of exercise on their physical and mental quality of life, as well as their ability to control their body weight. For future reference, the list of pros and cons should be written down in table form (Table 6.3).

Table 6.3 An example table of the pros and cons of change

Reasons not to exercise	Reasons to exercise
I will have to exercise even when I don't feel to like it	*I will lose more weight and keep it off*
I will have to overcome my laziness	*I will be in better shape*
I like to rest when I have free time	*I will improve my health*
I feel very tired when I exercise	*I will meet new people*
I will have less time to play chess—my hobby	*I will be happier*
I will be tired all the time	*I will be more physically attractive*
I will be embarrassed if other people see me exercising	*I will increase my self-confidence*

The pros and cons of change table should then be analysed in detail with the patient. During this discussion, the CBT-OB therapist should focus the patient's attention on their long-term goals, not just on their immediate future. Every reason to change should be reinforced. It is also important to deal with the cons of changing—the aim being to help patients to come to their own conclusion that exercise will be necessary to for them to control their body weight in the long-term and to reduce the medical and psychosocial complications associated with obesity.

6.2 Types of Exercise Recommended by CBT-OB to Increase Levels of Physical Activity

One of the primary goals of CBT-OB is to help patients to gradually develop an active lifestyle, concentrating on the physical activities that are part of everyday life (such as walking, standing, climbing, cleaning the house, gardening), as this helps to improve body composition and cardiorespiratory fitness and is associated with a better weight-loss maintenance [23]. However, lifestyle activities alone do not improve other important components of the physical fitness, such as muscle strength (i.e. the muscle's capacity to exert force against resistance), endurance (the ability to perform a specific muscular action for a prolonged period of time), body composition (the percentages of fat mass and fat-free mass), flexibility (the ability to move joints effectively through a complete range of motion) and neuromotor fitness (the ability of the nervous system to communicate with the musculoskeletal system, which affects balance, coordination and agility) [24]. For this reason, we recommend that patients associate an active lifestyle with simple exercises (see Sect. 6.2.2) selected to improve specific components of their physical fitness, bearing in mind the results of the previous assessment.

Formal exercise is the physical activity that involves effort and increases heart and respiratory rate (such as swimming, tennis, running, etc.). Although formal exercise is associated with improvement in general health conditions, it is suggested only to CBT-OB patients who are motivated to start it or that already do some.

6.2.1 Strategies for Developing an Active Lifestyle

Unlike diet, exercise adherence tends to increase the less structure is imposed—presumably through a reduction in the barriers to exercising (e.g. lack of time or financial resources) [25]. Hence, the exercise recommended as part of CBT-OB is primarily focused on helping patients to increase the level of physical activity involved in daily activities.

6.2.1.1 Reducing Sedentary Activities

The first strategy that we suggest to patients for developing an active lifestyle is reducing sedentary activities. There are many ways in which this can be achieved (see Table 6.4), and the strategy should be personalised on the basis of a patient's

Table 6.4 Strategies used to reduce sedentary activities

At home
• Reducing the use of labour-saving devices (e.g. using the body's energy to mix food, open cans, mow the lawn and so on)
• Walking up and down the stairs several times a day (if the house has more than one floor)
• Gardening
• Cleaning the house
• Washing cars by hand rather than at the car wash
At work
• Taking the stairs instead of the elevator
• Taking a walk during morning and mid-afternoon breaks
• Raising the body off a chair by bearing weight on the arms or hands (if they sit for many hours a day)
Transport
• Walking rather than driving a car
• Parking farther away in the parking lot
• Avoiding shortcuts and introducing detours when walking

lifestyle and habits. For example, a housewife with obesity could be encouraged to reduce the time she spends watching TV, to take the stairs instead of the elevator and to clean the house alone, without resorting to a housekeeper. Similarly, a person who always uses a car to get around should be encouraged to use the car as little as possible and begin to get around by bike.

Patients should be educated that developing an active lifestyle by reducing sedentary activities has several positive consequences. Moreover, it is easy to adopt, takes little time, does not require special clothes or equipment, easily becomes a habit over time and makes a person feel better both physically and mentally.

6.2.1.2 Increasing the Daily Step Count

The second strategy we suggest that patients adopt as part of developing an active lifestyle is to gradually increase the number of daily steps until they reach the goal of 10,000–12,000 steps per day. This will produce a calorie deficit of at least 400 kcal/day—an amount of exercise that promotes weight loss, maintains muscle mass and prevents weight cycling [26].

However, patients should be discouraged from increasing their step count too rapidly, as this may cause skeletal pain and a return to a sedentary lifestyle. An action plan that can be suggested to patients is using a pedometer to check their habitual daily step count (i.e. the number of steps at baseline) and then to gradually increase their daily steps each week (i.e. the first week 5000 steps per day, the second week 7500 steps per day and the third week 10,000 or more per day). As regards the intensity of walking, we suggest that patients walk without hyperventilating (they should be able to have a conversation while they are walking) and without feeling musculoskeletal pain.

It is also advisable to discuss with the patient when to walk during the day; we suggest that every moment of the day is suitable for walking (e.g. before breakfast, after lunch, during breaks, at the end of the day before returning home and/or after dinner or late in the evening before going to bed) and that patients should choose the time(s) compatible with their own lifestyle. As with changing eating habits, patients are also advised to plan in advance when and how long to walk and to adhere to this plan, without being influenced by thoughts, emotions and physical states, until this behaviour becomes a habit.

Walking can be also replaced by jogging (20–40 min/day), cycling or swimming (45–60 min/day), in accordance with a patient's individual preferences.

Vignette

The patient is employed in a post office but, even though he lives nearby, gets to work by car; after 8 h of sitting at a desk, he returns home and spends long hours watching TV or using the computer. At weekends, he spends most of his time at home engaged in sedentary activities. The therapist discussed with the patient the importance of developing an active lifestyle, and together they drew up a plan for him to reduce his sedentary activities and gradually reach the goal of walking 10,000 steps every day. Although initially reluctant, the patient began to travel to his office on foot and to use the stairs at work rather than the elevator. He also agreed to perform several body raises in his chair a day. This change in habits permitted him to increase his daily steps from 2500 to 10,000 in 4 weeks. When the therapist asked if he had still any doubts about the importance of an active lifestyle, he reported that, although he found it difficult in the first 2 weeks, he had started to feel better, more energetic and happier and that his improved fitness was associated with less difficulty in controlling his diet.

6.2.2 Strategies for Improving Physical Fitness

By careful assessment of a patient's functional exercise capacity (see Sect. 6.1.2), a personalised exercise programme and advice can be devised to focus the single components of physical fitness that they should add to lifestyle activity enhancement. However, since few clinical teams have the opportunity to collaborate with a physical activity specialist, our physiotherapist colleague has developed three simple exercises—described in Fig. 6.1—that can be recommended to most patients with obesity [27]. These exercises are easy to perform and include in their day-to-day lives, and patients are encouraged to do them several times during the day (e.g. exercise 1 every 30 min at work, to interrupt long periods of sitting in front of a computer screen). There are not an exact number of repetitions that should be done, but patients should continue each exercise until they feel that the muscles involved are a little tired. Once again it is important that not too much is attempted too soon.

Patients who are very motivated to improve their cardiorespiratory, musculoskeletal and neuromotor fitness should be assisted by a physical activity specialist (our team includes a physiotherapist trained in CBT-OB), who may suggest to them specific exercises for improving their physical fitness. Our physiotherapists recommend exercises derived from the guidelines published by the American College of

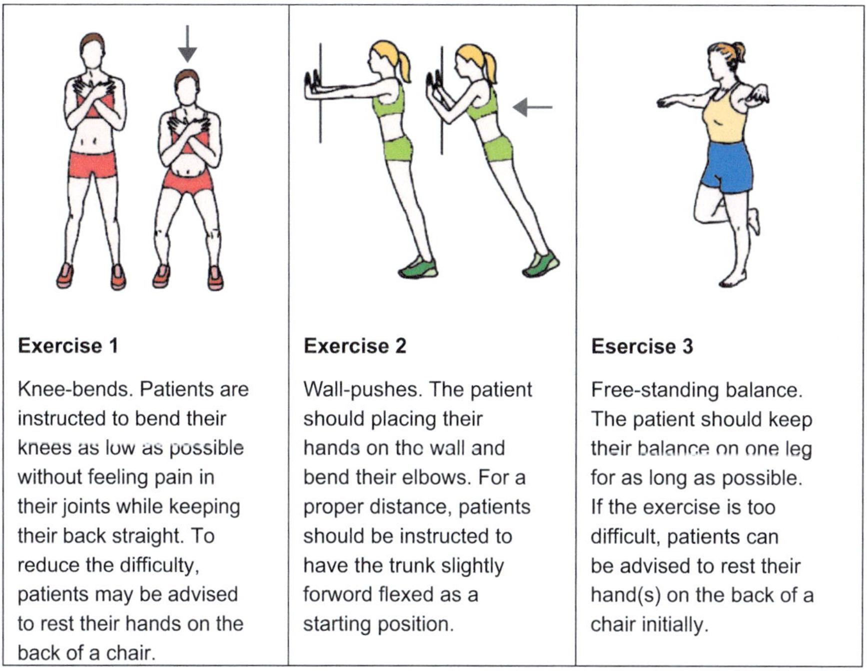

Fig. 6.1 Three simple exercises for improving physical fitness in patients with obesity

Sports Medicine (ACSM) Position Stand [7] but adapted specifically for patients with obesity, with particular regard to long-term weight-loss maintenance:

- Progressing to a moderate (3–5.9 METs) to vigorous level of cardiorespiratory exercise training (>6 METs), equivalent to 200–300 min/week (e.g. brisk walking). This should be completed in bouts of at least 10 min. In combination with a reduced energy intake, this amount of physical activity, which is greater than the ≥150 min/week recommended by the ACSM [7], enhances long-term weight loss and reduces the risk of weight regain [23].
- Resistance exercises for each of the major muscle groups and neuromotor exercises involving balance, agility and coordination ≥2 days a week. Although resistance does not have a significant effect on weight loss (in part because it may cause an increase in lean mass), it does have a favourable effect on cardiometabolic risk factors, as well as improving muscle strength and function [23].
- A series of flexibility exercises for each of the major muscle–tendon groups ≥2 days per week to maintain the joints' range of movement.

6.2.3 Strategies for Continuing or Commencing Formal Exercise

Most people with obesity find it difficult to do sports, often due to medical problems associated with their excess weight (e.g. arthrosis of the knees or hips) and/or because they are embarrassed to reveal their body to others. If our patients do not like the idea of doing sports, we do not insist, as formal exercise is not the goal of the programme. Indeed, patients can lose and maintain weight by adopting a more active lifestyle alone. However, if a patient is willing to take up a sport or already does one, it is a good idea to encourage this, because formal exercise, besides helping people lose weight, is very effective at improving health in general [28]. In any case, patients should be informed that once they do take up a sport, they should continue, because its abrupt suspension is often associated with weight gain.

Patients who wish to take up a sport but do not have a precise idea about of what type to choose should be invited to write down a list of the sports they would like to do and evaluate the pros and cons of each, thinking about the potential obstacles to address (e.g. lack of time, non-availability of adequate spaces for a certain type of exercise, the need to buy special clothes and equipment, etc.). It is also useful to encourage patients to exercise with a family member or friend, to register with a club or gym, to buy an exercise bike etc. or to engage a personal trainer, as these are all good strategies that can help patients to increase their adherence to regular sport.

6.3 Strategies for Increasing a Patient's Adherence to Exercise

As mentioned above, many patients with obesity may find it difficult to stick to a regular exercise regime. Nonetheless, CBT-OB has been designed with this in mind and includes several strategies and procedures that should maximise the chances of them doing so.

6.3.1 The Problem of Adherence to Exercise

Most individuals with obesity are sedentary, and changing their lifestyle to include consistent exercise is not easy. Indeed, they often display considerable aversion and low tolerance for exercise—one of the major reasons for the long-term failure of treatments for obesity. Hence, a patient's adherence to physical activity recommendations is one of the most important factors to address.

Available data suggest that the stage of change and the patient's self-efficacy, psychological wellbeing and expectations are the most important psychological predictors of adherence to physical exercise. The Stage of Change model—originally developed to guide the study of smoking behaviour [29]—can be used to classify five main stages in the path to initiation and maintenance of exercise as follows [30]: (1) pre-contemplation (no exercise now and no intention of exercising in the next 6 months), (2) contemplation (no exercise, but intention to do so in the next 6 months), (3) preparation (no exercise, but intention to do so in the next 30 days) and action (has been exercising for fewer than 6 months) and (4) maintenance (has been exercising for more than 6 months). This theory explains why some patients are more responsive than others to exercise counselling; for example, subjects at the contemplation or pre-contemplation stages (who have limited or no immediate intention to exercise) are generally less receptive than those in the preparation stage (who intend to exercise and may have already given it considerable thought).

Likewise, perceived self-efficacy is a consistent predictor of physical exercise adherence; it is defined as the degree of a person's belief in their capabilities to produce designated levels of performance [31]. In other words, perceived self-efficacy is the extent to which an individual believes they are capable of implementing a behavioural change—in this case increasing the level of physical activity. Self-efficacy therefore plays an important role in achieving healthy behavioural change [32] and should be encouraged by CBT-OB (building a trusting relationship, setting achievable goals, etc.).

The initial psychological wellbeing perceived by the subject seems to be another important psychological factor influencing exercise adherence. Indeed, poor initial psychological wellbeing and the mental stress associated with exercise (training) may reduce the limited energy normally available for self-change even further [33]. In addition, poor psychological wellbeing may have a negative influence on self-efficacy, thereby contributing to an increased likelihood of attrition [32].

Finally, unrealistic expectations also seem to be a major determinant of a failure to change behaviour. Several studies have shown that subjects scoring high on a measure of expectancy (but low on self-efficacy) displayed higher rates of attrition [34].

The interaction between these cognitive processes has been investigated by one study assessing the comprehensive role of expectation, self-efficacy, stage of change and psychological wellbeing in adherence to an exercise programme. This study revealed that participants who completed the course had lower baseline expectations of change, which made it easier for them to reach their targets, with respect to those who dropped out [35]. Unsurprisingly, this achievement led to an improvement in perceived self-efficacy in completers, a factor that tended to deteriorate in dropouts. These findings suggest that unrealistic and overly optimistic expectations may lead to dissatisfaction and attrition in exercise programmes. It is therefore essential to bear in mind these cognitive processes when suggesting to a patient with obesity that they increase their level of physical activity.

6.3.2 Tailoring Activity Goals to Individual Patients

The CBT-OB therapist should always assess whether the suggested exercise is physically and psychologically feasible for patients, taking into account all the relevant obstacles that emerged at the assessment stage. Accordingly, the therapist should actively assist patients in developing an achievable exercise plan and provide them with the cognitive and behavioural skills to enable them to modify their sedentary habits. Recommendations should not be given as generic prescriptions but tailored to each patient's preferences and ability. Indeed, as already mentioned in this chapter, exercise adherence tends to increase when less structure is imposed, presumably as this throws up fewer obstacles. The research shows that patients are more likely to engage in physical activity when instructed to do so on their own at home than when asked to attend supervised, group-based on-site exercise sessions. In addition, increasing lifestyle activity results in comparable weight loss but better maintenance than structured, planned activity. Finally, multiple short bouts of exercise (10 min each), rather than one long session, may help patients accumulate more daily minutes of exercise by providing them with more easily achievable goals. In summary, these data suggest that de-structuring helps patients to overcome both practical and psychological barriers to exercise [25].

6.3.3 Goal Setting

Patients should be encouraged to set specific and quantifiable weekly physical activity goals, which should be achievable but moderately challenging. Indeed, achieving goals is associated with a sense of accomplishment, which is self-reinforcing and enhances perceived self-efficacy—a construct associated with long-term weight-loss maintenance. The therapist should suggest that patients start with gentle exercising and gradually increase to a goal of 200–300 min per week [23]. As described in Sect. 6.2.1.2, walking is the preferred exercise, as it is a form of unstructured physical activity that may easily be included in the daily routine. When discussing this topic with the patient, unrealistic goals should be promptly discouraged because they are likely to cause attrition (see Chap. 1).

6.3.4 Self-Monitoring

Self-monitoring of physical activity, alongside food intake and body weight, is one of the core procedures of CBT-OB. Self-monitoring raises patients' awareness of their exercise habits, and helps them to identify ways in which they can maximise their energy deficit. As described in detail in Chap. 4, physical activity in the form of daily step count and minutes of formal exercise should be recorded on the Monitoring Record. Patients interested in having a more precise measurement of their daily energy expenditure may use an accelerometer—which measures not only total energy expenditure over a prescribed period but also the energy expended during a particular session of physical activity, the duration and the levels (in METs) of the session and the time spent sleeping.

Patients may also benefit from recording events, thoughts, moods and physical sensations associated with exercise in the Comments column of the Monitoring Record. This strategy may highlight obstacles to exercising, and self-monitoring can also be used to provide information for the identification of activity contingencies, which can be targeted for intervention.

6.3.5 Responding to Non-adherence

Long-term adherence to exercise and body weight control can be extremely difficult, due to a complex combination of biological, environmental and psychological pressures. The therapist should therefore congratulate patients on every success they achieve and never criticise failures. Indeed, criticism may produce guilt and loss of self-confidence, thereby increasing the likelihood of attrition. Unconditional acceptance of a patient's behaviour and the adoption of a problem-solving approach will safeguard the clinician–patient relationship, and the strategies and procedures to address obstacles to an active lifestyle are described in detail in the Chap. 7 (Module 4). This approach will also help patients understand that long-term success in body weight management is related to a set of skills rather than willpower alone.

References

1. Wu T, Gao X, Chen M, van Dam RM. Long-term effectiveness of diet-plus-exercise interventions vs. diet-only interventions for weight loss: a meta-analysis. Obes Rev. 2009;10(3):313–23. https://doi.org/10.1111/j.1467-789X.2008.00547.x.
2. Mayo MJ, Grantham JR, Balasekaran G. Exercise-induced weight loss preferentially reduces abdominal fat. Med Sci Sports Exerc. 2003;35(2):207–13. https://doi.org/10.1249/01.mss.0000048636.46744.01.
3. Wing RR, Phelan S. Long-term weight loss maintenance. Am J Clin Nutr. 2005;82(1 Suppl):222s–5s.
4. Manson JE, Greenland P, LaCroix AZ, Stefanick ML, Mouton CP, Oberman A, et al. Walking compared with vigorous exercise for the prevention of cardiovascular events in women. N Engl J Med. 2002;347(10):716–25. https://doi.org/10.1056/NEJMoa021067.
5. Richardson CR, Kriska AM, Lantz PM, Hayward RA. Physical activity and mortality across cardiovascular disease risk groups. Med Sci Sports Exerc. 2004;36(11):1923–9.
6. Katzmarzyk PT, Church TS, Janssen I, Ross R, Blair SN. Metabolic syndrome, obesity, and mortality: impact of cardiorespiratory fitness. Diabetes Care. 2005;28(2):391–7.
7. Garber CE, Blissmer B, Deschenes MR, Franklin BA, Lamonte MJ, Lee IM, et al. American College of Sports Medicine position stand. Quantity and quality of exercise for developing and maintaining cardiorespiratory, musculoskeletal, and neuromotor fitness in apparently healthy adults: guidance for prescribing exercise. Med Sci Sports Exerc. 2011;43(7):1334–59. https://doi.org/10.1249/MSS.0b013e318213fefb.
8. Canadian Society for Exercise Physiology. Physical Activity Readiness Questionnaire—PAR-Q. Revised 2002. www.csep.ca/forms.
9. Brooks D, Solway S, Gibbons WJ. ATS statement on six-minute walk test. Am J Respir Crit Care Med. 2003;167(9):1287. https://doi.org/10.1164/ajrccm.167.9.950.
10. El Ghoch M, Rossi AP, Calugi S, Rubele S, Soave F, Zamboni M, Chignola E, et al. Physical performance measures in screening for reduced lean body mass in adult females with obesity. Nutr Metab Cardiovasc Dis. 2018. https://doi.org/10.1016/j.numecd.2018.06.008.
11. Hamilton A, Balnave R, Adams R. Grip strength testing reliability. J Hand Ther. 1994;7(3):163–70.
12. Whitney SL, Wrisley DM, Marchetti GF, Gee MA, Redfern MS, Furman JM. Clinical measurement of sit-to-stand performance in people with balance disorders: validity of data for the Five-Times-Sit-to-Stand Test. Phys Ther. 2005;85(10):1034–45.
13. Duncan PW, Weiner DK, Chandler J, Studenski S. Functional reach: a new clinical measure of balance. J Gerontol. 1990;45(6):M192–7.
14. Dalle Grave R. Motivating patients with obesity to exercise. In: Hansen D, editor. Exercise therapy in adult obesity. New York: Nova Press; 2013. p. 167–82.
15. Ballor DL, Poehlman ET. Exercise-training enhances fat-free mass preservation during diet-induced weight loss: a meta-analytical finding. Int J Obes Relat Metab Disord. 1994;18(1):35–40.
16. Wing RR. Physical activity in the treatment of the adulthood overweight and obesity: current evidence and research issues. Med Sci Sports Exerc. 1999;31(11 Suppl):S547–52.
17. Jeffery RW, Wing RR, Sherwood NE, Tate DF. Physical activity and weight loss: does prescribing higher physical activity goals improve outcome? Am J Clin Nutr. 2003;78(4):684–9.

18. Jakicic JM, Winters C, Lang W, Wing RR. Effects of intermittent exercise and use of home exercise equipment on adherence, weight loss, and fitness in overweight women: a randomized trial. JAMA. 1999;282(16):1554–60.
19. Andersen RE, Wadden TA, Bartlett SJ, Zemel B, Verde TJ, Franckowiak SC. Effects of lifestyle activity vs structured aerobic exercise in obese women: a randomized trial. JAMA. 1999;281(4):335–40.
20. Campbell A, Hausenblas HA. Effects of exercise interventions on body image: a meta-analysis. J Health Psychol. 2009;14(6):780–93. https://doi.org/10.1177/1359105309338977.
21. Sherwood NE, Jeffery RW. The behavioral determinants of exercise: implications for physical activity interventions. Annu Rev Nutr. 2000;20:21–44. https://doi.org/10.1146/annurev.nutr.20.1.21.
22. Ekkekakis P, Lind E, Vazou S. Affective responses to increasing levels of exercise intensity in normal-weight, overweight, and obese middle-aged women. Obesity (Silver Spring). 2010;18(1):79–85. https://doi.org/10.1038/oby.2009.204.
23. Jakicic JM, Rogers RJ. Exercise in the management of obesity. In: Brownell KD, Walsh BT, editors. Eating disorders and obesity: a comprehensive handbook. 3rd ed. New York: Guilford Press; 2017. p. 546–50.
24. Caspersen CJ, Powell KE, Christenson GM. Physical activity, exercise, and physical fitness: definitions and distinctions for health-related research. Public Health Rep. 1985;100(2):126–31.
25. Fabricatore AN. Behavior therapy and cognitive-behavioral therapy of obesity: is there a difference? J Am Diet Assoc. 2007;107(1):92–9. https://doi.org/10.1016/j.jada.2006.10.005.
26. Dalle Grave R, Calugi S, El Ghoch M. Increasing adherence to diet and exercise through cognitive behavioural strategies. In: Lenzi A, Migliaccio S, Donini LM, editors. Multidisciplinary approach to obesity. Cham: Springer International Publishing; 2015. p. 327–35.
27. Soave F. Strategie per adottare uno stile di vita attivo e per migliorare la fitness fisica. Emozioni e Cibo. 2014;39:18–20.
28. Warburton DER, Nicol CW, Bredin SSD. Health benefits of physical activity: the evidence. Can Med Assoc J. 2006;174(6):801–9. https://doi.org/10.1503/cmaj.051351.
29. Prochaska JO, DiClemente CC. Stages and processes of self-change of smoking: toward an integrative model of change. J Consult Clin Psychol. 1983;51(3):390–5.
30. Marcus BH, Simkin LR. The transtheoretical model: applications to exercise behavior. Med Sci Sports Exerc. 1994;26(11):1400–4.
31. Bandura A. Social foundations of thought and action: a social cognitive theory. Englewood Cliffs: Prentice-Hall; 1986.
32. Strecher VJ, DeVellis BM, Becker MH, Rosenstock IM. The role of self-efficacy in achieving health behavior change. Health Educ Q. 1986;13(1):73–92. https://doi.org/10.1177/109019818601300108.
33. Muraven M, Baumeister RF. Self-regulation and depletion of limited resources: does self-control resemble a muscle? Psychol Bull. 2000;126(2):247–59.
34. Sears SR, Stanton AL. Expectancy-value constructs and expectancy violation as predictors of exercise adherence in previously sedentary women. Health Psychol. 2001;20(5):326–33.
35. Jones F, Harris P, Waller H, Coggins A. Adherence to an exercise prescription scheme: the role of expectations, self-efficacy, stage of change and psychological well-being. Br J Health Psychol. 2005;10(Pt 3):359–78. https://doi.org/10.1348/135910704x24798.

Module 4: Addressing Obstacles to Weight Loss

7

Module 4 starts the week after Modules 2 and 3, but the strategies and procedures that it introduces should be continued and reinforced until the end of the weight-loss phase. It is designed to help patients to identify and address their personal obstacles to weight loss. As such, patients are educated on the main mechanisms that maintain excessive eating and a sedentary lifestyle. Each obstacle will be incorporated into each patient's Personal Formulation and subsequently addressed, providing them with specific cognitive behavioural strategies and procedures designed to help the patient overcome them.

7.1 Educating Patients on Cognitive Behavioural Weight-Loss Obstacles

In Session 3, after in-session weighing and a review of the week's Monitoring Records, the CBT-OB therapist introduces the topic of weight-loss obstacles to the agenda. According to CBT-OB, these fall into the following three categories [1]: (1) antecedent stimuli, (2) positive consequences and (3) problematic thoughts.

7.1.1 Antecedent Stimuli

The CBT-OB therapist starts by explaining that the Western environment in which we live is full of stimuli that encourage excessive eating and promote a sedentary lifestyle. Such stimuli arouse physiological, behavioural, cognitive and/or emotional responses that make it difficult to lose weight. These are called "antecedent stimuli" because they produce a subsequent behavioural response—for example, excessive eating or the adoption of a sedentary lifestyle. Antecedent stimuli can be divided into eating and non-eating stimuli:

- *Eating stimuli*. These are produced by the presence of food in the environment in which we live. The mere sight of food is a stimulus that naturally determines a

R. Dalle Grave et al., *Treating Obesity with Personalized Cognitive Behavioral Therapy*, https://doi.org/10.1007/978-3-319-91497-8_7

physiological response: it is enough to see an ice cream or a pastry shop to experience an involuntary increase in salivation and desire for food—a response that is particularly strong in individuals on a diet [2].

- *Non-eating stimuli.* These include events and changes in mood that encourage eating to excess or sedentary behaviours. Examples include negative (i.e. anger, anxiety, sadness, boredom) or positive (i.e. joy, cheerfulness) emotions, times of day (i.e. the evening, after dinner) and places (i.e. the parents' house, the armchair), as well as doing certain activities (i.e. watching TV), experiencing physical symptoms (i.e. tiredness, muscle aches) or practical impediments to exercise (e.g. not having the proper clothes or equipment, not having much money, having to exercise alone, living too far from the gym). Other non-eating stimuli are less easily identifiable, but in some individuals, they are one of the biggest barriers to weight loss, favouring both excessive eating and a sedentary lifestyle, and should therefore be investigated by the CBT-OB therapist.

The therapist underlines that repeatedly associating an eating stimulus (food) with a non-eating stimulus (e.g. watching TV sitting in an armchair after work) eventually determines a learned response, called "classical conditioning" [3]. In other words, if a person gets into the habit of eating in front of the TV, they are triggered to want food every time they watch TV. Similarly, the repeated association between a sedentary lifestyle stimulus (i.e. tiredness) and sitting in an armchair encourages the person to always seek to resolve tiredness by sitting in an armchair.

7.1.2 Positive Consequences

Another element that can hinder weight-loss attempts is the gratifying effect of food intake and sedentary behaviours. The gratification and pleasure associated with food intake results from a complex interaction of biological (e.g. food intake—especially sweet foods—seems to stimulate the mesolimbic/mesocortical dopaminergic reward circuitry [4], the same systems stimulated by recreational drugs), cognitive (i.e. the positive expectation of the consequence of food intake [5]) and emotional (i.e. the positive or negative emotional consequences of food intake [6]) factors. However, the therapist should make patients reflect that some people tend to use food as an exclusive or predominant means of gratification and that this behaviour could be an important obstacle to weight loss.

To help the patients to understand better the concept of positive consequences, the CBT-OB therapist should make use of examples to illustrate that each behaviour produces certain consequences; if the consequence is positive, we tend to repeat the same behaviour (e.g. "I always go to that restaurant because I like the food and they give me large portions"; "Every night I lie on the couch watching TV because it relaxes me"), while if the consequence is negative we tend to avoid the behaviour (e.g. "I don't drink coffee because it gives me indigestion"; "Sitting down for a long time always makes me feel sluggish"). This process, called "operant conditioning" [7], is based on the concept of *reinforcement*, which can be positive or negative:

- *Positive reinforcement*. This occurs when a behaviour produces gratification or a positive subjective response (e.g. "I feel comforted when I eat food I like"; "I'm so relieved to be sitting down at last!") and increases the likelihood that the same behaviour will be repeated over time, in the search for the same gratification.
- *Negative reinforcement*. This occurs when a behaviour is practised to get out of an unpleasant situation or to eliminate a negative emotion (e.g. "If I eat something, I won't be so 'angry'"; "I won't be so tired if I sit down for a while").

7.1.3 Problematic Thoughts

After having explained the association between eating/non-eating stimuli and problematic behaviours (i.e. eating when stressed), the CBT-OB therapist should then start to describe the influential role that thoughts, beliefs and attitudes towards eating and exercise can have on emotions and behaviours [8], explaining that the way we think can facilitate or prevent the adoption of problematic behaviours.

Thoughts that hinder weight loss are also called "sabotaging thoughts" [9], because they lead to behaviours that sabotage any attempt to lose weight. These thoughts are mainly automatic, and the person is often unaware of them. They typically occur when a patient trying to lose weight by changing their behaviours perceives effort and frustration, which they use to justify the maintenance or recurrence of old habits.

The therapist should therefore educate patients about such sabotaging thoughts. These may have emerged in the first review of the Monitoring Records, but common problematic thoughts reported by patients that should be discussed are as follows [9]:

- *Justification thoughts*. There are many reasons that patients use to justify excessive eating or sedentary behaviour, but all have the effect of sabotaging the attempt to lose weight. Typically, these thoughts start with the phrase: "I eat because…" or "I'm not going to do any exercise because…". Here are some examples:
  - "I'm going to eat because I'm celebrating; it's a special occasion".
  - "I'm going to eat because I need the energy; it's been a tiring day".
  - "I'm going to eat because it's free; you shouldn't look a gift horse in the mouth!"
  - "This food isn't very fattening, I can eat a little".
  - "It would be a shame to let all this food go to waste".
  - "I'm going to eat this food because I spent money on it".
  - "I may as well eat because nobody is watching".
  - "I'm just going to have a snack because I'm stressed/tired/bored/sad/angry".
  - "Food is the only pleasure I have nowadays".
  - "I'm too tired to do any exercise tonight".
  - "I haven't got enough time to do any exercise today".
  - "I'm too fat to do any exercise".
  - "If I do any exercise I will only get hungry again".

- *Self-critical thoughts*. Besides hindering weight-loss attempts, self-criticism promotes deviation from the meal and/or exercise plan. Self-critical thoughts reduce self-confidence in the ability to lose weight and may lead to a person giving up their attempt entirely. Some examples of self-critical thoughts that may provoke this result are:
  - "I'm too weak-willed".
  - "I'm incapable of sticking to a diet".
  - "I have no willpower".
  - "I cannot control myself".
- *Negative predictions*. These thoughts are characterised by the prediction that the weight-loss attempt will fail. As such, they sabotage the adoption of the behaviours needed to lose weight. Typically, negative predictions arise when the patient sees that the weight loss they have achieved does not meet their expectations, in spite of all their effort. Here are some examples of negative predictions:
  - "I will never be able to lose the weight".
  - "Even if I manage to lose some weight, I'll only put it all back on again".
  - "If I am not losing at least one kilo per week, there is no sense in making all this effort to diet and exercise".
- *All-or-nothing thoughts*. This type of thoughts almost inevitably leads the patients to abandon any attempt to control eating and typically occurs when they break a rule that they have set for themselves (as regards eating or exercise) or do not see the results (in terms of weight loss) that they feel that they deserve or expect. Patients adopting an all-or-nothing style of thinking do not recognise half measures—either they diet or they eat to excess; either they are losing weight or they will put it on. Here are some examples of all-or-nothing thinking:
  - "If I don't manage to stick to the diet, I'll just give up and binge".
  - "If I don't lose at least X kilos a month/week, I'll stop bothering".
  - "I've already eaten a chocolate bar that I didn't intend to, so today may as well be a no-diet day".
  - "There is no way I will be able to walk for an hour, so I'd be better off just sitting here".

7.2 Introducing the Weight-Loss Obstacles Questionnaire

After having explained the principal cognitive behavioural obstacles to weight loss, the CBT-OB therapist can introduce the "Weight-Loss Obstacles Questionnaire" (see Appendix D). This is a self-report questionnaire that the patient should fill in once a week; it includes key questions that investigate whether or not they are applying the set strategies and procedures and if any other behaviours or attitudes that might hinder weight loss have occurred over the previous week. For every obstacle identified, the patients should report on the Questionnaire their opinion of why it arose and what mechanisms could be driving the problematic behaviours.

The Weight-Loss Obstacles Questionnaire also investigates an individual's attitudes to weight loss (i.e. satisfaction, self-efficacy and motivation) and the degree of family support they are receiving. These questions are designed to help the patient and therapist to intervene when a dysfunctional attitude regarding weight loss arises (see Chap. 8) or to intercede with a view to improving support from significant others (see Chap. 9).

7.3 Creating the Personal Formulation

From Session 4 onwards, until the end of the weight-loss phase, part of each session should be dedicated to helping patients identify and address their individual obstacles to weight loss. The patients are actively involved in this task through weekly compilation of the Weight-Loss Obstacles Questionnaire and collaborative review of their Monitoring Records.

With the aid of the therapist, the obstacles identified are incorporated by each patient into their Personal Formulation—a procedural tool that has been specifically adapted with a view to personalising CBT-OB. The "formulation" concept is widely used in other areas of CBT [10], but not generally in traditional BT-OB. It involves creating a visual representation (a flow chart) of the cognitive behavioural processes, previously described to the patient (see Sect. 7.1), that may hinder their adherence to the lifestyle changes needed to lose weight. Specifically, it includes [11] (1) antecedent stimuli, (2) positive consequences and (3) problematic thoughts (see Sect. 7.1, above).

The creation of the Personal Formulation has a number of purposes:

- It helps to engage the patients in the treatment.
- The process of creating the Formulation distances the patients from their problems. Rather than simply eating to excess or living a sedentary lifestyle, the patients are now encouraged to step back and try to understand the problem and why it persists, a procedure that can help the patients to develop an interest in their behaviours and subsequently to understand how to change them.
  The Formulation itself helps the patient to understand that their difficulties in losing weight are related to a variety of interacting, self-perpetuating mechanisms, rather than a simple lack of willpower.
- It provides a guide to what needs to be targeted by the treatment, by highlighting the main mechanisms that are maintaining the patient's excessive eating and sedentary lifestyle.
- Developing a Formulation is a key procedure in terms of personalisation of the treatment, which will determine the implementation of only the strategies and procedures that are potentially useful for addressing the patient's specific weight-loss obstacles.

An example of a CBT-OB Formulation is shown in Fig. 7.1, while Appendix B is a blank formulation that can be used as a template.

The Formulation should be constructed step by step in an unhurried manner, with the therapist taking the lead but the patient being actively involved [10]. The Formulation should focus only on the main mechanisms that appear to be maintaining the excessive eating and/or sedentary lifestyle in the individual patient. The therapist should stress that the Formulation is provisional and will be custom-modified as needed during the treatment.

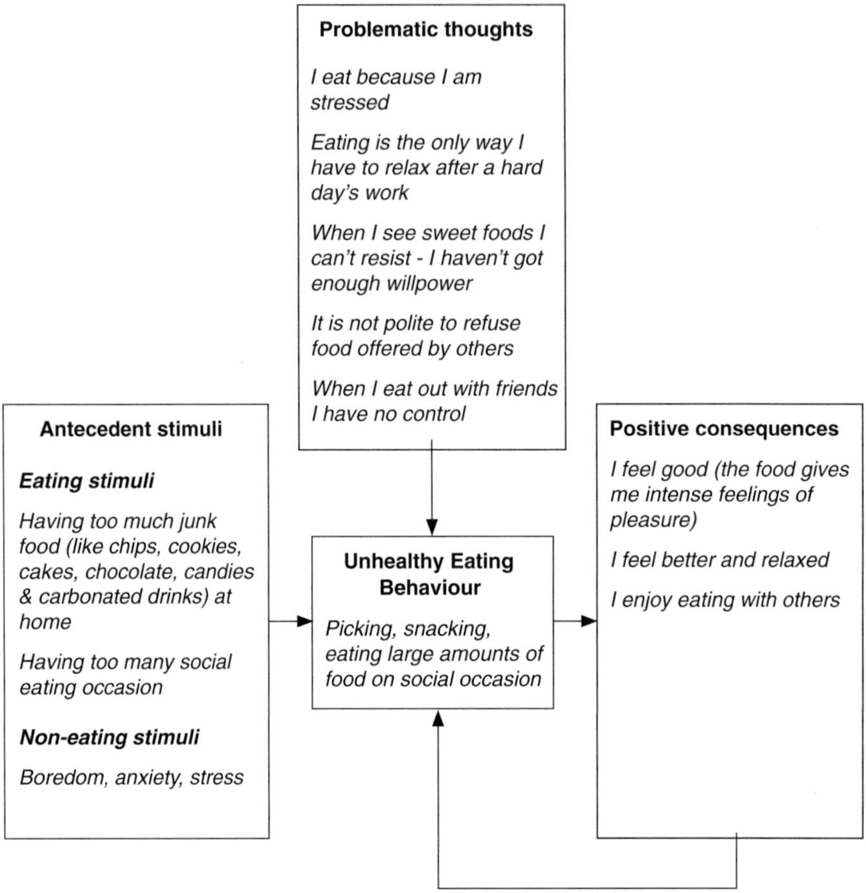

Fig. 7.1 An example personal cognitive behavioural Formulation featuring a patient's main obstacles to weight loss (based on this formulation, the treatment was focused on reducing eating stimuli; addressing boredom, anxiety, and stress; challenging problematic thoughts; and finding alternatives to food as a reward) (From Dalle Grave et al. [11]:1–11. Reprinted with the permission of Springer-Verlag Italia)

Once the Formulation has been created, the therapist should discuss its implications with the patient. One major point to emphasise is that control of neither eating nor physical activity is wholly dependent on their willpower. In fact, it can be improved by learning specific cognitive and behavioural skills designed to counteract the biological, environmental, cognitive and emotional pressures to eating excessively and adopt a sedentary lifestyle—the main goal of CBT-OB.

In collaboration with the patient, the therapist should decide which weight-loss obstacles to address and in which order. To this end, it is important to note that, like CBT-E for eating disorders [10], CBT-OB is administered bearing in mind two key principles: first, simple procedures are best, and, second, it is better to do a few things well rather than many things badly ("principle of parsimony").

At the end of the session, patients should be given a copy of their formulation and asked to review it before the next appointment, when it will be modified as necessary. At each subsequent session, just after collaborative weighing and Monitoring Record review, the therapist should ask the patients to complete the Weight-Loss Obstacles Questionnaire (when the sessions are held every 2 weeks, the patients should fill in the questionnaire at home in the week in which there is no session). When a new obstacle is identified, patients are invited to update their formulation to include any newly identified mechanisms hindering weight loss.

The following *Vignette* is an example of how a personalised formulation can be effectively constructed with a patient.

Vignette

Luisa is a 45-year-old high school teacher who began the CBT-OB weight-loss programme with enthusiasm but after 2 weeks felt demoralised and inadequate because of the difficulties she encountered adhering to the meal plan; as a result of this, she tended to overeat. A review of her Monitoring Records showed that she was eating more food than she planned at specific mealtimes—namely, Sunday breakfast and Tuesday and Thursday afternoon snacks. The therapist asked the patient to fill out the Weight-Loss Obstacles Questionnaire and used the resulting information to help her address this problem:

- *Therapist*: "Well, Luisa, if you agree, I would like to analyse with you what happened in the situations in which you were not able to stick to your meal plan. Can we refer to what you wrote in the Questionnaire?"
- *Patient*: "Yes, willingly. I feel terrible when I don't eat what I have planned".
- *Therapist*: "I understand what you mean, and that's exactly why I want us to discuss this issue. I would like to analyse these difficult situations together. If we can understand how they happen and why, we can find solutions".
- *Patient*: "That would be nice!"
- *Therapist*: "Well, let's start with the first episode, which occurred at breakfast on Sunday morning. You wrote that on that occasion you ate a slice of cake, instead of the crispbread you had planned. You report in your Monitoring Record that the reason was that there was some cake left over from dinner the night before in the kitchen. Can you tell me more about this situation?"
- *Patient*: "Of course! On Saturday night, my husband and I, just like always, had my sister and her husband to dinner. During dinner, I was able to maintain good eating control and stick to my meal plan—it was simple because I cooked the foods that I planned to eat. My sister, however, usually brings a cake. She bakes it herself, and we all love her cakes. I usually have no problem during dinner, as I have already eaten my meal and I do not need to eat a slice of cake. However, on Sunday morning, when I went to the kitchen to make breakfast, I caught sight of the rest of cake, sitting on the counter. I couldn't resist and had a big slice of cake instead of the crispbread I had planned. I'm just greedy!"

- *Therapist*: "I understand that this makes you feel bad, but let's take a look at your Personal Formulation (*the therapist indicates the Formulation, which is on the desk*); where should we put this slice of cake in the diagram?"
- *Patient*: "I think we should put it into the 'antecedent eating stimuli' box".
- *Therapist*: "Great! You are right! From what I understand, this is a stimulus you encounter every Sunday morning".
- *Patient*: "Yes, it is".
- *Therapist*: "Ok, now let's try to break this down; when you go to the kitchen on Sunday mornings, you always encounter tasty food that does not require any preparation. Right?"
- *Patient*: "Yes".
- *Therapist*: "This stimulus drives you to eat something that you had not planned and therefore to eat more than you would like. Is that right?"
- *Patient*: "Yes, just like that!"
- *Therapist*: "The sight of the cake every Sunday morning and the fact that it is a food that you like prompts you to repeat the same behaviour. It is very difficult to resist readily available food, especially the food that we like. We call this mechanism 'positive reinforcement'; do you remember? You planned to eat crispbread, but instead you ate a slice of cake, as you prefer that to crispbread. In the moment this made you feel good because the cake was delicious. This positive consequence reinforces your desire to do the same thing again next Sunday. Do you see?"
- *Patient*: "Yes, now it is clear, and it also seems simple to understand".
- *Therapist*: "Good! So, we can put this mechanism in the Formulation (*the patient writes it*)".
- *Therapist*: "Excellent! Now, before we review the whole thing, I would like to discuss with you the other situations in which you eat to excess that you have identified".
- *Patient*: "Are you talking about the afternoon snacks?"
- *Therapist*: "Yes, especially the episodes on Tuesdays and Thursdays that you noted as problematic. In the Weight-Loss Obstacles Questionnaire, I saw that you wrote that the snack you planned was not enough. Can you try to help me understand?"
- *Patient*: "Yes, just like that. On Tuesdays and Thursdays, I always go to the gym; I like it because I do an aerobics course with my friends—we have fun, and it's a way to spend time together. Since the course is at 6 pm, I plan my snack, usually some fruit, at 5 pm. But then I'm afraid that a piece of fruit will not be enough and I add a large slice of bread and jam, though I know

it's too much and I'll go over my calorie allowance. I feel guilty; I say to myself that next time I will stick to the plan, but then it always ends badly".

- *Therapist*: "Why do you think that some fruit is not enough?"
- *Patient*: "I'm afraid of feeling faint, my blood pressure dropping, and not having enough energy. Once it happened and it was terrible!"
- *Therapist*: "You are right. It is bad when you feel that you don't have enough energy. Can you tell me when that happened to you?"
- *Patient*: "It happened a couple of years ago; I'd had a bad chest infection so I was feeling a bit run down. I was still on antibiotics because my GP told me I had to finish the cycle. I was back at work, and a friend from my gym group called and told me there was a nice new teacher (*she smiles*), and I absolutely had to go to the gym. Although I wasn't completely well, I was feeling much better and so I decided to go. However, after about 15 min of physical activity, I felt my legs giving way—I got dizzy and had to lie on the floor. My friends all gathered round and took me home. It was a really awkward and embarrassing situation!"
- *Therapist*: "Since then, have you ever felt sick in the gym?"
- *Patient*: "No, but I have always prevented it, by eating something else before I go".
- *Therapist*: "So your reasoning is more or less this: 'If I do not eat enough before going to the gym I might be sick'. Am I right?"
- *Patient*: "Yes, that's right".
- *Therapist*: "Hmm… Thinking back over the last 2 years, have you ever had to go to the gym without having eaten an adequate snack?"
- *Patient*: "Now that you mention it… Yes! Sometimes, though not often, after dropping my son off at the swimming pool, I've been chatting with the other mothers and lost track of time. On those occasions, I was running late and I had to hurry to the gym without having a snack".
- *Therapist*: "Well… and on those occasions, did you have any problems during your exercise session?"
- *Patient*: "To tell you the truth, I do not remember any so… I suppose I was fine".
- *Therapist*: "Well, this tells us something important".
- *Patient*: … (*the patient reflects*) "Yes, it does. Maybe I can do physical activity without any physical problems even if I only eat fruit".
- *Therapist*: "If you don't try you will never find out. It is probable that when you felt sick other factors were the cause, not the lack of energy due to the lack of food".

- *Patient*: "Yes, I was probably weakened by illness and medicine… Now I'm physically fit".
- *Therapist*: "Right! Looking at your Formulation, where would you put this obstacle?"
- *Patient*: "It seems to me to be a problematic thought".
- *Therapist*: "I agree. Can we try to break it down? Try to think what went through your mind when you ate bread and jam after the fruit".
- *Patient*: "Probably something like this: 'I should eat more so I don't feel bad when I'm at the gym'… Of course, I like bread and jam…".
- *Therapist*: "That sounds accurate. It seems that you used this thought to allow yourself to eat a food you like without feeling too guilty. However, by analysing the situation in detail, we have seen that feeling bad during physical activity seldom actually happens and that continuing to maintain this way of thinking sabotages your attempt to lose weight rather than helping you increase your energy at the gym. Why don't you write this example of problematic thinking in your Formulation?"
- *Patient*: "I will (*the patient inserts the problematic though into her Formulation*)".
- *Therapist*: "Well done! Now, we have been able to identify some obstacles to your losing weight and incorporate them into your Formulation. As you can see, the Formulation helps us to understand what drives you to eat too much. We have identified an antecedent eating stimulus and a problematic thought, both of which are very powerful. Now, look at the Formulation again; where should you focus your efforts if you want to prevent new episodes of overeating?"
- *Patient*: "Undoubtedly by trying to address the obstacles—that is, Sunday morning cake and my problem thoughts".
- *Therapist*: "Exactly! We will have to find strategies that will help you to overcome these obstacles. This Formulation helps us to see that, in order to deal with eating to excess, it is necessary first to identify the mechanisms maintaining your unhealthy behaviour and then to find appropriate solutions. Your willpower does not come in to it!"
- *Patient*: "You are right. This makes me feel a lot calmer… (*she smiles*) Maybe I can do it!"
- *Therapist*: "I would say so! You can do it (*smiling*)".
  Afterwards, the therapist helps the patient to draw up an action plan to address the weight-loss obstacles identified in this way using the procedures outlined in the following paragraphs.

7.4 Addressing Weight-Loss Obstacles

In this section we report the strategies and the procedures recommended by CBT-OB for addressing the main weight-loss obstacles described in Sect. 7.1.

7.4.1 Reducing Environmental Stimuli

Unfortunately, our patients live in an environment that makes it difficult to control eating. Environmental stimuli, such as appetising food, that promote excessive eating are all around, and most people are very busy and surrounded by labour-saving devices, which make it difficult for them to get enough physical activity. It is therefore essential to train patients to adopt strategies that will reduce their exposure to excessive environmental stimulation and thereby facilitate their compliance with the treatment.

To this end, patients whose Personal Formulation indicates that environmental stimuli are an obstacle to their weight-loss attempt are provided with an exhaustive list of counteractive strategies, as shown Table 7.1. The list has been designed to include several everyday situations in which people typically encounter unhelpful environmental stimuli.

Table 7.1 Environmental stimuli that hinder weight loss and strategies for reducing them

Strategies for reducing eating stimuli
Doing the grocery shopping
• Plan in detail what to buy beforehand (e.g. based on a weekly meal plan) • Only do the grocery shopping on a full stomach • Stick to your shopping list and do not buy food that you do not need • Do not take more money than you need • Avoid the confectionary aisle and tempting shops • Stock up on food that requires preparation
Storing food
• Don't leave food in sight • Only keep food in the kitchen or pantry • Store food in pre-established places • Store food wrapped in foil or dull containers • Put tempting foods in inaccessible places
Preparing food
• Cook the exact amount of food you need and prepare single portions • Cook using as little fat as possible • Don't taste food during preparation • Don't cook when you are hungry • Chew gum while cooking • Put cooking utensils in soapy water as soon as you have finished using them

(continued)

Table 7.1 (continued)

Serving food
• Serve food on individual plates rather than serving dishes
• Don't put a basket of bread or "nibbles" on the table
• Wait 5 min before having second helpings
• Use small plates
During eating
• Take small bites and chew thoroughly
• Put your cutlery down between one bite and the next
• Always eat meals in the same place
• Always eat sitting at the table or breakfast bar
• Focus on what you are eating
• Focus on the taste of food
• Eat at the same time every day
• Eat according to your meal plan, not according to hunger or eating stimuli
After eating
• Get up as soon as you have finished your meal
• Clear the table right after you've finished eating
• If possible leave the kitchen
• If you have coffee after your meal, drink it in the living room
• Do not hoard leftovers
• Wrap usable leftovers in foil
Social occasions (restaurant, friends' houses, parties)
• Avoid these occasions if you do not feel ready or if you are having to deal with too many high-risk situations (a lot of dinner invitations)
• Plan calorie management ahead (e.g. eat fewer calories the day before and/or the day after the social situation in which you eat with others)
• Plan how to tackle the difficulties you will encounter in terms of limiting your calorie intake
• Order before the others
• Choose low-fat dishes
• Avoid the bread basket and appetisers
• Limit alcohol consumption
• Eat slowly
Strategies for reducing sedentary lifestyle stimuli
• Buy workout clothes
• Plan physical activity (what, who, when and how)
• Prepare your workout clothes the evening before, and put them where you will see them as soon as you get up
• Keep a gym bag in your car so you don't have to go home to get it
• Set an alarm to remind you it's time for exercise
• Arrange with a friend to exercise together
• Phone them to remind them of your exercise appointment
• Have a break if you get tired
• Reward yourself after you have done the physical activity you planned[a]

[a]Rewards should not be food-based (see Sect. 7.4.5)

Vignette

Returning to Luisa, the therapist addresses the "antecedent eating" stimulus, namely, the Sunday morning cake. Food availability, especially if the food is highly palatable and ready to eat, makes it difficult for her to maintain control overeating. With the aid of the therapist, and referring to the list in Table 7.1, the patient identified the following possible solutions for reducing that specific environmental stimulus: she could ask her sister to bring something other than the cake (e.g. a bottle of wine, which would not be a problem for the patient since she is teetotal) or bring a smaller cake that would be just enough for Saturday dinner; she could give her sister the rest of the cake to take home; she could put the leftover cake in an opaque container, in a less accessible place, and give it to other family members at Sunday lunch. After evaluating the pros and cons of each potential solution, Luisa decided to ask her sister if she would be willing to bring some wine instead and only on special occasions (e.g. a birthday or a party) to bring a—small—cake and to take home any leftovers. With these strategies to rely on, the patient felt very relieved and was able to deal effectively with her antecedent eating stimulus.

After looking at possible ways to reduce exposure to unhelpful environmental stimuli, patients are set the relevant homework; we ask them to compile a table of how they reacted to such stimuli before the treatment began and, based on the information discussed in the current session, what they will do from now on. The therapist should review this table (see example in Table 7.2) with the patient in the following session.

Patients are educated that in order to change dysfunctional behaviour, the replacement behaviour needs to be implemented consciously, until it becomes a new habit. This is why we recommend that patients periodically read their table and continue to systematically apply the new behaviours. Generally, patients realise that after a "training" period, the new behaviours become spontaneous. But, to help the patient better understand how a new behaviour can become a habit, we use the example of driving. Learning to drive a car is a very stressful activity because it requires the simultaneous implementation of a series of "unnatural" movements. For example, when we drive, we have to press down on the accelerator but also keep steering, looking ahead of us and in the mirrors, keep an eye out for road signs and be ready to brake. At first, we have to consciously think about every single behaviour before putting it into action, and this requires enormous concentration, but after we have driven for a while, the new behaviours become habitual, and we no longer realise how many simultaneous movements and gestures we are performing when we are driving—we just drive.

Table 7.2 Example of a completed table on reducing exposure to environmental stimuli

What I used to do	What I will do now
Doing the grocery shopping	
I used to go to the supermarket once a week and bought food (often junk food) without a shopping list	*I will now go to the supermarket three times a week. I will plan in detail what to buy and buy only food that requires preparation and that I need for my meal plan*
Storing food	
I used to place chocolates and sweets in a dish by the TV	*I will no longer leave any food in sight*
Preparing food	
I used to make a large amount of food, using a lot of fat and condiments, and often tasted the food while I was cooking	*I will cook the exact amount of food I need and prepare single portions. I will use the least amount of fat possible, and I will not taste food during preparation*
Serving food	
I used to put all the food on the table on large serving dishes, so that family members could help themselves	*I will avoid placing serving dishes on the table and instead serve food on individual plates, like in a restaurant*
During eating	
I used to eat very fast, and I was always the first to finish a meal	*I will take small bites and chew each one thoroughly. I will put my knife and fork down between bites and try to gradually increase the time it takes me to finish a meal*
After eating	
I usually stayed at the table after finishing the meal and often snacked on chocolates or walnuts afterwards	*I will avoid staying at the table for a long time, and I will stay out of the kitchen after meals*
Social occasions	
I often used to drink too much alcohol, and I ate all the food that was served	*I will cut down on (or even avoid) alcohol, and I will plan ahead what to eat; I will order first and eat slowly*
Sedentary lifestyle stimuli	
I always used to drive everywhere	*I will get to work by bike and plan daily physical activity*

7.4.2 Addressing Events Influencing Eating and Physical Activity Habits

Reviewing the Monitoring Record and the Weight-Loss Obstacles Questionnaire with the patients enables them to see whether changes in eating or physical activity have been preceded by certain events. If this is indeed the case, it is useful to analyse by which mechanisms the event might have influenced the behaviour, making reference to the Personal Formulation. This procedure has the aim of helping the patients to deal with "trigger" events and moods directly and effectively and to prevent them changing eating or physical activity habits. To this end, the therapist should introduce "proactive problem-solving" [10].

The proactive problem-solving procedure should be presented in the session in which an event associated with a change of eating or exercising habits comes to light. The sequence of events that led to this change should be reconstructed in detail, exploring the triggering event (e.g. pressure at work, tiredness, having nothing to do all day, etc.) and the subsequent feelings, thoughts and behaviours. The therapist should help the patients to see that this sequence could have been interrupted, with the aim of introducing the notion that such disruptions of eating or physical activity habits are not inevitable. For example, the sequence of events that led to excessive eating on a particular occasion could have been interrupted by someone calling the patient to invite him or her out to see a film or to take a walk. Moreover, it should be explained to patients that while many problems may seem overwhelming at first, if they are addressed systematically via a proactive problem-solving procedure, it is possible to resolve them in most cases. Effective problem-solving is a skill which, once learned, permits a person to address negative events without overeating or avoiding exercise.

Subsequently, the patient should be trained how to use proactive problem-solving techniques to address events that might trigger changes in eating or physical exercise habits in advance. Effective problem-solving involves the following steps:

- *Step 1. Identify the problem as early as possible.* Spotting problems early on is vital, as the great majority of problems are easier to deal with if they are pre-empted. For example, if you know you have nothing to do this evening, which will likely lead to overeating out of boredom, plan to go to the cinema with a friend. It is almost always easier to solve a problem earlier in the day than at the last minute.
- *Step 2. Understand the problem.* Working out the true nature of the problem is essential to finding the best solution. If it emerges that there are actually two or more co-existing problems, each problem should be addressed individually.
- *Step 3. Consider as many solutions as possible.* All possible solutions to the problem should be considered ("brainstorming"). Some solutions that come to mind may seem nonsensical or impractical but should nevertheless be included on the list. The more solutions generated, the more likely a good one will emerge. Patients who find it difficult to think of potential solutions should consider what they would suggest to a friend who is in a similar situation.
- *Step 4. Think of the pros and cons of each solution.* The likely effectiveness and feasibility of each solution should be evaluated.
- *Step 5. Choose the best solution or combination of solutions.* Interestingly, if Step 4 has been conducted thoroughly, choosing the best solution (or combination of solutions) is usually straightforward.
- *Step 6. Act on the solution.* The solution chosen should be applied without any hesitation.
- *Step 7. Review the process of problem-solving.* Patients should review how they solved their problem the next day to assess if the issue has been resolved and/or whether and how the problem-solving procedure could be improved.

Having explained this procedure, the therapist should encourage the patient to address an identified problem (using the first six steps of the problem-solving procedure) as if it had been spotted in advance. This is crucial practice, and the patient should be encouraged to take the lead whenever possible. If time allows, it is advisable to identify and address another recent event associated with a change in eating in the same way.

As homework, the therapist should ask the patient to practise problem-solving. Patients should be instructed to keep a look out over the following days for any potential events that could trigger a change in eating and address them in advance using the proactive problem-solving procedure. Specifically, once patients identify a problem they should write "Problem" in the right-hand column of the day's Monitoring Record and then turn the sheet over and write out the problem-solving steps required to address it. Patients should be also advised against problem-solving in their head alone, as this is much less effective. The homework should be reviewed in the next session and further practice encouraged. Table 7.3 shows an example of the proactive problem-solving procedure in action.

Table 7.3 Example of the problem-solving procedure being used to handle events associated with a change in eating

Problem!	
Step 1. Identify the problem as early as possible	
I eat too much when I get home from work	
Step 2. Specify the problem accurately	
I usually eat too much when I had a very hard day, I'm tired and I have no plans for the evening	
Step 3. Consider as many solutions as possible	***Step 4. Think about the pros and cons of each solution*** *(+ = pros, − = cons)*
Have a hot bath	*(+) It's a good idea; I'd relax and at the same time I'd get away from the temptation of food* *(−) None*
Watch television	*(+) None* *(−) There is nothing good on tonight, and in any case, I often want to snack in front of the TV*
Call friends to see if they are free	*(+) This is definitely a good idea. I know that when I feel alone, if someone calls or comes to see me, I feel better* *(−) Everyone might be busy*
Do some housework	*(+) The house would be cleaner* *(−) After a long day of work, I'd only be miserable and frustrated if I had to clean the house; it would only increase my sense of loneliness*
Take a walk	*(+) This is also a good idea; it would help me to stay away from food, relax and at the same time burn calories* *(−) None*

Table 7.3 (continued)

Step 5. Choose the best solution or combination of solutions
Having a hot bath, calling friends and taking a walk if they are not free
Step 6. Act on the solution (write the date, the day and the situation)
Tuesday January 20th. I came home from work. I first took a hot bath, then I called two friends, neither of whom was free, so I went out and took a 45-min walk; once I was back home, my desire to eat had faded, so I watched a little television and then went to sleep
Step 7. Review the process of problem-solving
I did a good job, but I have to think about taking up a hobby, preferably involving other people, that would keep me occupied in the evenings

7.4.3 Addressing Impulses and Emotions Influencing Eating and Physical Activity Habits

Applying the proactive problem-solving procedure helps to prevent predicable event-related changes in eating or exercising behaviour, but sometimes impulses or emotions are sudden and unpredictable and therefore need to be addressed using different strategies. CBT-OB adopts two main strategies for addressing sudden mood swings or impulses. The first of these strategies is using the Monitoring Record "Comments" column to report, in real time, the nature of the emotional state or impulse and a strategy to help "decentre" from these states without changing eating or deviating from planned physical activity. The second strategy, which should be associated with the first, is the "procedure of things to say and do" [1].

"Things to say" involves the patient learning to use phrases that help them maintain control whenever they feel they are at risk of deviating from their eating or exercise plan. Such phrases are designed to help a patient to tolerate the frustration of coping with the impulse and emotion without changing eating or physical activity habits and to see the craving for food/hunger/impulse to eat or desire not to exercise as transitory and tolerable states. To the same end, patients should also be instructed to use "things to do". To be an effective means of managing these impulses, the "things to do" should meet three main criteria: (1) help pass the time (after a while the impulse will fade—half an hour should be long enough for this to occur), (2) make it difficult to eat excessively from a practical point of view and (3) distracting and preferably pleasant. The procedure adopted to facilitate adherence to the physical activity plan should remind the patient of the commitment they have undertaken and stimulate the desire to persevere.

We usually furnish the patients with a list of example "things to say and do" in these situations (see Table 7.4) but ask them to create their own list as homework. This should be written on an index card (or similar) that they should always carry with them. The card should include the things to say and do that they think would be useful in helping them to cope with their impulse/mood change. When they feel at risk of deviating from their eating or physical activity plan, they should immediately get the card out and apply without hesitation the things to say and do that seem most appropriate on that occasion.

Table 7.4 Examples of things to say and do to handle sudden impulses to eat or deviate from the physical activity plan

Things to say
Eating
• *No choice (I cannot change my schedule)* • *Hunger is not an emergency; I can tolerate it* • *Think how healthy I will be when I reach my weight-loss goals* • *Reflect on the negative consequences of overeating* • *I do not want to let myself down* • *Desire for food is like a wave; it gets bigger and stronger until it reaches its peak, then diminishes in intensity* • *Think of the reasons that led me to stop eating too much* • *It's tough, but I can do it* • *I'm following a scientific programme that helps me to keep control over my eating* • *Hunger is powerful, but sooner or later, it will go away*
Physical activity
• *I want to be more physically active* • *If I overcome the initial difficulties of starting exercise, then I will feel better* • *The more I train, the easier it will be to do physical activity* • *I will start exercising now, and I will finish my set* • *Feeling fit is very pleasurable* • *I know I can do it!*
Things to do
Eating
• *I will immediately walk away from food stimuli* • *I will call a friend* • *I will take a walk* • *I will wait until the desire for food diminishes* • *I will not eat for 1 h* • *I will read a book* • *I will listen to my favourite music* • *I will slap a cushion* • *I will pick up an ice cube and focus on the physical sensation* • *I will brush my teeth*
Physical activity
• *I will put my sneakers on immediately* • *I will go out for a walk* • *I will not sit on the couch*

7.4.4 Addressing Problematic Thoughts

Patients are educated that the first step in addressing problematic thoughts effectively is to recognise them in real time. To this end, the therapist should first help the patients to identify thoughts that are hindering their weight loss whenever a Monitoring Record indicates that there is a deviation from the meal or physical activity plan. In this event, the therapist should ask the patient something like this:

"What was going through your mind before you overate/decided to lie on the couch instead of going for a walk?" In most cases the patient's answer will enable easy identification of the problematic thoughts associated with the change in behaviour. The therapist should then instruct the patient to ask themselves the same question in real time ("What is going through my mind") when they encounter any difficulties in sticking to their eating and/or exercise plan. With practice, patients usually learn to identify a thought that is likely to hinder their weight-loss attempt and "decentre" in advance, before it leads to a disruption in their planned behaviour. Patients should be asked to write the problematic thought that they have identified in the "Comments" column of their Monitoring Record, so it can be discussed in the next session, for example: "I eat sweets because it is the only pleasure I have in my life", or "I'm lying on the couch because I'm tired".

The last step in this procedure is to suggest that the patient "does the opposite" of whatever the problematic thought is encouraging them to do, for instance, to eat the apple they had planned to eat rather than the sweets they want or going for the walk they had planned to do rather than lying on the couch. If the problematic thoughts are recurrent, the therapist can advise the patient to write a personal reminder to themselves to decentre on a piece of card to carry with them, of the type: "This is a problematic thought, but losing weight is a very important goal for me. I will stick to what I have planned, and I will not be conditioned by what is going through my mind". The therapist could also help the patient to write the benefits that they hope to attain by losing weight on the card, which may help them deal more effectively with difficult situations.

Vignette

Returning to Luisa, she wrote the following reminder card to address her problematic thought of falling ill in the gym if she did not eat enough before: "I haven't been ill at the gym for a long time; why should it happen right now?"; "If I start feeling weak, I will stop exercising and rest"; "If I stick to my meal plan, I will lose weight and my health will improve"; and "When I exercise I feel better—it makes me stronger, not weaker!" Luisa made it a habit to read this reminder card every Tuesday and Thursday afternoon before eating her afternoon snack, and in this way, she was able to adhere to her meal plan before going to the gym. She did not feel a sense of weakness during or after physical activity, and this helped her to continue successfully on the CBT-OB programme.

7.4.5 Addressing the Use of Food as a Reward

Many patients use food as their main source of gratification in life. They take pleasure in organising evenings out with friends to try out new restaurants; they plan holidays according to the food they will discover and eat when there is nothing better to do or they are bored. Using food as a reward, however, is one of the most powerful obstacles to weight loss. To address this problem, the therapist should help the patients to identify—using their Monitoring Records and Weight-loss Obstacle Questionnaire—all the situations in which the prime purpose of the food they eat is as a reward. The patients are then asked to assess which other activities in their life are rewarding, in the search for alternatives.

7.4.5.1 Identifying Rewarding Activities and Their Consequences

This should start by discussing with the patient that the need for gratification is a fundamental element in anybody's life. The patient should therefore be helped to identify their particular "rewarding activities" and to draw them on a pie chart, in which the size of each slice represents the degree of gratification conferred by each rewarding activity (i.e. larger the slice, the more gratifying is the activity). Then the implications of the pie chart should be discussed and a plan devised for addressing any problems associated with the use of food as a main form of reward. Here follows an example dialogue between a therapist and patient addressing the issue of using food as a reward.

- *Therapist*: "So, taking a look at the course of our treatment, I think that it is becoming increasingly clear that you have an important obstacle to weight loss".
- *Patient*: "Yes, I realise that food is an important part of my life".
- *Therapist*: "I agree... Food seems to be an important form of gratification in your life".
- *Patient*: "That's right, I think that if I can't eat what I like or taste new or special foods, my day is ruined. After all, food is the spice of life!"
- *Therapist*: "Certainly! Food is one of the great pleasures in life. However, I would like to discuss with you if there are any other things that make you happy. All people are on the lookout for gratification... reward is something that keeps us going, even if the day is otherwise tedious or stressful. For example, some people get their kicks from doing a hobby, such as photography, others are gratified by the work they do, and others get their sense of reward from doing a sport, buying new clothes or gadgets or just chatting with friends. Of course, as we said before, food is very rewarding, but many people do several types of rewarding activity, not only eating, and this enables them to get more pleasure out of life. Do you agree?"
- *Patient*: "Yes. Yes, I do".
- *Therapist*: "So I think we should explore what other options you have. To understand if you find an activity rewarding, we have to consider some parameters. The first is your desire to do it, the second is the pleasure you experience while you are doing it, and the third is the frustration you feel if you can't. Is that clear?"
- *Patient*: "Yes, I think so. For example, there is a colleague of mine who can't wait to go home to build his model aeroplanes—it's his passion".

- *Therapist*: "Exactly! I am sure that for him building model aeroplanes is a rewarding activity. Now let us try to understand what your rewarding activities are at this time of your life. A good way to represent them is to draw a pie chart in which each slice represents the activities that you perceive as rewarding and the size of each slice as how gratifying you rate them. Before we start, however, I suggest we write a list of all the activities you find rewarding".

The therapist helps the patient to generate a list of rewarding activities. If patients have difficulties in identifying rewards other than food, the therapist should explain to them that rewarding activities may have become part of their life without them noticing them anymore. To elucidate what these are, the patient should be asked to focus on their typical days, to figure out whether stopping some routine activities—such as having a coffee break with colleagues, taking a child to school or listening to music in the car—would cause frustration and a general decline in daily satisfaction. The more examples the therapist provides to the patients, the easier it will be for them to recognise some of their own rewarding activities.

Once the list of rewarding activities has been created, the pie chart should be drawn—the more rewarding an activity, the larger the corresponding slice. Patients should be told that the best way to understand the size of the slice that represents the rewarding activity is thinking of the intensity and duration of frustration when they are not able to do it—the more frustrating the consequence, the bigger the slice should be.

The therapist should then ask the patients about their views on their pie chart. Figure 7.2 shows an example of a dysfunctional pie chart dominated by a large slice representing the reward obtained from food, which is accompanied by few other less rewarding activities, and a functional pie chart with a larger number of rewarding activities and none predominant. Many patients whose pie chart is like the

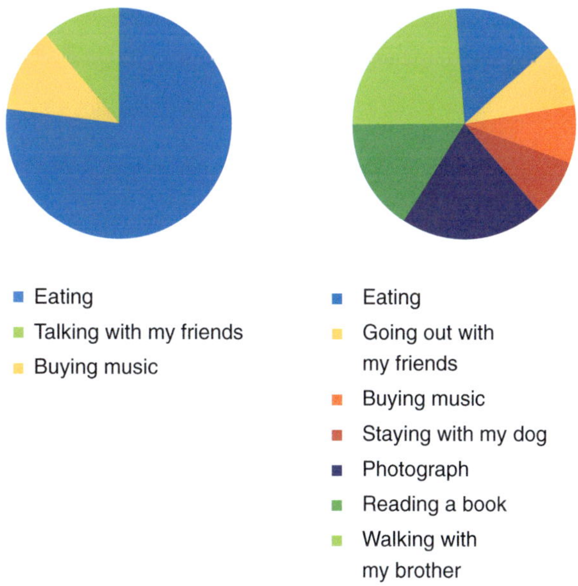

Fig. 7.2 A dysfunctional pie chart (on the left) and a functional pie chart (on the right) of rewarding activities

former are embarrassed and ashamed about the importance they place on food. They should, however, be reassured that this is common to many people and is something that they can change.

As homework, the patient should be asked to review their pie chart each day and think about whether it accurately represents the true state of their rewarding activities based on their day-to-day attitudes and behaviours. It may be helpful for them to redraw their pie chart at the end of each day (on the back of the day's Monitoring Record), and at the next session, the pie chart should be further discussed and the size of the slices adjusted as needed.

Once the pie chart has been produced, the therapist should discuss with the patient the implications of their rewarding activities and prompt them to think about whether there might be any problems with it. This discussion should lead to the identification of the main adverse consequences of using food as main form of gratification. At this stage the therapist should explain to the patient that having a pie chart with a dominant slice can be risky. This is because when gratification is predominantly represented by a single activity, it is likely that all will be well as long as it can be put into practice, but when for some reason it cannot, life seems less significant and satisfactory. Another problem with having a pie chart dominated by a single slice is that this narrow interest is self-perpetuating and marginalises other activities. As a consequence, interests, attitudes and relationships can get reduced to situations in which food must be present. Finally, if the predominant rewarding activity, like eating or sedentary behaviour, is practised to excess, it may have negative consequences for health and represent a factor that promotes the onset and maintenance of obesity.

Vignettes

A patient stated that eating with friends and trying out new dishes in exotic restaurants were very rewarding for him, but he realised that when he went out to dinner with his friends, they only talked about food and shared few other topics of conversation. He said: "It's crazy! I've only just realised that we meet each other to eat, and then we spend all evening taking about food… the food we ate at other restaurants, the food we would like to try, or how one of us has a new recipe… it's as if there's nothing else in our life. In the past, we did all sorts of other things together… I miss that".

Another patient admitted that she thought of food as both her best friend and worst enemy, saying "When I have a stressful day at work or I'm tired, I start thinking that I'll feel better when I get home and tuck into my favourite food. Then I go home, I eat, and I feel better. Food is my great companion, sometimes I think of it as my best friend… it is always available and does not ask for anything in return. But it is also true that it does not really help me, because I am continuing to gain weight, and this makes me increasingly tired and stressed out".

7.4.5.2 Enhancing the Importance of Other Rewarding Activities

Once the patients become aware of the importance of addressing the use of food as their main form of gratification, two strategies can be adopted. First, the patient should be encouraged to break the link between pleasure-seeking and food by using the previously described procedures for managing events, emotions and impulses that influence eating (i.e. proactive problem-solving, "things to say and do"). Secondly, the possibility of finding rewards other than food should be explored and encouraged. We stress to our patients that this strategy has the advantage of making life more pleasurable, creating and maintaining new opportunities for gratification and not having the food as a primary form of reward.

The first step in helping a patient to engaging in other rewarding activities is to explain the rationale behind it. For example, the therapist might say something like this: "We know that weight loss is an important goal in your life. However, together we have noticed that you often seek reward through food, and that this is a major obstacle to weight loss. One way to address this obstacle is to engage in other rewarding activities. Investing time doing other activities will permit you to discover that food is only one of several rewarding activities, and may in fact be the least useful for you".

Subsequently, the second step should be to identify new activities which the patient may be interested in doing. Clues to these may come from activities or interests that the patient used to do in the past but gave up and/or consideration of what their friends or work colleagues do in their free time. A "brainstorming" approach is best here, with all possibilities being listed, even if they seem (to the patient) silly or intimidating. In patients who report that they have no time for other activities, as they are too busy with family and work, etc., the therapist should remind them that to achieve a good outcome in weight loss and maintenance, it is essential to consider the treatment as a priority in life, and finding new sources of reward could be a very important step in this process.

The third step is to agree on one, or possibly two, activities that the patients will try to include in their life. These can be anything, as long as they are feasible and habitual. It is best if the patient involves others (especially significant others) in these activities and the decision to take them up, as that way they will be more likely to become self-perpetuating.

Once the patient has agreed to take up a new hobby, the fourth step is to ensure that they actually start engaging in the identified activity. The therapist should ask the patients to use the last column of their Monitoring Record to document this activity and in particular any barriers. These should subsequently be reviewed and solutions sought. The therapist should not be shy about actively encouraging hesitant patients get started. For example, if the patient is considering enrolling in a photography course, it would be quite appropriate for the therapist to help them work out ways of identifying suitable courses and talking them through the registration process. Indeed, getting the patient started should be the main priority at this stage. The patient's progress should also be reviewed week by week (as a permanent item on the session agenda), and the therapist should be encouraging and facilitative. Patients should be helped to use problem-solving to overcome any difficulties

Vignette

A 43-year-old patient reported that he found food extremely rewarding. He likes to eat and has a social life that is predominantly focused on social occasions at which food is present. He also says that after a busy day at work, he says to himself, "What could be better than a nice aperitif with something to nibble on? It makes me feel good just thinking about it!" Understandably, the patient had a hard time giving up this habit because, even though he recognised it as an obstacle to weight loss, he thought that he would feel deprived and would miss this source of gratification. However, with the aid of the therapist, the patient tried to understand what other activities, other than drinking and eating, would make him feel good. Upon reflection, the patient identified two evening activities that might be rewarding: reading his favourite comic books and going to a movie club with his friends. In this way, he would avoid "happy hour" and meet his friends after dinner. Although not without some initial difficulty, the patient learned to see the benefit of his new "hobbies", which he not only enjoys, but allow him to avoid "happy hour", and therefore limit occasions to indulge in alcoholic drinks and energy-rich snacks.

they encounter. It is important to bear in mind that the rewarding activities may change over the course of treatment, as unsuitable ones are dropped and additional activities identified and adopted.

7.4.5.3 Using Non-food Rewards

It is well known that a behaviour followed by a reward will have a good chance of being repeated, but if it results in a punishment, it is less likely to be repeated. For example, we reward children with sweets or chocolate when they are "good", but we punish or scold them when they misbehave. In our society, food is often used as a reward; many mothers use it as an expression of love and affection, and it is how we celebrate when we pass an exam or get a job promotion. We like to eat together to mark a special event or even when we just need cheering up. If it is other people celebrating, it may be difficult to refuse, but patients who are trying to lose weight should avoid using food as a reward for their own behaviour.

Hence, when it emerges from a patient's Monitoring Records that this is occurring, the therapist should help the patient to create a list of non-food rewards to employ instead. These rewards should be personalised, enjoyable and take little time, money or effort. The more positive the consequences, the easier it will be to commit to this strategy long term. Patients are encouraged to use one of the non-food rewards on the list when they reach a personal goal. For example, when they achieve their weekly CBT-OB target (e.g. losing 0.5 kg/week, filling out the Monitoring Record every day or doing 10,000 steps on at least 5 days a week) or other personal goals (involving work, school, family or friends), they should reward themselves with a non-food reward from the list. Similarly, they can use the same strategy when they have succeeded in dealing effectively (i.e. without deviating from their eating plan) with a negative emotion, like anger after a quarrel or frustration at work.

The system works best if the non-food reward is awarded immediately after the behavioural goal has been achieved. There are three types of rewards that the patient should consider:

1. *Favourite activities*, for example, going out, shopping, doing a hobby, chatting with friends, calling a loved one, taking a trip to the cinema, listening to music, doing physical activity, having a massage and going dancing or going to a spa.
2. *Saying nice things to themselves*, for example, "I'm proud of myself", "I handled that situation well", "I'm doing great", or "I'm a good person".
3. *Thinking about nice things*, for example, "It'll be great when I reach a healthy weight".

At the next session, when the patients have created a list of non-food rewards, the therapist should recommend that they reward themselves often, even once a day, saying "the more you reward yourself, the easier it will be to succeed".

Patients should also learn how to use "cognitive credits" once they reach their exercise goals, metaphorically patting themselves on the back by using phrases such as "I've done well", "I'm doing great", and "I can achieve my goals". The regular use of such cognitive credits may help patients reduce the frustration associated with exercise and strengthen their confidence in their being able to control body weight and maintain an active lifestyle.

7.4.6 Addressing the Patient's Rational Excuses for Not Adopting an Active Lifestyle

At first, physical exercise is hard; the more sedentary the lifestyle, the more difficult it is to exercise. Patients with obesity may find it more enjoyable to sit in front of the television than to go for a walk, but those who have started treatment may feel a certain amount of guilt about this. It is common for patients to combat these feelings by reporting rational excuses for not having an active lifestyle to the therapist. The following paragraphs contain some of the common rational excuses for not exercising that we have heard and how the therapist should best respond.

- *Patient*: "I work long hours and when I get home in the evening, I'm too tired to do any physical activity".
- *Therapist*: "I can image that you are tired after a long day of work; however, the fatigue accumulated during the day is mainly due to nervous tension, and physical activity helps to reduce stress-related fatigue".

- *Patient*: "I have no time to do physical activity".
- *Therapist*: "20–30 min is a tiny fraction of your day. If you do not find this time, it means that your daily commitments are too stressful and you certainly need to do some physical activity to reduce stress".
- *Patient*: "I'm too fat to be running and jumping about".
- *Therapist*: "I suggest you start slowly and gradually increase the intensity of your physical activity. If you persevere with the programme we have designed, you will see that it will get easier and more enjoyable as you go along. Moreover, doing exercise regularly will help you to keep the weight off in the long term".
- *Patient*: "I can't do any physical activity because there's no one else to look after my child".
- *Therapist*: "I know that this is an obstacle to exercise. However, why don't we try to find some solutions together to resolve this problem?"
- *Patient*: "Hmm… Maybe I could take a walk with my child using a running stroller, like my friend Anna does".
- *Therapist*: "Great! Any other ideas?"
- *Patient*: "I suppose I could get a babysitter for a few hours a week, so I can go for a walk".
- *Therapist*: "That is an excellent idea, and the money you spend on the babysitter will not be wasted, because you will be investing it in improving your health".
- *Patient*: "I'm too old to start an exercise programme".
- *Therapist*: "Why don't you try to start gradually by increasing your daily step count? Walking is a physical activity that is suitable for all ages, and regular physical activity also helps to slow down the aging process".
- *Patient*: "I'm too depressed to do any sport".
- *Therapist*: "I know that it may be difficult to exercise, especially when you are feeling low. However, several studies have shown that a good way of improving mood is doing regular physical activity".

7.5 Getting Back on Track

Patients should be aware that most people experience setbacks. Engaging in behaviour that hinders weight loss is very common, but if they are to succeed in losing weight, they need to be able to get back on the track after a lapse—an episode in which they have deviated from their meals or exercise plan. It is common that patients who are doing well in treatment hope that they will not resume their problematic behaviours. However, this is unlikely in the majority of patients, and without being unduly negative, the therapist should ensure that their expectations are more realistic, as they will otherwise be prone to react negatively to any small setback.

The final goal of CBT-OB is for patients to develop a stable weight-loss mindset, but this will require time, effort and an effective strategy for dealing with setbacks. To help the patient confront these difficult situations, the therapist should agree with them in advance some phrases that they could use on such occasions. For example, they might say to themselves, “Okay, I should not have eaten that much; I made a mistake. However, if I stick to my meal for the rest of the week, I am unlikely to put on weight”, or “I ate something that I did not plan to, but it is not the end of the world. I can stick to my meal plan again now. Just because I had a slip, I do not have to give up. That would not make sense. There are far more reasons to stop overeating now than to continue”.

References

1. Dalle Grave R, Sartirana M, El Ghoch M, Calugi S. Personalized multistep cognitive behavioral therapy for obesity. Diabetes Metab Syndr Obes. 2017;10:195–206. https://doi.org/10.2147/DMSO.S139496.
2. Tepper BJ. Dietary restraint and responsiveness to sensory-based food cues as measured by cephalic phase salivation and sensory specific satiety. Physiol Behav. 1992;52(2):305–11.
3. Cambiaghi M, Sacchetti B. Ivan Petrovich Pavlov (1849-1936). J Neurol. 2015;262(6):1599–600. https://doi.org/10.1007/s00415-015-7743-2.
4. Vucetic Z, Reyes TM. Central dopaminergic circuitry controlling food intake and reward: implications for the regulation of obesity. Wiley Interdiscip Rev Syst Biol Med. 2010;2(5):577–93. https://doi.org/10.1002/wsbm.77.
5. De Young KP, Zander M, Anderson DA. Beliefs about the emotional consequences of eating and binge eating frequency. Eat Behav. 2014;15(1):31–6. https://doi.org/10.1016/j.eatbeh.2013.10.012.
6. Desmet PM, Schifferstein HN. Sources of positive and negative emotions in food experience. Appetite. 2008;50(2–3):290–301. https://doi.org/10.1016/j.appet.2007.08.003.
7. Skinner BF. The behavior of organisms: an experimental analysis. New York: Appleton-Century-Crofts; 1938.
8. Beck AT, Rush AJ, Shaw BF, Emery G. Cognitive therapy of depression: a treatment manual. New York: Guilford Press; 1979.
9. Beck JS. The Beck diet solution: train your brain to think like a thin person. Birmingham: Oxmoor House; 2007.
10. Fairburn CG. Cognitive behavior therapy and eating disorders. New York: Guilford Press; 2008.
11. Dalle Grave R, Calugi S, El Ghoch M. Lifestyle modification in the management of obesity: achievements and challenges. Eat Weight Disord. 2013;18(4):339–49. https://doi.org/10.1007/s40519-013-0049-4.

Module 5: Addressing Weight-Loss Dissatisfaction

8

Our studies have found that a key cognitive factor involved in weight maintenance is patient satisfaction with the weight lost [1, 2]. In addition, we have recently shown that a decline in weight-loss satisfaction from around the week 19 of the programme, specifically a cut-off score of 7 or less on the weight satisfaction item of the Weight-Loss Obstacles Questionnaire (Appendix D), may help to identify patients who will be unable to maintain the weight they have lost [3]. As discussed in Chap. 1, it is feasible that dissatisfaction with the results obtained in the weight-loss phase of treatment may cause patients to decrease their motivation and reduce adherence to the lifestyle modification needed to maintain the weigh lost in the long term. To address this problem, CBT-OB Module 5 specifically aims to help the sub-group of patients who manifest weight-loss dissatisfaction 4–5 months after the beginning of treatment. The aim is to help the patient to arrive at the start of the weight-maintenance phase satisfied and positively accepting of the weight they have lost and therefore with the right attitude to develop a long-term weight-maintenance mindset.

8.1 Detecting Weight-Loss Dissatisfaction and General Strategies to Address It

The degree of satisfaction with weight loss is assessed by the therapist, session by session, conducting a review of the patient's response to the first item in the "Attitudes" section of the Weight-Loss Obstacles Questionnaire (Appendix D). For this item, the patient is asked to assess their satisfaction with the weight they have lost on Likert scale (0–10). If the patient assigns a score of 7 or lower to this item, the issue of weight-loss dissatisfaction should be included in the session agenda.

CBT-OB addresses weight-loss dissatisfaction by means of two different general strategies. If dissatisfaction occurs in the first 12 weeks of treatment, and is associated lower with a rate of weight loss than the weekly CBT-OB goal (i.e. 0.5 kg/week), it is addressed via the strategies and procedures described in Module 4

R. Dalle Grave et al., *Treating Obesity with Personalized Cognitive Behavioral Therapy*, https://doi.org/10.1007/978-3-319-91497-8_8

(see Chap. 7); these aim to help the patient to identify and address the obstacles to weight loss and thereby improve their adherence to the eating and physical activity plan. It is important to address this early weight-loss dissatisfaction promptly, as it is often associated with dropout [4, 5]. However, if weight-loss dissatisfaction occurs after week 12, it should be addressed using the specific strategies and procedures described in the following sections. Dissatisfaction with the results achieved at this late stage is likely to be due to unrealistic expectations, problematic primary goals for losing weight and/or negative body image, rather than weight-loss obstacles, which should have already been largely overcome.

8.2 Identifying Reasons for Weight-Loss Dissatisfaction

It is essential to identify the reasons why a patient is dissatisfied with the amount of weight loss that they have managed to achieve. To do so, the therapist may ask something like this: "I noticed that in the Weight-Loss Obstacles Questionnaire, you reported a score lower than 7 on the question regarding weight-loss satisfaction. Is there some specific reason why you are dissatisfied with your weight loss?" Commonly, patients initially report generic reasons, such as that they want to lose more weight and/or they thought they would have lost more by this stage. However, if the therapist investigates these feelings in more detail, it usually emerges that the reasons behind this dissatisfaction fall into one or more of the following broad categories [6]:

1. *Unrealistic weight goals*
2. *Dysfunctional primary goals for losing weight*
3. *Negative body image*

Investigation of unrealistic weight goals and dysfunctional primary goals may be facilitated by asking the patient to fill in the "Weight and Primary Goals Questionnaire" (see Appendix E). The questionnaire has three sections, the first of which asks the patient to fill in the following three weight goals:

1. *Dream weight*—the weight they would ideally like to be (even if it may be unrealistic and unattainable)
2. *Desired weight*—the weight that they want to achieve and think is attainable
3. *Acceptable weight*—the highest weight that they think they could accept

For each of the above weight goals, the patient should report a number in kilograms. Sometimes, patients have no specific goal in terms of weight but want to get to a desired clothing size or lose as much weight as possible. Even if this is the case, they should be invited to quantify their desired size, etc. with a precise number in kilograms.

The second section of the Weight and Primary Goals Questionnaire includes specific items about the desired weight—which can be considered the "true" weight-loss goal. Patients are also asked to report the reasons why they have selected that desired weight, if this has changed at all, and why this variation has occurred (if that is indeed the case). Another question in this section asks the patient to think about the difficulty they think they will have reaching and maintaining their desired weight and how long in the past they had been able to maintain it. Finally, the third section of the questionnaire includes questions about the primary goals for losing weight, what they expect to achieve by losing weight and whether this necessarily entails losing weight.

Identification of negative body image is a more complex task and requires a sympathetic and accepting approach, as patients with obesity are generally very sensitive about this issue. This assessment can be facilitated by asking patients to fill in the "Body Image Inventory" reported in Appendix F. The inventory includes the following four sections: (1) body concerns, (2) body avoidance, (3) body checking and (4) feeling fat.

The Body Image Inventory should be reviewed in detail with the patient in order to get a good picture of their body image and to discern which of the four principal areas are necessary to address. In our practice, at this point we also ask patients if they are exposed to some individual specific social pressures, such as family attitudes to body weight and shape (e.g. living with significant others that criticise their body weight and shape or that overvalue thinness), job requirements (e.g. the need to travel by plane or bus, etc. or to give public presentations or wear revealing clothes) or other social contexts that serve to maintain their body image concerns. Finally, we also explore with the patients if their attitudes and behaviours associated with body image impair some aspects of their life, such as psychological wellbeing, interpersonal relationships and/or work or school performance. If this review indicates that patients report expressions of negative body image very frequently, and that these seem to impair their quality of life, the therapist should suggest that they address it together (see Sect. 8.6). On the other hand, if the therapist realises that the patient does not have a negative body image, there is no reason to address it.

8.3 Which Reasons for Weight-Loss Dissatisfaction to Address First?

As general strategy, if patients do not report a negative body image, the intervention should address unrealistic weight goals and eventually some specific reasons associated with their desired weight. However, if their responses indicate a negative body image, this should be addressed as a priority, as it will be difficult to help patients not to pursue unrealistic amounts of weight loss if they are unable to accept their new weight and appearance. Naturally, the body image intervention should be integrated on a case-by-case basis, using the procedures to address unrealistic weight-loss goals and any associated primary goals that will be helpful to the patient in question.

8.4 Addressing Unrealistic Weight Goals

CBT-OB does not address unrealistic weight-loss expectations at the beginning of the treatment, as these are associated with greater weight loss [2]. That being said, since high weight-loss expectations are also associated with a higher rate of dropout [4, 5], the patients are encouraged from the beginning to focus on achievable short-term weight-loss goals (e.g. a weight loss of between 0.5 and 1.0 kg per week), rather than their long-term weight-loss goal. However, when the weight-loss phase is winding down, it is essential to ensure that patients are ready to embark on the weight-maintenance phase, which will entail them setting aside their long-term weight-loss goals, at least for the duration. Hence, unrealistic weight-loss goals are addressed, by means of the procedures described in the following sections, after week 12 if a related decline in weight loss-dissatisfaction is detected. The goal is to help patients to be satisfied with a reasonable and healthy weight loss, balancing what can be changed with what can be accepted.

8.4.1 Educating the Patients on Body Weight Regulation

The first step towards acceptance is educating the patient about body weight regulation and results generally obtained by treatments for obesity based on lifestyle modification. The principal points to discuss are the following:

- Some aspects of obesity can be changed, others cannot.
- Body weight is partially controlled by genetics, and there is therefore only so much a person can do to change it.
- There are currently no treatments (with the exception of bariatric surgery) that determine a mean weight loss greater than 10–15% of the initial body weight.
- Even people who lose a lot of weight have difficulty maintaining it in the long term.
- Most people, if they do not adopt specific weight-maintenance strategies, regain one third of the weight lost after 1 year and the entire weight lost after 5 years.
- Most people who start a weight-loss treatment want to lose more than 10–15% of their body weight, and these unrealistic expectations may lead them to abandon the programme or not engage in weight-loss maintenance, because they consider the achievable result unsatisfactory.
- A 5–10% weight loss has many health benefits, and this can have a positive effect on quality of life, as well as reducing the major medical complications associated with obesity.
- A good treatment helps to change what can be changed and to accept what cannot. A balance between change and acceptance is a common goal in medicine, especially in other chronic medical conditions such as diabetes mellitus.

Based on these facts, the patient should be asked to discuss and consider the following three points [7]:

1. Some changes (i.e. weight loss) are possible, and although maybe less than ideal, they can bring significant benefits.
2. The treatment can successfully address other primary reasons associated with personal weight goals, and this will result in an improvement in quality of life. However, to succeed it is essential to accept what cannot be changed (acceptance as self-affirmation).
3. If there is no acceptance of what cannot be changed, there is a high risk of relapse. This is because there is a tendency to underestimate what has been achieved during treatment and reduce commitment to maintaining the weight lost, as it is not considered important.

8.4.2 Questioning the Desired Weight

The second step towards preparation for the weight-maintenance phase is to help patients accept and be satisfied with the weight that can be achieved by the weight-loss phase. To this end, they should be questioned on their desired weight goal, taking care to address the following topics [7]:

1. *Sources of the desired weight.* The therapist should ask the patient about the origins of their desired weight. In our experience, the most common answers patients give are doctor's recommendations, the ideal weight chart, the desire to return to a lower weight they had been at a certain period of life or the belief that a particular weight is needed to achieve the primary goals.
2. *Variability of the desired weight.* The therapist should explore whether their desired weight has changed over the years. If the answer is yes, as is often the case, they should explore together the reasons that led to a change in their desired weight.
3. *Previous weight-loss attempts.* The patient should also be asked whether they were able to reach their desired weight in previous weight-loss attempts. If not, what were the obstacles that they met? If so, why were they not able to maintain that weight?
4. *Difficulties and risks in pursuing the desired weight.* The patient should be helped to reflect upon the difficulties they will have to overcome in order for them to reach their desired weight and whether there are any risks associated with wanting to reach it at all costs.
5. *Consequences of achieving the desired weight or not.* The therapist should also ask the patients what they think will realistically happen if they do, or do not, reach their desired weight. How will they interpret this result? What will they do? Will their life really change?

8.4.3 Reviewing the Causes of Poor Weight-Loss Maintenance in Previous Attempts

Another strategy that can help patients to accept a higher weight than that desired is to review with them in detail the causes that led to past failures to maintain the weight they had lost. To this end, the therapist should help them analyse both the weight-loss and weight-maintenance phases of previous weight-loss attempts as follows:

- *Weight-loss phase*. The patient should be asked about their initial weight, how long the weight-loss phase lasted, how much weight they lost and whether or not they reached their desired weight. It is also important to encourage patients to come to some conclusion about their previous experience.
- *Weight-maintenance phase*. The patient should be asked if they intentionally decided to start weight maintenance. If so, why? If not, why not? It is also useful to ask how long their weight maintenance lasted and which factors affected their subsequent weight regain. In this regard, the therapist should invite the patient to consider three main processes [7]: (1) having unrealistic weight-loss goals and being dissatisfied with the weight that they had achieved made them abandon the commitment to maintaining the weight lost; (2) not knowing how to maintain weight; and (3) having difficulties adhering to an excessively restrictive diet for a long time.

8.4.4 Identifying the Benefits of Current Weight

Positive acceptance of a higher weight than that desired can be facilitated by helping the patient to assess the benefits of a modest weight loss and the positive changes that they have already achieved through the treatment. To this end, it may be useful to encourage the patients to consider their improvement in following areas:

- Physical appearance and reduced clothing size
- General wellbeing
- Self-confidence
- Obesity-related medical complications (the therapist can suggest that patients repeat the laboratory blood tests they had before the weight-loss phase to assess any objective improvements)
- Physical fitness (e.g. climbing the stairs with less fatigue, feeling more agile, lacing up shoes more easily)

8.4.5 Evaluating the Pros and Cons of Aiming for the Desired Weight

The next step is to encourage the patients to write the pros and cons of continuing to aim for their desired weight in a table; they should consider the potential advantages but also the disadvantages and risks.

Vignette

The patient is a 50-year-old woman who started CBT-OB with a body weight of 95 kg. At baseline she also suffered from hypertension, diabetes and high cholesterol, which were being kept under control by several medications. After 5 months of treatment, she had reached a body weight of 81 kg, but her personal goal was to reach a weight of 65 kg, which she had at the age of 20 years, when she had an unforgettable sentimental relationship. After educating the patient on body weight regulation, the therapist asked her to re-examine her desired weight by reviewing her previous weight-loss attempts (she had never been able to go back to 65 kg). Highlighting her achievement of a 14 kg weight reduction, the therapist asked the patient to identify any benefit that she perceived at her current weight. Without hesitation, the patient replied that she had obtained many physical benefits. In particular, she had reduced the number of medicines she needed to take to control her blood pressure, glucose and cholesterol; she felt more agile—able to walk for several kilometres without panting and no longer experienced the excessive sweating that had previously caused her embarrassment on social occasions. However, she was still dissatisfied with the weight loss she had achieved and by the fact that her body weight had remained stable over the last 2 weeks. She was determined to increase her dietary restriction in order to reach her desired body weight of 65 kg. The therapist therefore set her the homework of filling in the table of pros and cons of reaching her desired weight. In the next session, a review of this table revealed that the patient had reported no cons of reaching the desired weight but only pros (such as feeling better physically, having a greater choice of clothes and being able to go jogging) with her friend. Here is the dialogue that took place between the therapist and patient:

- *Therapist*: "Thank you for filling in the table. How did you feel doing this homework?"
- *Patient*: "Good! However, I could only find advantages to losing more weight".
- *Therapist*: "I see (the therapist indicates the pros of the table). You wrote that if you reached your desired weight you would have a greater choice of clothes and be able to go running with your friend".
- *Patient*: "I would like to wear a medium… it would be a pretty good goal. And I would love to go jogging with my friend".
- *Therapist*: "Ok, I understand. I see that your weight-loss satisfaction score is currently 6".
- *Patient*: "Yes, it is! I think that if I manage to reach 65 kg, with its positive effects, it would be a nine or ten".
- *Therapist*: "Let us analyse the fact that you did not write any disadvantages of reaching your desired weight; what do you plan to do to achieve your 65 kg goal?"

- *Patient*: "What do you mean? I'll do the same as I am already doing!"
- *Therapist*: "Are you sure? In the last 2 weeks, your body weight has remained stable".
- *Patient*: "That's true (*frowning*)".
- *Therapist*: "This is a common event. Weight loss tends to reach a plateau after 5–6 months. This because the weight lost produces a progressive decrease in energy expenditure".
- *Patient*: "That's bad. So, I need to eat fewer calories or do more exercise".
- *Therapist*: "Yes, that is correct. However, but before you decide whether or not you should increase caloric restriction or energy expenditure, we should talk about the consequences of doing so. For example, now you are following a meal plan containing about 1500 calories per day. If you want to continue to lose weight and reach 65 kg, that means you may have to reduce your energy intake to 1000 or 800 calories per day".
- *Patient*: "Yes, that is so".
- *Therapist*: "Have you thought about the consequences of following a very restrictive diet?"
- *Patient*: "What do you mean?"
- *Therapist*: "For example, how you will cope in social situations. I know that you go out to eat with your friends twice a week, and you like to spend this time with them".
- *Patient*: "I'll eat very little during the day so I can relax in these social situations. Either that or I'll choose what to eat in the restaurant very carefully… Hmm… perhaps, it would be better to increase physical activity".
- *Therapist*: "How do you think you would organise your day? Last month, work commitments made it very difficult for you to do 10,000 steps every day".
- *Patient*: "That's true".
- *Therapist*: "And doing more exercise would not make it any easier for you to control what you eat in social situations; if you can only eat 800–1000 calories per day, and your plan is to reduce what to eat during the day and do a lot of exercise, by dinner-time you will be very hungry indeed. How do you think you will manage the eating stimuli you are exposed to in the restaurant—the delicious food on the menu, and seeing your friends and enjoying the food they eat, for example".
- *Patient*: "I will have to control myself".
- *Therapist*: "Don't you think that excessive control might condition you or have negative consequences?"
- *Patient*: "Hmm… Maybe yes. My friends will probably see that I am not happy-go-lucky and too uptight. However, it will be worth it in the end".

8.4.6 Reviewing and Adjusting the Desired Weight

The above vignette illustrates the very common occurrence that discussion of the pros and cons of pursuing the desired weight does not end with the patient concluding that they should adjust their goals. Nevertheless, the aim of this intervention is to instil some doubt about the potential risks and disadvantages of achieving overly challenging weight-loss goals. The therapist should also ask the patient to rewrite the pros and cons of achieving their desired weight as homework and to assess whether or not it would be advisable to adjust it to a higher, more realistic level, considering the problems that could arise if they did not. As always, the homework should be reviewed in the following session.

Vignette

In the next session, the patient, who had previously expressed a desired weight of 65 kg, reported that she had identified several disadvantages of achieving that goal. Her pros and cons table now included the negative influence on interpersonal relationships and the risk of overeating—as she had experienced in the past when she had adopted rigid and extreme dietary rules. She also realised that it would be unrealistic to maintain an excessive dietary restriction for the rest of her life to avoid weight regain and, considering the benefits already obtained in the weight-loss phase, decided to focus her efforts on maintaining a body weight of 81 kg.

8.5 Addressing Dysfunctional Primary Goals for Losing Weight

We can consider the goals driven by the patient's main reasons for losing weight as their "primary goals"—what the patient most hopes to achieve through weight loss. These should already have been identified in the third section of the Weight and Primary Goals Questionnaire (see Sect. 8.2 and Appendix E) and do not necessarily require a large weight loss or, in fact, any weight loss at all. Some primary goals, such as improving health and fitness, improving physical appearance and modifying body shape, may be achieved through a modest weight loss and/or other factors, and others, like improving interpersonal relationships and/or self-confidence, are not necessarily linked to weight loss [7]. The association of psychological and interpersonal goals with weight loss is in part linked to the positive stereotyping of thinness in Western society and the notion of an "ideal" weight. The media in particular fosters the purported association, particularly in women, of this physical characteristic with important values such as happiness, control, competence, intelligence and romantic success.

As suggested by Cooper et al. [7], the first step in addressing dysfunctional primary goals is to review with the patient which of them they have already achieved—and are therefore likely related to weight loss—and those that they have not; they should be asked to consider whether additional weight loss would solve these "problems" or whether different strategies (other than weight loss) will be required. Depending on the reasons the patient reports for wanting to lose weight (i.e. their primary goals), there are several interventions that can be attempted by the therapist.

8.5.1 Improving Physical Appearance

Most patients are satisfied with a moderate weight loss; however, a subgroup maintains a significant degree of body dissatisfaction, despite the weight loss they have already achieved. In this case, the therapist should help the patient to understand that the problem is not their body weight per se (i.e. an objective number) but rather their (subjective) opinion of their physical appearance. If they can understand this, they should be able to see that losing weight is not the only solution to their "problem". Alternatively, it may be useful to suggest that the patient tries to develop a different way of thinking about their weight and to consider whether or not they judge other people in the same way as they judge themselves. Conclusions such as "a person's value does not depend on their weight" and "I can look nice at this weight" should be elicited if possible, and other solutions for improving physical appearance should be discussed. For example, we routinely suggest that patients treat themselves to a haircut or new clothes and make-up, without waiting until they reach their desired weight to make these changes. In our clinical experience, this strategy helps the majority of our patients to reduce their body dissatisfaction and to accept a reasonable body weight. However, this intervention has a limited effect on those with a negative body image (see Sect. 8.6).

8.5.2 Improving Health

One of the most common reasons why patients seek treatment for obesity, especially those who are older or have already developed some medical complications—such as diabetes, hypertension, cardiovascular disease or arthrosis—is to improve health. In most cases, it is not necessary to directly address this primary goal, because patients will achieve a significant improvement in health with a weight loss of 5–10% and the adoption of a lifestyle similar to that recommended by the programme. However, if patients still express some doubt about the progress they have made in terms of improving their health, despite a reasonable weight loss, it may be useful to prescribe repeat laboratory blood tests. Generally speaking, results will show that there has been a positive shift in the main metabolic indices (glycaemia and lipid profile, hepatic function, etc.)—an objective demonstration of how a moderate weight loss has produced a considerable improvement in their health status.

8.5.3 Improving Physical Fitness

A common primary goal of many patients is to improve their physical fitness. In most cases the goals are to overcome some of the difficulties they encounter in their daily lives, such as walking upstairs without panting, lacing up shoes, etc., or to take up sport. Adopting an active lifestyle, such as that indicated by the CBT-OB, is a strategy that helps improve physical fitness regardless of the overall amount of weight lost. Moreover, an active lifestyle exerts positive effects on other primary goals such as body image, self-confidence and, when performed with others, interpersonal relationships. To provide an objective demonstration of the improvement in physical fitness, it is useful to repeat the measurements of functional exercise capacity done at baseline (i.e. 6MWT, handgrip test, five times sit-to-stand test and functional reach test; see Sect. 6.1.2).

8.5.4 Improving Interpersonal Relationships

A subgroup of patients seeking treatment for obesity has the goal of improving their interpersonal relationships, as they (irrationally) think they have no friends or unsatisfactory relationships due to their excess weight. If the patient expresses this reason for losing weight, the best thing to do is to encourage them to try to become more socially active from this point forward, without postponing this until they achieve their desired weight. Patients should be advised to break down this process and set themselves small, specific, achievable goals (e.g. calling a friend and inviting them to go for a walk or have a coffee). To address the obstacles, patients should be advised to use a proactive problem-solving procedure, which they should already be familiar with (see Sect. 7.4.2). It may also be of use to ask them whether they would shun someone because they were overweight. If patients have marked long-term interpersonal difficulties (e.g. interpersonal conflict or interpersonal deficits), they should be referred to a psychology specialist for dedicated treatment.

8.5.5 Improving Self-Confidence

If improving self-confidence is a primary goal for losing weight, this can be a complex goal to achieve. In a person with adequate self-esteem, low self-confidence usually derives from general demoralisation, whereas other patients may suffer from long-standing low self-esteem. Neither of these states are necessarily linked to body weight, but self-confidence can be enhanced through several mechanisms targeted by CBT-OB, such as weight loss, greater eating control, increased levels of physical fitness, improved physical appearance and better health. As with other primary goals for losing weight, it is crucial to suggest that patients consider trying other means, in addition to weight loss, of improving their self-confidence. However, these changes will have a limited effect on subjects who suffer from low self-esteem that is not dependent on their weight. In such cases, the patient should be referred to a psychology specialist to address this issue.

8.5.6 Making Life Changes

Some patients seeking treatment for obesity think that weight loss will allow them to make important and beneficial life changes. Some examples of changes that patients cite are getting a better job or a promotion, taking up a new hobby, interrupting an unsatisfactory relationship, starting a new relationship and/or taking up a sport. As a rule, such patients tend to put off initiating these life changes until they reach their desired weight. In this case too, therefore, the strategy should be to suggest that the patient implements the desired changes straight away, without waiting until they achieve their primary goal.

8.6 Addressing Negative Body Image

Body dissatisfaction is very common, particularly among women living in Western societies, who may be suffering from "normative discontent" [8]. Body dissatisfaction is almost always a factor in patients seeking weight-loss treatment and is one of the main goals for weight loss. However, it is also associated with a higher dropout risk in comparison with patients whose primary reason for losing weight is health concerns [5].

Available studies show that patients with obesity who lose weight, either through BT-OB [9] or bariatric surgery [10], report a significant improvement in body image, but these results are largely independent of the amount of weight lost and may in fact occur without any appreciable reduction in body weight [11]. Indeed, we confirmed this finding in a study which assessed 473 treatment-seeking patients with obesity across 13 medical centres [12]. At 6-month follow-up, the mean percentage of weight loss was about 9% in men and 7% in women. Both men and women displayed a significant improvement in body image, but this was correlated with improvements in measures of psychological distress and binge eating—not with the amount of weight lost. It is also our clinical experience that most patients with body dissatisfaction may be helped to accept a reasonable and healthy weight loss by means of the CBT-OB procedures described in Sects. 8.4 and 8.5 of this chapter; these address unrealistic weight goals and the primary goals (e.g. improving physical appearance) for aiming for the desired weight.

However, there is a subgroup of patients who reports no improvement in body image, even though they have lost weight. This becomes a major obstacle to the acceptance of a reasonable and healthy weight loss and makes it less likely that the patient will acquire and practise weight-maintenance skills [6, 7]. Hence a negative body image needs to be addressed, in parallel with the work on unrealistic weight goals and dysfunctional primary goals for weight loss, and should often be continued in the weight-maintenance phase.

Vignette

Emma started CBT-OB at a body weight of 129.3 kg and a BMI of 39.9. During the weight-loss phase, she never really felt satisfied with her weight, despite having an average loss of 0.7 kg per week. She often reported a weight-loss-satisfaction score under 7 on the Weight-Loss Obstacles Questionnaire and was very upset on the few occasions that her weekly weight loss had been less than 0.5 kg per week. At the time, the therapist encouraged the patient not to focus on a single reading but instead to consider the 4-week trend in her weight loss and the improvement in her overall wellbeing. Unfortunately, however, this intervention had little impact on her attitude, and the improvement in quality of life she perceived was minimal at best. Compounding the issue, after about 5 months, her 4-week weight-loss trend revealed a plateau, when she had reached the weight of 98 kg (BMI 30.0). This resulted in her weight-loss-satisfaction score decreasing to 4. The therapist asked her why she felt so unhappy about her weight loss, as she had lost 30 kg, and the patient responded that she was still very dissatisfied with her physical appearance and embarrassed by her weight, especially when she met new people. She linked this embarrassment to the fear of being seen as a weak person with no willpower and reported avoiding situations such as taking her 3-year-old child to the water park; she did not want to be ridiculed or experience the usual disgust she felt when parts of her body wobbled. Concerns about her body shape also prevented her from doing previous hobbies such as horseback riding, as she believed that a horse would not be able to bear her weight. The patient took little care of her physical appearance, wearing no make-up and dark, loose clothing. Her negative body image also caused her to avoid social situations such as throwing a birthday party for her child or stopping off for a coffee after taking him to kindergarten. When the therapist asked if she might consider addressing this type of avoidance, she replied that the only chance of her doing so would be if she continued to lose weight and reached a weight of 60 kg.

As the above *Vignette* illustrates, addressing negative body image in patients with obesity is challenging for both the therapist and the patient. The therapist, in particular, needs to be very sensitive to the attitudes that fuel the patient's unrealistic weight-loss expectations. It is essential that the therapist accepts the patient unconditionally, with no preconceptions or prejudices against people with obesity, if they are to have any change of helping them improve their body image and self-esteem. It is also vital that the therapist truly understands how patient with obesity experiences their body shape in a culture that associates excess body weight with a lack of willpower and sends the message that the solution to obesity is the commitment of the individual.

When the therapist explores the patients' weight-loss dissatisfaction, it is inevitable that he or she develops a feeling of discomfort and impotence while listening to their emotional suffering. Patients often report upsetting experiences that reinforce their sense of feeling discriminated against, such as not being able to fit comfortably in a movie theatre or aeroplane seat, having difficulty finding clothes that fit and/or being blamed by significant others and health professionals for their excessive weight. For these reasons, the therapists should be empathetic, showing that they understand how difficult it is for patients with obesity to live in our society. Empathy is skill crucial for validating a patient's negative feelings about their body shape and weight and for helping them attain a cognitive shift—from adopting the negative societal prejudices against obesity to the positive acceptance of themselves that promotes the behavioural changes needed to improve self-esteem without pursuing unrealistic weight-loss goals.

8.6.1 Explaining the Differences Between Body Image and Physical Appearance

Patients should be educated on the concept of "body image" as distinct from "physical appearance". The therapist should explain that body image is not the actual "objective" physical appearance but the mental picture that people have about their own body. To explain this concept clearly, the therapist should explain that many adolescents, but also some adults, feel fat and overweight, even if they are not considered so objectively; at the other end of the spectrum, some people who have obesity feel good about their body and have good self-esteem and interpersonal relationships, despite their excess weight. The therapist should also explain that many people with body dissatisfaction might like how they look after a moderate weight loss and making changes to other aspects of their appearance; body dissatisfaction does not have a negative influence on their self-evaluation or their ability to function in social situations. However, as we have seen, in some people, body image concerns continue to have a negatively impact on self-esteem and their everyday functioning despite a healthy weight loss, and in such cases it will be necessary to address these concerns to achieve successful weight maintenance.

8.6.2 Engaging the Patients in the Decision to Address Negative Body Image

Generally, the difference between body image and physical appearance is immediately understood by most patients, and some of them admit admiring people who are able to accept or even like their own body, even if they are overweight, but they really do not believe that this could happen to them. In such cases, it is important to instil hope in patients by informing them that there are specific strategies and procedures that, by addressing the cognitive and behavioural mechanisms maintaining a negative body image, can help to promote a positive acceptance of body shape, irrespective of the amount of weight lost.

Even if patients understand the difference between body image and physical appearance, however, some will persist in the belief that an improvement in the former will only be possible if they reach a normal weight. In such cases, the therapist should review with the patient their previous weight-loss attempts and the effect that these had on their physical appearance and body image. It is common that, in spite of losing a large amount of weight and achieving significant change in their physical appearance, such patients report that this resulted in no improvement in their body image. In the event of this disclosure, the therapist should explain that these previous experiences underline the differences between physical appearance and body image and that it might be interesting to understand—and then address—the mechanisms maintaining a negative body image that are not linked to physical appearance. The patient should also be informed that the maintenance of body image concerns may be an obstacle to weight maintenance, because it maintains dissatisfaction with weight loss and may prompt the adoption of severe dietary restriction. This is usually impossible to maintain over time and can therefore make the individual more vulnerable to weight regain in the future. Moreover, continued pursuit of weight loss would prevent them from taking the opportunity afforded by the programme to learn the skills needed to maintain the weight they have already lost in the long term.

If a patient reports that past weight loss improved both their physical appearance and body image, the therapist should review with them why they failed to maintain the weight lost. This discussion should persuade the patient to conclude that one of the major causes of their weight regain was that they were unable to stick to an excessively restrictive diet over a long period of time, as it was not compatible with everyday life.

At the end of this discussion, the therapist should ask the patient to evaluate the pros and cons of addressing body image concerns directly and to emphasise that this will be conducted while they continue to work on losing weight (i.e. until the end of Phase 1). This is important, as it will obviate anxiety about having to immediately abandon any attempt at weight loss in favour of focusing on improving body image. In our clinical experience, most patients agree to address this topic as part of their treatment, as they report that negative body image is one of the major reasons that led them to seek help for weight loss.

8.6.3 Discussing the Maintenance of Negative Body Image

The first step in attempting to overcome a patient's negative body image is to tell them that the key strategy is to address the cognitive processes that are reinforcing it. For this reason, the therapist should describe the main maintenance mechanisms behind negative body image—focusing in particular on those that emerged in a review of the Body Image Inventory—and the pertinent pressures exerted by society at large and the individual's surroundings (see Sect. 8.2).

General and individual social pressures. The therapist should explain that "general" and "individual" social pressures may contribute not only to the development of a negative body image but also to its maintenance. General social pressures are those that lead a person to want to conform to the prevailing social standard of beauty based on thinness. Patients with obesity live in a society that perpetuate body concerns, as it overvalues thinness and fosters negative judgements about individuals who are overweight. Furthermore, some patients are exposed to specific individual social pressures—in the family or at work, for example—that magnify the effect of the general pressures in contributing to maintain a negative body image (see Sect. 8.2).

Body concerns. There are a wide variety of body concerns that patients with obesity can suffer from, on a continuum of severity from slight body dissatisfaction to extreme self-loathing. This range of severity is primarily mediated by the degree of importance that the individual attaches to body shape and weight in their self-evaluation and at its extreme is characterised by what is termed the "overvaluation of shape and weight". If this is found to be the case (as is common in patients with BED, see Chap. 13), the individual will judge themselves predominately or even exclusively in terms of their shape and weight. Such body concerns explain the main expressions of negative body image, such as body checking, body avoidance and feeling fat.

Body avoidance. This is a typical behavioural expression of body concerns, and it is very common among patients with obesity. It refers to the avoidance of situations in which patients think they will feel very self-conscious about their physical appearance [7]. Body avoidance has a positive short-term effect by reducing the distress associated with body exposure, but in a long term it tends to maintain and intensify body concerns through the mechanisms described in Sect. 8.6.7.2.

Body checking. This behavioural expression of body concerns is manifested by a subgroup of patients with obesity. It involves the frequent checking of body shape and weight—by pinching, weighing, looking in the mirror and comparing one's own body with that of others. As with body avoidance, body checking, in some cases, may have a positive effect in the short term, reassuring the individual that they have not put on weight, but in the long term, it has a negative impact—serving to maintain body concerns through the mechanisms described in Sect. 8.6.7.1.

Feeling fat. Another expression of body concerns is feeling fat. This sensation is frequently reported by patients with obesity, but it is not necessarily related to their actual body weight, since it is also reported by many normal or low-weight individuals and not by some individual who are overweight. Moreover, it is not present all the time, being triggered by certain body-related experiences and emotions; this too serves to maintain the body concerns, via the mechanisms described in Sect. 8.6.7.3.

Figure 8.2 illustrates the main maintenance mechanisms of negative body image. These should be explained to any patient that displays this feature.

8.6.4 Devising a Plan to Address Negative Body Image

The next step in addressing negative body image is devising a personalised action plan. This should be focused on the main maintenance processes operating in the patient that emerged from the review of the Body Image Inventory and individual social pressures (see Sect. 8.2). That being said, in the majority of cases, the plan will employ three complementary strategies designed to (1) address social pressures, (2) enhance the personal significance of other self-evaluation domains and (3) address the expression of body concerns (i.e. body checking, body avoidance and feeling fat).

8.6.5 Addressing Social Pressures

Unfortunately, there is little we can do to reduce the general social pressure to be thin that a patient is subject to, and it is also often difficult to address the individual social pressures they experience. Nevertheless, the therapist should help the patient to become aware of these social pressures and the negative effect they have on people that are not naturally normal weight. It is also important to help the patient to understand that negative social attitudes towards people with obesity are unjustified—merely the result of prejudice and ignorance, since several scientific findings indicate that obesity is often the result of a complex interaction between genetic and environmental risk factors. As suggested by Cooper et al., patients should be encouraged to ask themselves "Is it my problem or a problem with society in general?" [7].

If the patients agree that it is society that has the problem, they should be encouraged to distance themselves from these prejudices and to avoid being negatively influenced by them. It is also useful to discuss with patients some possible strategies for coping with social pressures. These may be as simple as ignoring them and responding to criticism assertively, or more active, for example, writing a letter to a newspaper and/or joining a group that fights prejudice against people with obesity.

If the patient is experiencing social pressure from within the family, the therapist should evaluate with them whether it would be helpful to involve significant others in their treatment. In this way, their major critics could be educated and discuss how they could temper their judgemental attitude the patient's eating, shape and weight (see Chap. 10).

8.6.6 Enhancing the Personal Significance of Other Self-Evaluation Domains

As described in Sect. 8.6.3, negative body image is primarily mediated by the importance that the individual attaches to their body shape and weight in their own evaluation of themselves. For this reason, a CBT-OB strategy for indirectly reducing the degree of importance attributed to shape and weight is to help the patient enhance the personal significance of other self-evaluation domains.

The first step in this process is to educate the patient about the abstract concept of self-evaluation. Here we report a dialogue between the therapist and Emma (the patient introduced in the previous *Vignette*) on this topic.

- *Therapist*: "Today I think we should talk about the way people evaluate or judge themselves".
- *Patient*: "That is interesting topic. I like the idea".
- *Therapist*: "Well, you know that all of us have a way of judging ourselves. If we are fulfilling our expectations in the areas of life we value, we feel quite good about ourselves, but if not, we feel bad".
- *Patient*: "I agree".
- *Therapist*: "Typically, people judge themselves according to various domains; one example domain could be how they are doing in their relationships with a partner and/or friends. Other things that may be important to their self-evaluation could be how they are performing at work and the quality of their performance in their pastimes—for example, sports or hobbies. However, largely due to the negative messages that our society sends regarding obesity, people who do not feel that they fit into the "normal" stereotype often judge themselves harshly on their shape and weight, which they feel are very important".
- *Patient*: "I know; this is my problem".
- *Therapist*: "If someone feels very bad if one area of their life is going badly, this indicates that that particular aspect of their life is probably very important to them".
- *Patient*: "I understand. So, when I see my body and I feel terrible, this means that my body is very important to me. You know, I feel so bad about myself that some days I don't go out".
- *Therapist*: "Exactly. This indicates that your shape and/or appearance are a very important part of how you judge yourself. A good way of looking at the criteria you use to judge yourself is to draw a "self-evaluation pie chart"; the various slices in the pie chart represent the areas of life that you use to determine your self-worth, and the bigger the slice, the more important it is to you".
- *Patient*: "Yes, I understand".
- *Therapist*: "Before you draw your own pie chart, we should first list the things that factor into the way you judge, or evaluate, yourself. What might they be?"

The therapist then helps the patient generate a list of "self-evaluation domains". Once the list has been drawn up, the therapist explores with the patient the relative importance of each, ranking them and drawing a provisional pie chart. Each slice of the pie represents the relative importance that the patient attributes to that area in their self-evaluation schema. The self-evaluation pie chart produced by Emma—the patient from the above vignette, who has a negative body image—is shown in Fig. 8.1 (on the left) alongside one pertaining to another patient with obesity but without a negative body image.

The self-evaluation pie chart provides the patients with a handy visual representation of the excessive importance that they may give to shape and weight and is used by the therapist to elicit the advantages and disadvantages of using a system of self-evaluation in which shape and weight have excessive importance [13]. This analysis should help the patient to conclude that having one large self-evaluation domain is a dysfunctional form of self-evaluation, as it marginalises other important aspects of life (e.g. relationships, school, work, hobbies, etc.) and leads to some behaviours (e.g. body avoidance and body checking) that characterise and

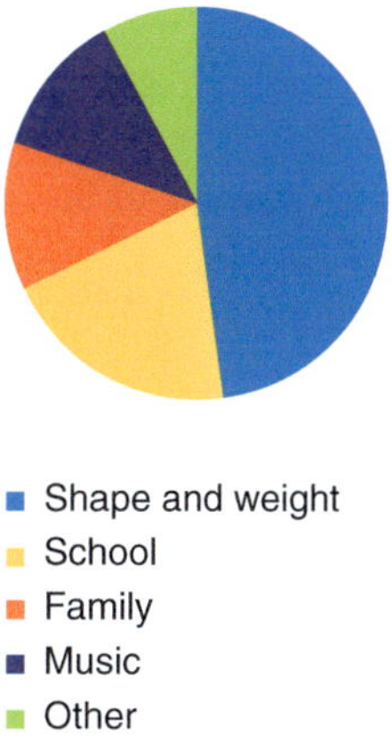

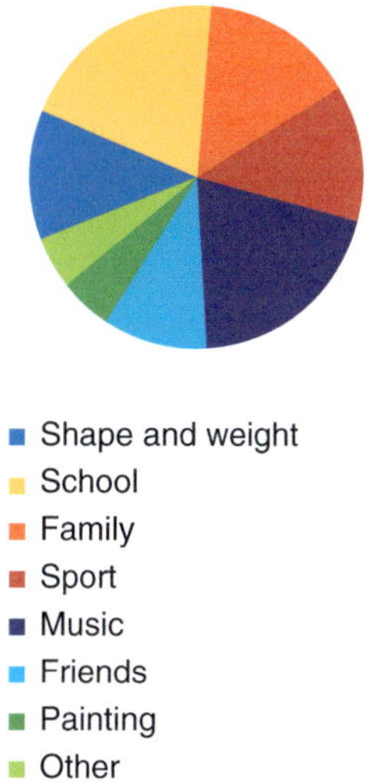

Fig. 8.1 A pie chart pertaining to a patient with obesity and negative body image (on the left) and one of a patient with obesity without negative body image (on the right)

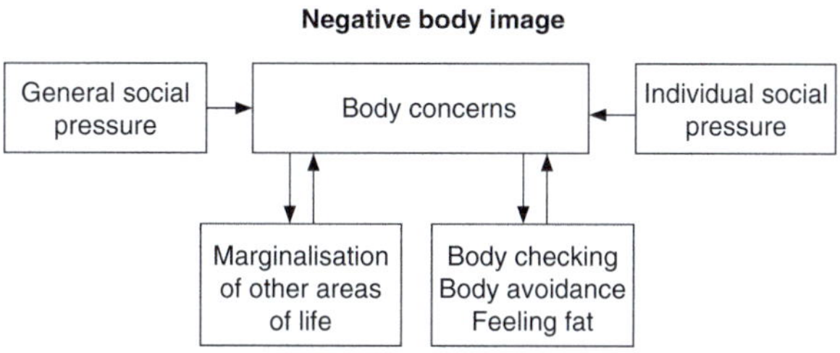

Fig. 8.2 An example of a body image Personal Formulation

maintain a negative body image. Furthermore, if something goes wrong (e.g. weight gain or not being able to reach the desired weight), it could cause self-worth to collapse entirely. Finally, it drives a person to pursue an excessive weight loss, which is not only difficult to achieve but also to maintain—they will never be satisfied with their weight.

Then, after the patient has agreed that a smaller slice devoted to weight and shape would be preferable, the therapist should help them to address any direct expressions of negative body image that they report, specifically the marginalisation of other life areas, the body checking, body avoidance and feeling fat [13]. Through several mechanisms, these expressions serve to maintain a negative body image and, therefore, need to be addressed by the treatment (see Fig. 8.2).

Hence the next steps are to help the patient to address the marginalisation of other areas of life and directly enhance the importance of other self-evaluation domains. Negative body image, especially if extreme, inevitably marginalises other areas of life, which might otherwise contribute positively to self-evaluation. However, even if the expressions of negative body image are not extreme, they may nevertheless have a strong influence on the patient's quality of life and their self-evaluation, having a negative impact on interpersonal relationships and/or limiting participation in some social activities, hobbies or sports that involve body exposure and therefore distress.

This type of marginalisation is generally manifested in two ways [13], both of which can be ascertained from the self-evaluation pie chart. First, self-evaluation domains not related to body image are few in number (i.e. there are few unrelated slices in the patient's pie chart) with respect to those that patients without body concerns might have. Second, they may be of limited importance (i.e. the slices are small in size), particularly in patients with extreme body concerns (i.e. those with overvaluation of shape and weight). The goal therefore is to help patients develop other areas of life that should take on more importance in their self-evaluation schema and thereby indirectly reduce the patient's overvaluation of shape or weight.

The strategy involves encouraging patients, using a "brainstorming" approach, to identify any activities or areas of life that they would like to work on, and assisting them to do so [13]. Possible areas to suggest are hobbies, etc. that the patients had in the past but gave up due to their obesity. Activities that they have always wanted to do but have never got round to may also help in this regard. Sometimes good ideas can come from considering what other people of the same age do in their spare time. In general, it is advisable to agree on one or possibly two activities that the patient will try and ensure that they actually start to engage in the activity identified. The last column of the Monitoring Record should be used to record and review any progress or obstacles in this area on a weekly basis, and any barriers that arise should be addressed through a problem-solving approach.

Vignette

Emma, with great reluctance, decided to enrol in a riding school, as to ride a horse had always been her dream. To her surprise, she was welcomed with kindness and warmth by the teacher and other members of the school. Attending the riding school gave her the opportunity to meet some nice new people and to spent enjoyable times at the clubhouse after the end of her riding lesson. She started to take more care of her physical appearance, buying new make-up and more colourful clothes. She also started to accept invitations to the birthday parties held by the mothers of her son's classmates.

8.6.7 Addressing Other Expressions of Negative Body Image

It is crucial to encourage the patient to target the other major expressions of negative body image directly. This strategy should be applied at the same time as enhancing the importance of other self-evaluation domains and involves tackling body checking, body avoidance and feeling fat. In most cases, it is advisable to address body checking first, as this tends to increase the body dissatisfaction that maintains body avoidance and triggers feeling fat. However, in some patients, body avoidance is the first expression to address, as they do not report significant body checking behaviours. Usually feeling fat is the last expression to address, although in some cases the order can be reversed if this expression of body concern is extreme.

8.6.7.1 Addressing Body Checking

As described in Sect. 8.6.4, a common direct expression of negative body image is body checking. The aim of this behaviour is usually to keep an eye on the shape of the body and/or to check whether it has changed. Body checking is common among people in general, but in those with a negative body image, it manifests more frequently and in very unusual ways [13]. Common body checking behaviours of patients with obesity are the following:

- Frequent weight checking (e.g. measuring the body weight frequently)
- Visual checking (e.g. frequent self-examination of specific parts of the body in the mirror, or any reflective surface, with a hypercritical attitude)
- Measurement checking (e.g. measuring the circumference of the body, for example, waist, hips, thighs and/or wrists)
- Tactile checking (e.g. pinching the folds of fat to gauge their size, wearing tight clothes to see how they feel)
- Comparison checking (e.g. looking at leaner people or particular features of others, such as a flat belly, slim, long or muscular legs; looking at models or actors in the media; taking interest in the weight and body size of others)
- Reassurance checking (e.g. asking other people for reassurance about the shape of their own body).

The first step in addressing these behaviours is to describe to the patient the main forms of body checking and how these maintain and intensify body dissatisfaction through the following main mechanisms [13]:

1. Checking weight too frequently favours negative interpretations of minimal weight changes (which are generally due to changes in the body's hydration status).
2. Constantly scrutinising, touching and measuring the body means that the "problem" is never out of sight or out of mind.
3. Focusing on disliked parts of the body amplifies the perceived defects.
4. Superficial observation of the body parts of atypical people (e.g. models or actors), a subgroup of lean people or those with "special" features (e.g. a flat belly) only intensifies the misperception that one's own body is the wrong shape.

The second step is to explain to patients that people are often unaware that they themselves are engaging in these behaviours, and they should therefore monitor any episodes that they notice over a 2-day period in the last column of their Monitoring Record. This will enable assessment of their frequency and implications and exploration of associated thoughts and emotions.

The third step is to review with the patients the motivation behind the body checking behaviours they have made note of and what they perceive to be the consequences. The following questions may be of assistance in this regard [13]:

- Why did you check your body?
- Why did you check your body so frequently?

- Which part of your body did you look at?
- Do you usually feel better after checking your body?
- Do you think that body checking has any negative effects?

This should lead to the conclusion that body checking increases body dissatisfaction, and the fourth step is therefore to discuss with patients which dysfunctional body checking behaviours (e.g. weight checking, mirror use, comparison checking) to address. The aim is to reduce the frequency and nature of these behaviours in order to obtain a functional control of body shape and weight.

During this period, the target behaviour should be monitored in real time, with the patient writing why they were doing it in the last column of the Monitoring Record. This should make it easier for the patient to learn to stop this behaviour at the outset and understand what they are trying achieve through this behaviour. As with weight checking (addressed in Module 1, see Sect. 4.4), preoccupation with shape may transiently increase, but it then tends to decrease as the patient gains control. However, if a patient finds it difficult to stop body checking, they should be encouraged to identify the trigger situations (e.g. after eating, when getting undressed) and to devise and practice strategies that will enable them to resist the urge (e.g. undressing in front of a mirror, handling an object instead of pinching their fat folds).

When it is suggested to patients that they attempt to change the frequency and nature of their body checking [13], the therapist should discuss the appropriate use of mirrors and in particular the purpose of looking in the mirror, as well as a normal frequency and time spent doing so. Patients should be advised to look in the mirror to check their hair and clothes in the morning when they get up or before they go out. There are no other healthy or useful reasons for looking in a mirror!

With patients that report frequent comparison checking, the therapist should suggest that this is addressed by targeting the two typical biases associated with this behaviour [13]: (1) subject bias (i.e. comparing oneself with someone who is young and attractive) and (2) evaluation bias (i.e. looking at other people's bodies in a superficial and uncritical way but being meticulous and critical when they check their own). Patients are encouraged to reduce the frequency of such comparisons, to become aware in real time of the two biases, to widen their focus of attention (e.g. hair, shoes) and to observe people's other characteristics (e.g. personality). It is also useful to stimulate patients to become aware of body diversity. In the event that comparison is focused on celebrities in magazines or other media, one useful strategy may be to point out to patients that such images are not representative of realistic body models, as the vast majority, if not all, have been retouched (there are numerous examples of "the Photoshop Effect" on the internet which may help them appreciate this).

8.6.7.2 Addressing Body Avoidance

Body avoidance is another typical expression of negative body image and is common in patients with obesity [12]. Avoiding situations that may cause distress due to the need to expose the body perpetuates body dissatisfaction. Although avoiding these situations prevents distress and discomfort in the short term, it does not give patients a clear idea of what they actually look like, or to learn to overcome their anxiety when swimming, exercising in public or other occasions in which they feel exposed [7]. The result is that patients become completely dependent on their own judgement about how they or others will see them, and as a consequence these negative predictions and fears are never put to the test. Body avoidance is also a huge obstacle to healthy socialisation, intimacy with a partner and everyday activities such as buying new clothes or going out with friends. Typical body avoidance behaviours include (1) avoiding checking body weight, (2) avoiding looking at one's own body, (3) avoiding touching one's own body and (4) avoiding exposing one's body to others.

The first step in addressing body avoidance is for the CBT-OB therapist to illustrate this process to the patient, taking the lead from some of their own experiences and explaining how it acts to reinforce body dissatisfaction. The therapist should help the patients to conclude that it is better to confront the situations they would rather avoid, if only to test their predictions and the negative consequences that they foresee [7].

Next the therapist should help plan specific behavioural tasks that the patient feels that they will be able to achieve. The plan should involve progressively exposing specific body parts, beginning with those that cause less discomfort (e.g. going out in three-quarter-length rather than long sleeves). Patients should also be encouraged to predict the consequences of body exposure, writing their predictions in the Monitoring Record, and, with the help of the therapist, plan in advance how to achieve the task and cope with the anticipated negative consequences [7].

The third step is to ask how the attempt went and whether the predicted negative consequences in fact occurred. The therapist should emphasise the positive aspects of the outcome, including the fact that the patients overcame their reticence to try it, and review with the patients what they have learned from the experience [7]. In this way, patients are assisted to gradually become accustomed to the sight and feel of their own body and ultimately to become comfortable exposing it in the presence of others. Usually, this process does not require many sessions and leads to a marked reduction in harmful body avoidance, as well as secondary benefits such as increased opportunities for socialising.

8.6.7.3 Addressing Feeling Fat

Many people report feeling fat, even if they are of normal or low weight, but the experience is extremely intense and frequent among those with obesity—especially in those with overvaluation of shape and weight and intense body concerns. Feeling fat seems to be consequence of "mislabelling" three main experiences [13]:

1. *Negative physical states* (e.g. the sensation of body fat wobbling—which is common in women and people who have excess body weight—and feeling tired, full, bloated or sluggish)
2. *Negative emotions* (e.g. anxiety or depression)
3. *Accentuated body awareness* (through body checking, wearing tight clothes and/or receiving comments on the body)

Research indicates that excessive feeling fat could be a consequence of patients' long-standing and prolonged preoccupation with body shape [13]. As feeling fat, like other expressions of negative self-image, increases body dissatisfaction, it must also be addressed by the treatment.

Patients are encouraged to identify when feeling fat "peaks" (i.e. when the sensation is more intense). They should then seek to identify the experience associated with that feeling by asking themselves questions such as, "Has something happened over the last hour or so that may have triggered my feeling fat?", or "What else am I feeling at this time (in addition to fat)?". Finally, they should address the circumstance directly (e.g. wearing looser clothes to address accentuated body awareness, problem-solving to cope with negative emotions and tolerating negative physical states by being aware that they are only transitory) [13].

8.7 Accepting a Reasonable and Healthy Weight

The interrelated and complementary strategies and procedures used to address negative body image in CBT-OB should produce a gradual erosion of its main expressions (i.e. weight checking and avoidance, shape checking, body avoidance and feeling fat). Together with an enhancement of the importance of other life domains, this acts to progressively reduce the patient's body concerns and the significance they place on shape and weight in their own self-evaluation. This process is also consolidated by addressing unrealistic weight-loss goals and dysfunctional primary goals or losing weight.

The final strategy of this type of intervention is to encourage the patient to reach positive acceptance of the body shape and weight they have achieved at the end of the weight-loss phase. The emphasis should be on balancing change and acceptance, i.e. changing what can be changed (lifestyle) and accepting what cannot (i.e. attaining an "ideal" body shape and weight) [14].

The patients should be helped to accept that extreme weight-control measures such as extreme dietary restriction and strenuous physical activity are counterproductive in the long term. Such extreme and unhealthy behaviours will not help them to achieve the ultimate goal of maintaining an "ideal" shape and weight and can in fact destroy self-confidence and self-esteem. The negative implications of an attempt to change what cannot be changed must be balanced with trying to consider the existing weight and body shape in a more positive light. Ideally, self-acceptance should become an active process of self-affirmation rather than a passive process of resignation or "surrendering to fate" [14]. The goal is to expand the patient's definition and sense of self. To achieve this, they should be encouraged to compile a list of personal strengths that do not depend on their body shape and weight. It may be also helpful to help patients to identify famous people that meet the current social criteria for physical beauty but actually have had a miserable life. Sometimes it is also helpful to ask the patients to give themselves the advice they would give to a friend in a similar situation.

Acceptance of obesity can be facilitated by exploring the origins of the patient's negative beliefs about body shape and weight. Among the factors involved, the therapist should discuss with the patients the social pressures, prejudice, discrimination and mockery that people with obesity are often subjected to in our society. The patient should be encouraged to think that if people with obesity are discriminated against, it is because they are perceived to belong to a certain category of people (all those who do not match the "ideal"), not due to their individual personality, and therefore it is no fault of their own.

The ultimate goal of this intervention is not to get the patient to "love their body" but instead to reduce the overemphasis on body shape and weight in their self-evaluation, especially in cases in which a patient's self-worth is primarily based on an idealised image of physical appearance. Patients are not forbidden from being unhappy with their body; in fact, as already described in Sect. 8.6, such discontent is "normal" in Western culture [8]. As Cash (1995) described, a useful analogy of body dissatisfaction is chronic interpersonal conflict [15], as follows: if you are unhappy with your partner, you can decide to separate, but the only option with your own body is to make peace with it. This includes reaching a compromise and accepting less than what might be considered ideal.

Vignette

Emma worked hard to address her negative body image. In addition to successful attempts to increase the importance of other self-evaluation domains, as previously described, she stopped some dysfunctional body checking entirely, such as repeatedly pinching herself, looking critically at her body shape in the mirror (in particular her legs and hips) and comparing herself with younger and slimmer women. Taking up horse riding helped her to become more self-confident about herself and to expose herself in situations that she had previously avoided, such as going to the beach with her son. Nevertheless, she still found it difficult to address feeling fat, which tended to become more accentuated before her period—when she also had a low mood—and when she rode a horse. In the latter situation, she partially overcame the unpleasant sensation of her body wobbling by using a sports bra, and, perhaps more importantly, she was able to label the sensation of feeling fat as a transitory phenomenon stimulated by her interpretation of negative emotions and body awareness. At the end of the weight-loss phase, although Emma was still dissatisfied with her body shape, she did agree to start weight-loss maintenance; she realised that her quality of life had already much improved thanks to the weight loss she had achieved to date and that her self-evaluation had also improved due to the effort she had put into addressing her negative body image.

References

1. Dalle Grave R, Melchionda N, Calugi S, Centis E, Tufano A, Fatati G, et al. Continuous care in the treatment of obesity: an observational multicentre study. J Intern Med. 2005;258(3):265–73. https://doi.org/10.1111/j.1365-2796.2005.01524.x.
2. Calugi S, Marchesini G, El Ghoch M, Gavasso I, Dalle Grave R. The influence of weight-loss expectations on weight loss and of weight-loss satisfaction on weight maintenance in severe obesity. J Acad Nutr Diet. 2017;117(1):32–8. https://doi.org/10.1016/j.jand.2016.09.001.
3. Calugi S, Marchesini G, El Ghoch M, Gavasso I, Dalle Grave R. The association between weight maintenance and session-by-session diet adherence, weight loss and weight-loss satisfaction. Eat Weight Disord. 2018. https://doi.org/10.1007/s40519-018-0528-8.
4. Dalle Grave R, Calugi S, Compare A, El Ghoch M, Petroni ML, Tomasi F, et al. Weight loss expectations and attrition in treatment-seeking obese women. Obes Facts. 2015;8(5):311–8. https://doi.org/10.1159/000441366.
5. Dalle Grave R, Calugi S, Molinari E, Petroni ML, Bondi M, Compare A, et al. Weight loss expectations in obese patients and treatment attrition: an observational multicenter study. Obes Res. 2005;13(11):1961–9. https://doi.org/10.1038/oby.2005.241.
6. Cooper Z, Fairburn CG. A new cognitive behavioural approach to the treatment of obesity. Behav Res Ther. 2001;39(5):499–511.
7. Cooper Z, Fairburn CG, Hawker DM. Cognitive-behavioral treatment of obesity: a clinician's guide. New York: Guilford Press; 2003.
8. Rodin J, Silberstein LR, Striegel-Moore RH. Women and weight: a normative discontent. In: Sonderegger TB, editor. Nebraska symposium on motivation: psychology and gender. Lincoln: University of Nebraska Press; 1984. p. 267–307.
9. Foster GD, Wadden TA, Vogt RA. Body image in obese women before, during, and after weight loss treatment. Health Psychol. 1997;16(3):226–9.
10. Adami GF, Meneghelli A, Bressani A, Scopinaro N. Body image in obese patients before and after stable weight reduction following bariatric surgery. J Psychosom Res. 1999;46(3):275–81.
11. Cash TF. Body-image attitudes: evaluation, investment, and affect. Percept Mot Skills. 1994;78(3 Pt 2):1168–70. https://doi.org/10.2466/pms.1994.78.3c.1168.
12. Dalle Grave R, Cuzzolaro M, Calugi S, Tomasi F, Temperilli F, Marchesini G, et al. The effect of obesity management on body image in patients seeking treatment at medical centers. Obesity (Silver Spring). 2007;15(9):2320–7. https://doi.org/10.1038/oby.2007.275.
13. Fairburn CG. Cognitive behavior therapy and eating disorders. New York: Guilford Press; 2008.
14. Wilson GT. Acceptance and change in the treatment of eating disorders and obesity. Behav Ther. 1996;27:417–39.
15. Cash TF. What do you see when you look in the mirror? New York: Bantam Books; 1995.

Module 6: Addressing the Obstacles to Weight Maintenance

9

Maintaining the weight lost is the most challenging problem of overweight and obesity treatment. There are many ways to lose weight, but none has thus far proved wholly effective in preventing future weight regain. To address this issue, Module 6 introduces several strategies and procedures specifically designed to help patients maintain their lower body weight. It coincides with the beginning of Phase 2 of the CBT-OB programme and lasts 48 weeks. In most cases, it is begun after the 24-week weight-loss phase, when the weight-loss rate has slowed or reached a plateau. However, the start of Module 6 may be delayed for several months if a patient wants to lose more weight and displays a constant weight-loss rate of 0.5 kg/week without adopting extreme weight-control behaviours. This is because studies have found that the more weight lost, the more satisfied the patients are with the treatment, and the greater the likelihood of them being able to maintain the weight lost over time [1]. However, the therapist should carefully evaluate with the patient the pros and cons of delaying the start of the weight-maintenance phase; whatever their decision at this stage, they should understand that weight maintenance is an integral part of treatment and cannot be postponed indefinitely.

Before starting Phase 2, one or two sessions should be dedicated to preparing patients for weight maintenance, since it is crucial that they agree to commit to a lifestyle and mindset oriented towards weight maintenance (not weight loss) for at least 48 weeks. As part of this phase, patients will attend one session every 4 weeks, and these sessions will be structured similarly to those in Stage 1.

9.1 Preparing the Patient for Weight Maintenance

By analysing our patients' past weight-loss attempts, we realised that in almost all cases, they never practised lasting maintenance of the weight lost. Indeed, from their accounts, it emerged that they had adopted weight-control behaviours with

R. Dalle Grave et al., *Treating Obesity with Personalized Cognitive Behavioral Therapy*, https://doi.org/10.1007/978-3-319-91497-8_9

the sole aim of losing weight and commonly went back to their previous eating habits when they stopped. As suggested by Cooper et al. [2], one of the reasons for poor long-term outcomes in obesity treatment is the failure of therapists and patients to appreciate the importance of establishing and practising weight-maintenance skills, which are different from those required to lose weight. For this reason, it is crucial to dedicate one or two sessions to preparing patients to start the weight-maintenance phase well. Usually, it is advisable to address this topic by reviewing collaboratively the amount of weight lost and the improvements achieved in the quality of the patient's physical and psychosocial life. Then the patient should be educated on weight maintenance. Finally, the therapist should actively involve the patient in the decision to start the weight-maintenance phase and only then start to address it.

9.1.1 Reviewing the Changes Achieved Through Weight Loss

A review of the changes in a patient's physical and psychosocial wellbeing associated with the weight they have lost is a good way to introduce the topic of weight maintenance, as it may help them to appreciate the importance of maintaining the weight lost. As part of this review, the therapist should ask the patient to compare their current lifestyle, physical condition and health with how they were before the beginning of CBT-OB. In most cases, patients report that now they adopt healthy eating and an active lifestyle; they have stopped overeating or binge eating; they sleep better, are less tired, have less pain in the joints and can get upstairs easily; and their physical fitness has dramatically improved. In some patients, the physical improvements can be confirmed by the normalisation of blood test results and a reduction in the medicines used to treat some comorbidities associated with obesity (e.g. hypertension, diabetes, dyslipidaemia, etc.). The therapist should also ask the patient if their weight loss has been associated with any psychosocial improvements. In many cases, the patients report that their self-confidence, mood and body image have improved, they are no longer excluded from things due to their weight, and they feel more confident during social occasions.

Once their achievements have been listed, the next step is to ask the patient if they consider it important to maintain the benefits obtained through weight loss. In most cases patients report that they do not want to go back to how they were because they feel much better now. The therapist should then draw the patient's attention to previous weight-loss attempts, asking them whether they had resulted in similar benefits, which were subsequently lost when they regained weight. Patients frequently respond "yes" to this question and conclude that their main problem is maintaining the weight lost. At this point, the therapist should ask the patients if they are interested in receiving some general information about weight-loss maintenance. Most patients respond that they would, and the therapist can therefore start to educate them on this topic.

9.1.2 Educating the Patient on Weight Maintenance

A fundamental step for helping patients to accept the weight-maintenance phase weight is to educate them on three main themes: (1) weight maintenance is more difficult than weight loss; (2) some people are able to maintain the weight lost in the long term; and (3) to maintain weight, it will be necessary to learn and practise the appropriate skills.

9.1.2.1 Weight Maintenance Is More Difficult Than Weight Loss

The therapist should explain that weight maintenance is more difficult than weight loss for the following reasons [2]: (1) one has to accept a weight that might previously have been considered unacceptable; (2) weight loss has a definite duration, while weight maintenance is an indefinite process that lasts forever; (3) during weight maintenance, people tend to receive little encouragement from significant others (indeed, sometimes they are criticised for not trying to lose more weight); (4) the positive results of weight loss can be evaluated each week, but assessment of weight maintenance requires months or years; and (5) during weight loss, the goal is to improve (e.g. weight, health, appearance, etc.), while during weight maintenance the goal is to preserve what has been achieved.

The therapist should also emphasise that relapse after weight loss is an insidious process, very different from that observed in substance misuse. Foremost in the minds of former substance misusers (e.g. alcohol, smoke, cocaine, etc.) is the possibility of "falling off the wagon", but this is generally not the case in weight maintainers. For instance, a person who has given up smoking knows that one cigarette will likely lead to relapse and is therefore very careful to avoid even minimal transgression and maintain a lasting abstinence. However, in weight maintainers, the first steps on the road to relapse are less obvious. In this case, the process of relapse usually begins with small but persistent changes in eating (e.g. eating food rich in fat, grazing, etc.) or physical activity habits (e.g. no longer walking 10,000 steps a day). At the beginning, these changes do not necessarily produce an immediate increase in weight, because to gain 1 kg it is necessary to eat about 7000 kcal more than those burned. This fact may lead the individuals to develop the false confidence that they can eat more and move less without gaining weight. Even when they regain 2 kg, they often remain unaware that a relapse is underway and tend to think that they will be able to lose this weight easily "whenever they want". In reality, however, this amount of weight regain is often the sign that old habits have been reactivated and re-established over a persistent period of time, and the patient is already on the slippery slope that will almost inevitably lead to gradually putting back on all the weight that they had lost. This means that in the weight-maintenance phase, it is essential for the patient to learn to pay attention to the early signs of relapse (i.e. changes in eating and/or physical activity habits), and to nip transgressions in the bud, even before their weight begins to creep up. In short, they must be taught how and when to get back on track.

9.1.2.2 Some People Are Able to Maintain the Weight Lost in the Long Term

The therapist should reinforce the notion that some people are able to keep their weight off in the long term by describing to the patient the results of analysing the National Weight Control Registry (NWCR). This scientific study was designed to follow people (18 years or older) who had lost at least 13.6 kg (30 lbs) and kept it off for at least 1 year. Over 10,000 people enrolled in the study, completing annual questionnaires about their current weight, diet and exercise habits and behavioural strategies for weight-loss maintenance, and in 2014 the study reported a 10-year observation of self-reported weight-loss and behavioural change in 2886 participants, recruited primarily through newspaper and magazine articles. The mean weight loss of these participants was 31.3 kg at baseline, 23.8 kg at 5 years and 23.1 kg at 10 years. Of note, 87% of participants were still maintaining at least a 10% weight loss after 5 and 10 years. The therapist should emphasise that the impressive NWCR data shows that long-term weight-loss maintenance is possible. The therapist should inform the patient that weight maintainers in the NWCR study adopted the following behavioural strategies [3]: (1) high levels of physical activity (about 1 hour per day); (2) eating a low-energy, low-fat diet; (3) eating breakfast regularly; (4) self-monitoring weight frequently; and (5) maintaining a consistent eating pattern across weekdays and weekends. Moreover, the chance of longer-term success increased in those who managed to keep their weight off for 2 years or more.

That being said, the therapist should inform the patients that the NWCR study was not, unfortunately, designed to answer the central question, namely, why some individuals do manage to continue to practise weight-control behaviours, and therefore maintain weight loss in the long-term, while others do not. Some have suggested that the driving force behind weight regain is the biological pressure on individuals to overeat in order to restore their original weight (the set-point theory) [4], while others implicate the exposure to an environment that promotes overeating and sedentary behaviours. Whatever the case, the NWCR study clearly shows that many individuals are able to overcome these pressures in the long term and to maintain significant weight loss through lifestyle modification.

If biological pressures are not entirely to blame, the therapist should suggest that it is conceivable that cognitive mechanisms interacting with specific changes in diet and physical activity may play a pivotal role in long-term weight maintenance. Indeed, the complex behaviours involved in lifestyle modification—in this case adopting and persisting with strategies required to lose and maintain weight—are in part influenced by conscious cognitive processes. Our research, for example, has found that weight maintenance is associated with greater satisfaction with the weight loss achieved and its attendant benefits [1, 5], while a decline in weight-loss satisfaction over the weight-loss phase is associated with weight regain in the long run (see Chap. 1) [6]. This indicates that cognitive processes strongly influence the likelihood of persisting with weight-maintenance behaviours. In particular, for long-term success, it is necessary to appreciate the weight loss achieved—even if it is less than that expected—and to develop a long-term weight-control mindset.

9.1.2.3 The Need to Develop and Practise Weight-Maintenance Skills

Patients should be informed that, after about 6 months (in most cases), weight loss tends to slow down and then stop. For this reason, CBT-OB initiates the maintenance phase at 24 weeks, after which it will focus on minimising the risk of relapse. It is important to stress to the patient that it will be necessary for them to dedicate time and effort to learning how to maintain the weight lost. In the maintenance phase, it is essential to stop any attempt to lose weight because this is incompatible with acquiring the cognitive and behavioural skills required to keep it off long term. The maintenance period should be at least 48 weeks long and could be followed by another cycle of weight loss and maintenance, if indicated.

9.1.3 Involving the Patient Actively in the Decision to Start Weight Maintenance

After having analysed the benefits achieved through weight loss and educated patients on weight maintenance, the next step is to evaluate collaboratively the pros and cons of initiating the weight-maintenance phase. Using the same strategy adopted in the Preparatory Phase (see Chap. 2), the therapist should ask the patient to think about their reasons for and against starting weight maintenance. It is best to begin by asking patients to list the cons, and whether continuing to pursue weight loss would provide them with any advantages that they would be afraid or unwilling to give up. Subsequently, patients should be asked to evaluate the pros, and at this stage, the therapist should prompt them to reflect on the possibility that the failure of previous weight-loss attempts could have been due, in part, to their not having learned and practised weight-maintenance skills. The list of pros and cons and the conclusions the patient draws from this discussion should be written down in table format (see Table 9.1).

If, despite this analysis, the patient is reluctant to begin the maintenance phase, the therapist should accept their decision on a temporary basis but emphasise the risks of continuing to pursue weight loss. In such patients, the therapist should use the following sessions to intensify their efforts to help them to address the obstacles to accepting body weight maintenance, employing the procedure described in Module 5.

Table 9.1 Pros and cons table of starting weight maintenance

Reasons for not starting weight maintenance	Reasons for starting weight maintenance
I want to lose other 10 kg *I am still obese* *I will be more attractive and happier if I lose more weight* *If I control my eating better I will lose more weight, and I then I will be more satisfied*	*I haven't lost any weight for 4 weeks* *I have already obtained several benefits from weight loss (I feel much fitter now, I have more energy, I can wear clothes that I like, my health has improved)* *In the past, I have never tried to maintain weight, and I have always regained the weight I had lost* *I really don't know how to maintain weight—either I lose weight or I gain weight*

Conclusions: *I want to start weight maintenance because I have already obtained several benefits from weight loss, and I need to learn how to maintain the weight*

9.1.4 Addressing Concerns and Questions About Starting Weight Maintenance

Patients should always be asked if they have any concerns or questions about starting weight maintenance. Here are some examples.

- *PATIENT:* "I am a little bit worried about starting weight maintenance. In the past, I have always regained the weight I had lost".
- *THERAPIST:* "It is not so bad that you are worried about weight maintenance, because as you know from your past experience, and as we discussed before, it is the most difficult part of treatment. However, this programme has been specifically designed to help you to develop skills to maintain weight in the long term. Moreover, your past experience may help alert you to the first signs of relapse and prevent you putting the weight back on".

- *PATIENT:* "I know that it is important to start weight maintenance, but my husband told me that I still need to lose weight".
- *THERAPIST:* "I am happy that you agree that it is important to start weight maintenance. Maybe we can meet with your husband to explain why you should be starting weight maintenance, and ask for his help".
- *PATIENT:* "Yes. I think that's a good idea".

- *PATIENT:* "What should I do if I start to put on weight?"
- *THERAPIST:* "Good question. With the treatment you will learn specific skills to prevent weight regain and to return to an acceptable weight-maintenance range if this occurs".

- *PATIENT:* "Can I change my mind and decide to lose more weight later on, after a month or so?"
- *THERAPIST:* "Of course. You are free to decide what you want to do. However, I do not think that would be a good idea, because you need time to learn and practise the skills required to maintain weight".

- *PATIENT:* "I feel I am able to lose more weight. Why do I have to start maintaining?"
- *THERAPIST:* "If you are confident in your ability to lose more weight you can choose to continue the weight-loss phase for a couple of months. However, before making this decision we should carefully evaluate the pros and cons of delaying the start of weight maintenance. Whatever your decision, you should be aware that weight maintenance is an integral part of the treatment, and will be necessary sooner or later if you are to succeed in keeping the weight off".

- *PATIENT:* "Will it be possible for me to lose more weight after the end of the weight-maintenance phase?"
- *THERAPIST:* "Yes, of course. We will address this issue towards the end of treatment".

Vignette

The patient, a 35-year-old single woman working as a lawyer, achieved a weight loss of 15 kg after 24 weeks of treatment (from 85 to 70 kg). However, over the last month, she only lost 1 kg. She reported that the weight loss she had achieved to date made her feel much better both physically and psychologically. Moreover, she had received many compliments from her clients and friends and also has a new "beau". Despite these gains, she was very reluctant to start weight maintenance because her goal was to reach a "normal" weight. Nonetheless, after receiving information about the need to learn and practise skills for weight maintenance and reviewing the failure of previous weight-loss attempts, in which she never practised a period of weight maintenance, she agreed to start Phase 2. When interviewed after 48 weeks of weight maintenance at 69 kg, she stated that the decision to interrupt the attempt to lose weight and to focus her attention only on maintenance was a good one. She reported great appreciation for her current lifestyle and physical fitness (she was routinely able to play tennis for 1 h without feeling tired) and acceptance of her body shape.

9.2 Procedures for Weight Maintenance

9.2.1 Establishing Weekly Self-Weighing and a Weight-Maintenance Range

Research has shown that one of the most important procedures involved in long-term weight maintenance is regular weighing and that people who stop doing this tend to recover all the weight they had lost [3]. It has been suggested that regular self-weighing has the potential to allow individuals to detect an energy imbalance early on, before these changes produce substantial weight regain [7] (although as we have seen, this may, in fact, be a relatively late sign). Regular weighing, most commonly once a week, has also been reported by the majority of the long-term successful weight-loss maintainers in the NWCR [8]. Hence, the therapist should inform the patient that weighing themselves once a week is a key procedure for weight maintenance and should become a lifetime habit, like washing or brushing teeth.

Patients have been trained in home self-weighing from the start of the treatment, during the in-session collaborative weighing (see Module 1 in Chap. 3), and they should now be experts in interpreting any changes in their weight. In the weight-maintenance phase, the patient should be firmly advised to continue the weekly self-weighing procedure at home, even though the frequency of in-session weighing will be reduced from every 2 weeks to every 4 weeks. For this purpose, the therapist should provide the patient with a "weight-maintenance graph" (see Fig. 9.1) with 48 weeks on the *x*-axis (i.e. the duration of Phase 2); a weight-maintenance range of

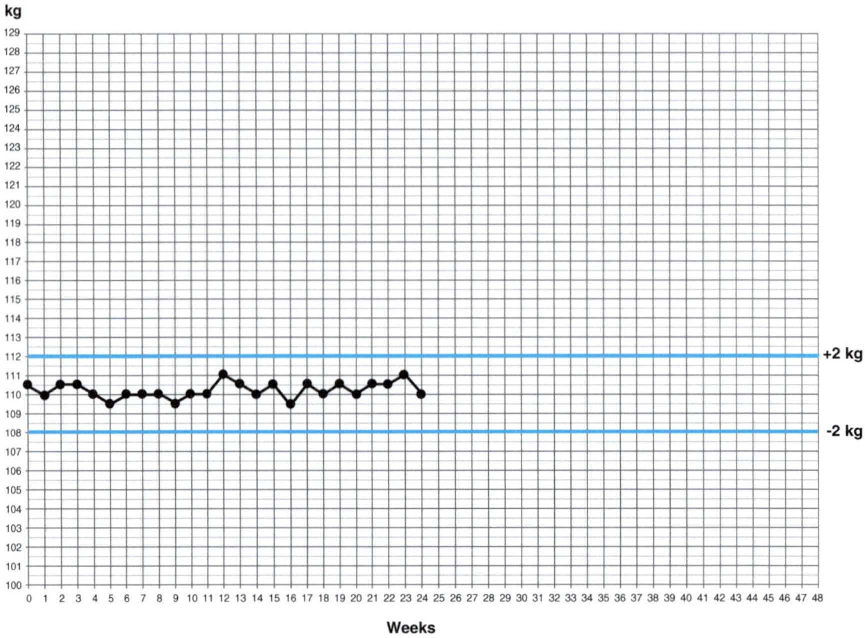

Fig. 9.1 An example weight-maintenance graph

2 kg either side of the patient's current weight (i.e. the mean of the last 4 weeks) should be traced or highlighted, to show them the outer limits of their individual weight-maintenance range—from the maximum (2 kg above the average weight) to the minimum (2 kg below the average weight). A range of 4 kg has been chosen because the body weight tend to fluctuate as consequence of normal alterations in body hydration [2].

In addition to analysing 4-week changes in weight rather than a single reading (the indication given to patients in the weight-loss phase), the patient should be instructed to look out for the following two situations when interpreting their weight-maintenance graph (see Fig. 9.2):

1. *The weight goes beyond the weight-maintenance range*. If the weight increases above the maximum weight in the acceptable range, they should immediately implement a pre-prepared action plan that will allow them to get back on track (see Sect. 9.2.7). Similarly, if their weight goes under the minimum in the maintenance range, it is important that the patient assesses whether or not this weight loss was intentional. If this is the case, they should be advised against pursuing further weight loss, because the goal of Module 6 is to learn to maintain weight, not to lose it—a necessary part of long-term success. If, however, the weight was not intentionally lost, it will be necessary to adjust the calorie intake to keep the weight within the maintenance range.

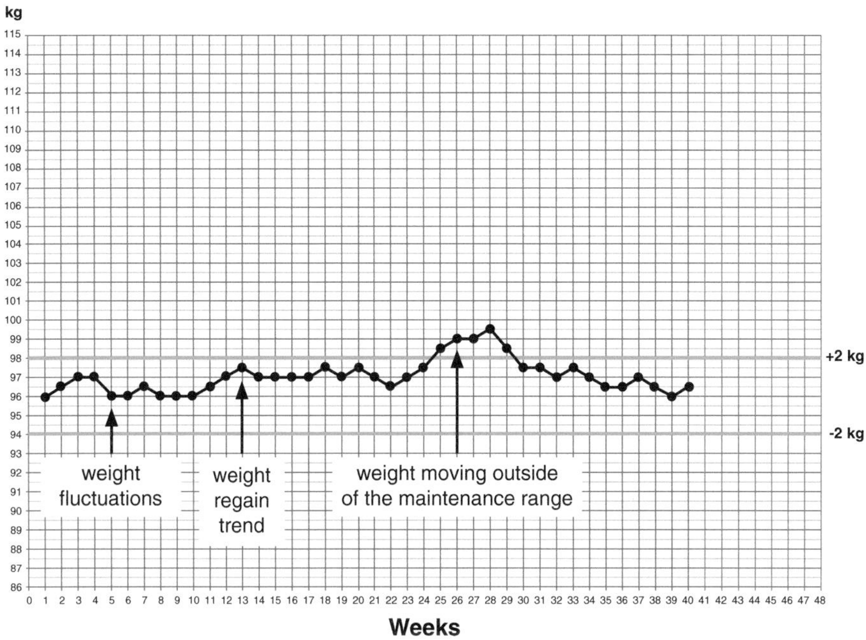

Fig. 9.2 An example of a weight-maintenance graph showing weight fluctuations, weight gain trend, and weight that goes beyond the effective maintenance range (dotted lines)

2. *Their weight seems to be increasing*. In this event, the patient is advised to assess whether their weight gain is related to normal weight fluctuations or is, in fact, the beginning of a weight regain trend (see Fig. 9.2). In order to resolve this issue, the patient should consider how their weight has changed over the last 4 weeks, rather than at a single weighing. Weight fluctuations are normal and can occur due to both physiological factors (e.g. in the premenstrual phase) and variations in the energy balance. If their weight shows an increase over 1 or 2 weeks, the patient should not worry, because the weight variation may be transitory and secondary to changes in their hydration status. However, if a trend of increasing weight develops over 4 weeks, the patient should put their contingency plan into action without hesitation.

9.2.2 Adopting Eating Habits Conducive to Weight Maintenance

The specific strategies that the therapist should suggest that the patient adopt to maintain weight will depend on the trend in their weight over the preceding 4 weeks. If a patient's weight seems to be stable—as is often the case—no energy balance modification is required. If, on the other hand, the patient's weight is showing a tendency to decrease, and they have agreed to start the weight-maintenance phase, the calorie intake should be increased on the basis of the amount of weight lost (e.g. an increase of 500 kcal per day for loss of 2 kg over 4 weeks, because 1 kg of weight loss corresponds roughly to an energy deficit of approximately 7000 kcal).

On a related note, the therapist should also generally recommend that patients seek to maintain the same nutritional composition as the meal plan they adopted for weight loss. However, if a patient lost weight by eating a low percentage of protein (e.g. less than 25%) but a relatively large proportion of carbohydrates, the therapist should inform them about the findings of a large randomised controlled trial that observed better weight maintenance with an ad libitum high-protein and low-glycaemic-index diet with moderate fat content [9]. On the basis of these findings, it is advisable that such patients increase their protein intake and limit foods with a high glycaemic index.

The therapist should also remind patients to maintain the eating habits they adopted during Phase 1, particularly regular eating (i.e. three meals and two snacks a day), and to follow a flexible healthy eating plan.

9.2.3 Adopting Physical Activity Habits Conducive to Weight Maintenance

Studies have consistently found that regular physical activity is associated with long-term weight loss maintenance [10, 11], but how much exercise is needed, and are particular types of exercise better than others for weight-loss maintenance?

A response to this question comes from the data pertaining to participants in the NWCR. This indicates that successful weight-loss maintainers do higher levels of physical activity (burning on average about 2600 kcal/week, which translates to ~60–75 min of moderate intensity activity, such as brisk walking, per day) than the traditional medically recommended target for body weight control (1000 kcal/week) [12]. In particular 75% reported expending >1000 kcal/week in physical activity; about half (54%) >2000 kcal/week; and 35% burned >3000 kcal/week, although 25% did report burning <1000 kcal/week [12]. Walking was a favourite activity among NWCR participants, but about 29% also reported some form of resistance training. Although resistance training is not required for successful weight-loss maintenance [12], it may contribute to enhancing the daily energy expenditure by promoting an increase in muscle mass [12]. That being said, about 92% of NWCR participants who reported doing resistance training also engaged in other physical activities.

The amount and type of exercise practised by NWCR success stories is similar to that recommended in Module 3 of CBT-OB (see Chap. 6). For this reason, the therapist should encourage patients to continue with the exercise plan that they had adopted during the weight-loss phase—if it was sufficiently intense (e.g. at least 10,000 steps a day). Otherwise, patients should be persuaded to gradually increase their physical activity to reach an energy expenditure of at least 2600 kcal/week, as this will improve their ability to maintain the weight lost in the long term. Any obstacles to physical activity should be addressed with the procedures described in Module 4 (see Chap. 7).

9.2.4 Constructing a Weight-Maintenance Mindset

Cognitive processes are strongly involved in the maintenance of the behaviours involved in maintaining the weight lost. In particular, our research indicates patients that were either satisfied with the results they had achieved or confident in their ability to control their body weight without additional professional help were more likely to succeed in long-term weight maintenance (3 years on). This finding highlights the importance of a construct similar to the concept of self-efficacy, which is associated with greater adherence to weight-loss treatment, and it is surprising that cognitive strategies are not exploited more often in standard body weight-control programmes. Working under the assumption that this may be one of the reasons for their limited effectiveness, CBT-OB Phase 2 includes specific procedures designed to help patients control their weight in the long term by developing a "weight-maintenance mindset". The first step in this process is to collaboratively create a list of the patient's personal reasons for sticking with their current body weight. To help them create this list, the therapist should encourage the patient to focus on the four main domains of their life—health, psychological wellbeing, interpersonal relationships and work performance—taking both a short-term and a long view (see Table 9.2). The patient should be encouraged to consult this list when their resolve starts to waver, in order to train their mind to focus on body weight control and adhering to the eating and physical activity habits necessary for long-term success.

Table 9.2 An example list of personal reasons for maintaining weight

Health domain:
• I feel fitter • I can get up the stairs without getting tired • My cholesterol is in the normal range • My blood sugar is in the normal range • My blood pressure is normal without the pills
Psychological domain:
• I have more confidence in myself • I am happier with my body shape and I can finally wear the clothes I like • I feel good and no longer get depressed
Interpersonal domain:
• I feel more confident around others • My sex life has improved • I can do things with others (e.g. going for a walk in the mountains) which I could not do before
Work domain:
• I feel less tired and more focused at work

The therapist should encourage the patient to maintain the eating and physical activity habits that led to these positive changes, but in most cases these will have already become ingrained and do not require a strong cognitive effort. However, patients should also be cautioned against readopting their old lifestyle habits—looking out for any hint of "backsliding"—as this would almost certainly promote weight regain. Patients should be informed that more a person persists in practising a behaviour, the more it becomes automatic and easy to do, whereas the opposite occurs when one is lazy and takes up the old dysfunctional habits. It may be useful to compare the control of eating to the physical training when explaining this concept; specifically, the more a person trains their muscles, the less fatigue they experience, while if they take time out from exercising, they will have to work hard to regain their former fitness.

Another important strategy for patients is to adopt a weight-maintenance mindset geared to their personal reasons for keeping off the weight. They will need to keep a constant focus on weight control and conduct daily self-awareness reviews of their eating and exercising. In particular, they should be sure to practise the following cognitive skills, which they learned during the weight-loss phase:

- Mentally planning at the beginning of the day when, what and where to eat.
- Eating consciously—appreciating the smell and taste of the food—and sticking to the meal plan without being influenced by external (e.g. the sight of food, events) or internal stimuli (e.g. cravings, need for gratification, hunger, thoughts of food, changes in mood) that may negatively influence their adherence.
- Awarding cognitive credits each week if the goal to maintain their weight within the weight-maintenance range has been achieved, using phrases such as "I've been good", "I'm doing great", and "I can achieve my goal of maintaining weight". The regular use of cognitive credits may help patients reduce the frustration associated with maintaining a lifestyle oriented to long-term weight control and strengthen their confidence in being able to control their body weight.
- Using proactive problem-solving to address events that might influence eating.
- Using the procedure of "things to think and do" to address changes in mood, impulses to overeat and cravings for high-calorie foods.
- Using a decentring procedure to address thoughts that could promote the adoption of old eating and physical activity habits.

9.2.5 Identifying and Addressing High-Risk Situations

The situations that put patients at a high risk of weight regain can be divided into three main categories [2]: (1) phases of life, (2) behaviours and (3) thoughts. Patients should be taught to recognise these situations and to address them appropriately. For example, to address high-risk "phases" (e.g. holidays, forced periods of inactivity, illness, etc.), the patient should implement two main strategies:

1. Have a contingency plan ready.
2. Evaluate the respective pros and cons of (1) trying to prevent weight gain or (2) suspending weight maintenance for the interim and then taking compensatory action once the high-risk phase is over.

As regards the latter, the therapist should suggest that the patient analyse their past experiences of option (2)—if whether after regaining weight they were in fact able to return to their habitual weight. The example of physical training may also help them decide to continue their weight-maintenance efforts throughout the high-risk phase, i.e. taking time out from exercising will make it harder to regain their former fitness—a concept that also applies to eating control.

Common behaviours that increase the risk of weight regain are the following:

- Eating foods rich in fats and calories in general or eating more in stressful periods
- Doing less exercise in general or in winter (e.g. less than 2600 kcal/week)
- Overeating during the holidays
- Overeating when eating out or in social occasions

Each of these problematic behaviours should be addressed by means of the pro-active problem-solving strategies described in Module 4.

Finally, there are several problematic thoughts that may promote the abandonment of controlled eating and physical activity habits and lead to weight regain, but the two most common are the following:

1. *Dysfunctional reactions to weight regain.* Examples include giving up weekly weighing ("ostrich" dysfunctional thinking), hoping that the problem will resolve itself ("vain hope" dysfunctional thinking) and abandoning any further attempts to control weight ("all or nothing" thinking).
2. *False confidence.* Example: "I can eat what I want without gaining weight". This attitude tends to develop when a person has not observed a weight regain after a short period of laxity. Unfortunately, it is axiomatic that maintaining a positive energy balance for prolonged period of time will inevitably lead to weight gain.

To address problematic thoughts and attitudes, the therapist should encourage patients to apply the procedures described in Sect. 7.4.4 (i.e. decentring and doing the opposite).

9.2.6 Preventing a Lapse Becoming a Relapse

At this stage, it is also important to emphasise to patients that their attitude to any setback is crucial in determining what happens next. Specifically, they are encouraged not to view any setback as a "relapse"—a passive, hopeless attitude highly likely to result in their regaining all the weight lost [13]. Rather they should identify any setback as a temporary "lapse", a strategy that should make them more likely to successfully address the problem. In particular, the therapist should discuss with the patient the following concepts:

1. The need to have realistic expectations regarding eating, because it is almost impossible to eat healthily at all times
2. The importance of recognising high-risk situations immediately and applying appropriate responses in order to pre-empt a lapse (e.g. planning in advance, eating consciously, things to say and do, proactive problem-solving and decentring from problematic thoughts)
3. The importance of reacting constructively when a lapse occurs and to get immediately back on track to prevent a lapse becoming a relapse
4. The importance of analysing and addressing the underlying reason(s) for the lapse using the proactive problem-solving procedure

9.2.7 Addressing Weight Regain

Weight maintenance requires balancing the caloric intake with the energy expenditure. Although the role of physical exercise in weight maintenance should not be underestimated, controlling energy intake is the most important aspect of maintaining this balance (see Sect. 9.2.3). Nevertheless, weight regain is commonly due to changes in energy intake or energy expenditure or both. The therapist should therefore tell patients that if weight regain occurs, they should immediately implement an action plan involving the following steps [2]:

1. Identify the type of weight variation: is it a "blip" or a trend (see Fig. 9.2)?
2. Identify the reason for the weight regain (in terms of energy balance): is it due to an increase in energy intake (more common), a decrease in energy expenditure or both?
3. Identify the underlying causes: is it due to poor management of a high-risk phase (e.g. holidays, work stress, disease), the adoption of dysfunctional behaviours (e.g. eating junk food, eating too much on social occasions, grazing, binge eating, drinking too much alcohol, etc.) or the effect of problematic thoughts (e.g. a dysfunctional reaction to weight regain or false confidence)?
4. Design and implement a contingency plan to address weight regain, based on the reason it occurred. Reducing energy intake and/or increase energy expenditure to create a negative energy balance of between 500 and 1000 kcal/day until the weight returns to the weight-maintenance range. Once that occurs, readjust the energy input and/or energy expenditure to the prior weight-maintenance levels.
5. Design and implement a plan to address the underlying causes. Use the proactive problem-solving procedure (in Module 4, see Chap. 7).

The therapist should also suggest that the patient use proactive problem-solving in the event of these three possible scenarios [2]:

1. An increase in body weight (e.g. upon return from holidays, during the pregnancy or after a period of inactivity due to illness)
2. A situation that might increase the risk of weight regain (e.g. stopping smoking, retiring from work, changing jobs, experiencing a family crisis, becoming unemployed, spending a period of time at the hospital, starting the menopause)
3. A situation where it is not possible to do the weekly weighing (e.g. because the scales are broken or being in a place for a long time where there aren't any)

Patients are encouraged to explore these potential scenarios and find effective solutions for them in advance. As these sections show, the style of the therapist–patient interaction begins to change during these sessions, on the one hand, becoming more and more oriented toward the future and, on the other, stimulating the patients to solve their problems independently.

Vignette

The patient, a 35-year-old divorced office worker, achieved a weight loss of 20 kg in CBT-OB Phase 1 and began Phase 2 without reluctance because she was very satisfied with both the weight loss achieved and the improvement in her control over eating and physical fitness. During the weight-maintenance phase, however, she experienced several recurrent episodes of weight regain, as she tended to eat large amounts of chocolate and sweets in the first half of her menstrual cycle. However, by implementing her personal action plan, she was always able to lose the weight that she had gained and to return to within the weight-maintenance range. Using proactive problem-solving, she discovered that by avoiding scheduling any stressful obligations, not drinking alcohol and planning meals and snacks high in unrefined complex carbohydrates in advance, she was able to reduce and deal with the craving for chocolate and sweets she habitually experienced before her period.

9.3 Discontinuing Real-Time Monitoring of Food Intake

Towards the end of treatment, the patient is asked to discontinue the use of Monitoring Records, because it would not be realistic to expect to continue food monitoring for the rest of their life. It is better to stop real-time self-monitoring during treatment rather than doing so suddenly when the programme is over, as this would likely increase the risk of relapse [2]. As always, suspension of self-monitoring should be controlled and approached in three steps:

1. The patient should stop counting calories but continue to write what they eat.
2. The therapist and patient should review the impact of this change on eating control and weight—if the patient has not experienced rapid weight gain or overeating, they are ready to stop real-time self-monitoring.
3. The therapist and patient should then review the impact of not monitoring on eating control and weight.

Even though the Monitoring Records will no longer be used, the therapist should suggest that the patient continues to mentally plan where, what and where to eat in advance and use the device that they have been using to count their daily steps. If a patient is very reluctant to suspend the use of their Monitoring Records, the therapist should ask them to do so as an experiment and remind them that this procedure is always available to them for use in case of necessity. Although they should be encouraged to suspend real-time self-monitoring, refusing to do so is not a barrier to successful weight maintenance. Indeed, some of our patients continue self-monitoring for several years, because this procedure helps them to maintain the weight lost. One of these, when asked why they continued to use self-monitoring 2 years into the programme replied: "You see, I know many people had to have bariatric surgery to lose a large amount of weight. I achieved and maintained a similar amount of weight loss using real-time monitoring of eating—a procedure that has no side effects and enables me to eat in a flexible way and stay in control".

9.4 Evaluating Possible Future Weight-Loss Attempts

In patients who still wish to lose more weight in the future, the therapist should suggest that they think very carefully about their reasons for and the potential risks of doing so. For example, will further weight loss really provide the desired result? What are the chances that attempting to stick to a very-low-energy diet will increase the risk of binge eating and/or disruption of the habits necessary for healthy weight maintenance? Even if they are determined to persist in a further weight loss attempt, they are encouraged to wait for an appropriate period of time (i.e. 48 weeks), which will give them the opportunity to learn and practise weight-maintenance skills, as these will eventually be necessary for long-term success.

9.5 Preparing a Weight-Maintenance Plan

The last procedure provided by the programme is to help patients plan effectively for weight maintenance. Their individual "weight-maintenance plan" should be collaboratively agreed upon and written down. The therapist should inform patients about the value of this plan, pointing out that it provides them both with a useful reminder of what has been learned during Module 6 and a handy guide to what to do in the future. Compiling a draft weight-maintenance plan should be set as homework, and to this end, the patient should be provided with a handout that includes the following sections:

1. The weight-maintenance range
2. Reasons to maintain the weight lost
3. Procedures for maintaining the weight lost
4. Procedures for preventing weight regain

Table 9.3 An example weight-maintenance plan

Weight-maintenance plan
1. My weight-maintenance range:
87–91 kg
2. Reasons I want to maintain weight: *(a) I have more confidence in myself at this weight* *(b) My health is good at this weight* *(c) I can wear some clothes that I like* *(d) I feel more comfortable with others at this weight* *(e) I like the healthy lifestyle I am adopting to maintain the weight* *(f) If I will regain weight, I will harm my health and my psychological wellbeing*
3. Procedures for maintaining weight:
(a) Weekly weighing:
• *I will check my weight every Monday morning (my official weighing day)* • *I will plot my weight on the weight-maintenance graph* • *I will interpret any change in weight by looking at the last 4 weeks (never a single reading)*
(b) Eating habits:
• *I will regularly eat three meals and two snacks* • *I will not eat between meals and snacks* • *I will accurately plan the food to buy so I can easily stick to my healthy eating plan* • *I will follow a healthy Mediterranean diet* • *I will limit animal fats (cheese, biscuits, cakes, pastries, pies, burgers, fried foods, crisps)* • *I will cook meat and fish without adding fat* • *I will use olive oil for seasoning* • *I will eat vegetable and fruits at all main meals* • *I will choose whole-grain bread, pasta and rice* • *I will limit red meat, and I will mainly choose fish, white meat, eggs and pulses as protein sources* • *I will avoid sugar and sugary drinks* • *I will limit my use of salt* • *I will drink at least 1.5 L of water every day* • *I will follow my meal plan in a flexible way, periodically introducing some of my favourite foods*
(c) Exercising habits:
• *I will try to walk at least 10,000 steps every day* • *I will do calisthenics exercises twice a week*
(d) Weight-maintenance mindset:
• *I will read my weight-maintenance plan every week* • *I will mentally plan when, where and what to eat every day* • *I will address the impulse to eat non-planned foods using the "things to say and do" procedure* • *I will use proactive problem-solving to address phases, events (e.g. holidays, social occasions, stressful periods, illness, etc.) and changes in mood that might negatively influence my eating behaviour* • *I will decentre immediately from thoughts that may negatively influence my eating behaviour* • *I will reward myself with cognitive credits (e.g. "I've been good", "I'm doing great") every week if I achieve my goal of keeping my weight within the weight-maintenance range* • *I will not view setbacks as a relapse, but as a lapse from which I can learn to improve my eating control. I will not think the worst, and I will remain in control, analysing the reasons for the lapse and using proactive problem-solving to get myself immediately back on track*

(continued)

Table 9.3 (continued)

4. Procedures for preventing weight regain:	
(a)	*To identify any early signs of weight regain, I will ask myself:*
	• *Are my old eating and physical activity habits creeping back in?* • *Is my weight outside the weight-maintenance range?* • *Does my weight-maintenance graph show a weight regain trend?*
(b)	*To identify explanations for any weight regain (in terms of energy balance):*
	• *I will look at any changes in my eating and exercising habits in recent weeks*
(c)	*To identify the underlying causes of weight regain:*
	• *I will look at any events, thoughts or emotions that may have negatively influenced my eating and exercising habits*
(d)	*To address weight regain*
	• *I will restart real-time self-monitoring* • *I will follow a 1500 kcal meal plan until my weight returns to the weight-maintenance range. I will then adjust my meal plan with the aim of maintaining weight*
(e)	*To address the underlying causes:*
	• *I will use proactive problem-solving to address the underlying causes*

The therapist should suggest that the patient review all of the CBT-OB procedures they have practised and to include those that they found useful for maintaining weight and preventing relapse. They are also encouraged to think whether some procedures that they have not yet implemented may be useful in the future.

In the following session, the therapist should review the draft collaboratively with the patient, point by point, and help them to prepare a detailed weight-maintenance plan (see an example in Table 9.3). This can be given or sent to them, and the patient should be asked to consult it periodically to ensure that they maintain focus on the procedures required to maintain weight and prevent relapse.

9.6 Bringing the Treatment to a Close

Towards the end of the Phase 2, patients are explicitly instructed in self-efficacy. They are reassured that they now have all the tools they will need to be able to maintain their lower weight by themselves and told that it is time to apply the procedures learned throughout treatment without the therapist's supervision.

The therapists should do their best to ensure that the treatment ends well, and should congratulate the patient for the results achieved, attributing their success to their own efforts and ability. Then the patient should be asked how they feel about the fact that the treatment is at an end and encouraged to continue to apply the following key procedures:

- Periodically reviewing their weight-maintenance plan
- Weekly weighing and analytical interpretation of any change
- Maintaining the eating and physical activity habits required to control weight
- Keeping the weight-maintenance mindset active at all times

Finally, patients are invited to attend post-treatment review sessions at 3-month intervals after the end of treatment for at least 1 year. These sessions will be focused on discussing their progress, and any obstacles that they have met while attempting to maintain weight, adjusting their weight-maintenance plan as appropriate.

References

1. Calugi S, Marchesini G, El Ghoch M, Gavasso I, Dalle Grave R. The influence of weight-loss expectations on weight loss and of weight-loss satisfaction on weight maintenance in severe obesity. J Acad Nutr Diet. 2017;117(1):32–8. https://doi.org/10.1016/j.jand.2016.09.001.
2. Cooper Z, Fairburn CG, Hawker DM. Cognitive-behavioral treatment of obesity: a clinician's guide. New York: Guilford Press; 2003.
3. Klem ML, Wing RR, McGuire MT, Seagle HM, Hill JO. A descriptive study of individuals successful at long-term maintenance of substantial weight loss. Am J Clin Nutr. 1997;66(2):239–46.
4. Keesey RE, Hirvonen MD. Body weight set-points: determination and adjustment. J Nutr. 1997;127(9):1875s–83s.
5. Dalle Grave R, Melchionda N, Calugi S, Centis E, Tufano A, Fatati G, et al. Continuous care in the treatment of obesity: an observational multicentre study. J Intern Med. 2005;258(3):265–73. https://doi.org/10.1111/j.1365-2796.2005.01524.x.
6. Calugi S, Marchesini G, El Ghoch M, Gavasso I, Dalle Grave R. The association between weight maintenance and session-by-session diet adherence, weight loss and weight-loss satisfaction. Eat Weight Disord. 2018. https://doi.org/10.1007/s40519-018-0528-8.
7. Pacanowski CR, Linde JA, Neumark-Sztainer D. Self-weighing: helpful or harmful for psychological well-being? A review of the literature. Curr Obes Rep. 2015;4(1):65–72. https://doi.org/10.1007/s13679-015-0142-2.
8. McGuire MT, Wing RR, Klem ML, Hill JO. Behavioral strategies of individuals who have maintained long-term weight losses. Obes Res. 1999;7(4):334–41.
9. Larsen TM, Dalskov SM, van Baak M, Jebb SA, Papadaki A, Pfeiffer AF, et al. Diets with high or low protein content and glycemic index for weight-loss maintenance. N Engl J Med. 2010;363(22):2102–13. https://doi.org/10.1056/NEJMoa1007137.
10. Pronk NP, Wing RR. Physical activity and long-term maintenance of weight loss. Obes Res. 1994;2(6):587–99.
11. Jakicic JM, Winters C, Lang W, Wing RR. Effects of intermittent exercise and use of home exercise equipment on adherence, weight loss, and fitness in overweight women: a randomized trial. JAMA. 1999;282(16):1554–60.
12. Catenacci VA, Ogden LG, Stuht J, Phelan S, Wing RR, Hill JO, et al. Physical activity patterns in the National Weight Control Registry. Obesity (Silver Spring). 2008;16(1):153–61. https://doi.org/10.1038/oby.2007.6.
13. Marlatt GA, George WH. Relapse prevention: introduction and overview of the model. Br J Addict. 1984;79(3):261–73.

Involving Significant Others

10

Optimal management of obesity requires long-term maintenance of lifestyle modification, which is more difficult to sustain if a person does not receive adequate support [1–3]. Nonetheless, many treatments for obesity fail to establish a supportive social and interpersonal context that could help to reinforce and maintain behaviours conducive to weight loss [4]. Support occurs most readily in a social environment that facilitates healthy eating and health-promoting exercise, and family is the social context most likely to influence healthy behavioural changes of patients with obesity. Fortunately, dietary and exercise behaviours are well suited for family interventions, because meals and recreational activities often involve other members of the family.

Several studies have identified spousal support as an important factor influencing weight reduction among women with type 2 diabetes and obesity [5]. Moreover, familial support has been reported as being effective at producing health-promoting behaviours among patients with cardiovascular disease [6] and in chronically ill family members' adherence to physical activity guidelines and better dietary behaviours [7]. Indeed, family support has been shown to correlate positively with physical activity levels [8].

10.1 Involving Family Members in the Sessions

Although CBT-OB does not necessarily rely on the involvement of others, it is our practice to involve family members (e.g., spouse, partner, parents) that live in the same house as the patient if this is likely to facilitate treatment. We do this with the aim of creating the optimum environment for facilitating change. As mentioned above, there are two specific indications for involving significant others:

1. If they could help the patient to make positive changes
2. If they are currently making it difficult for the patients to change—for example, by commenting adversely on their body weight and/or eating habits

R. Dalle Grave et al., *Treating Obesity with Personalized Cognitive Behavioral Therapy*, https://doi.org/10.1007/978-3-319-91497-8_10

Typically, joint meetings with significant others are held as part of Module 4 and take place immediately after a routine individual session. In general, we plan three or four such sessions, each lasting about 30 min, in about half of our patients.

If patients agree to involve their significant other(s), it is important that the joint sessions are prepared thoroughly in advance. The therapist should outline the aims and content of these sessions to the patient, explaining that they will be focused on discussing how the significant other(s) can create a home environment that will facilitate their attempt to lose weight. It is important to stress that no topics outside the focus of CBT-OB will be addressed.

Generally, the first joint session begins with an introduction by the therapist and a statement about the aims of the meeting. The patient is then invited to explain the nature of treatment, all the positive changes in eating and physical activity they have achieved so far, and the obstacles that they are seeking to overcome.

The next step is for both patient and therapist to listen to the points of view expressed by the significant other(s), providing answers to any questions they may have. Generally speaking, the most common question is about the attitude to adopt towards the patient who is trying to lose weight. In particular, significant others usually ask whether it is helpful for them to comment upon or check the food that the patient is eating and how they could encourage them to follow the diet and physical activity plan. All questions raised should be addressed in the same session, with the therapist encouraging the patient to state how they would prefer to receive help from their significant other(s). Indeed, while some patients prefer to receive support and advice about what food to eat and encouragement for exercising, others tend to perceive comments about eating and physical activity as criticism and would therefore prefer that their significant other(s) refrain from making such comments.

Based on this information, the subsequent part of the joint session should be dedicated to discussing how significant others could be of practical aid to the patient. In general, the support that patients may like to receive from significant others can be divided into three main categories:

1. *Dealing with a crisis*. Significant others may be asked to intervene when the patient displays some change in mood that could influence their adherence to the eating and exercise plan.
2. *Creating an environment that promotes positive changes in eating and physical activity habits*. Significant others may be recruited to help plan meals and do the grocery shopping, as well as reduce the availability of high palatable and ready-to-eat foods. They may be involved in helping the patient change the way they cook and limiting the use of condiments and/or reinforcing positive behaviours, adopting a positive attitude and accepting any setbacks that the patient may experience.
3. *Helping to apply the programme procedures*. Significant others may contribute by doing physical activities and/or meal planning and counting calories together with the patient.

Some family members are very critical towards patients with obesity and their eating and physical activity habits. In these cases, it is important to address their criticism, as it may create negative emotions and reactions in the patient and, paradoxically, promote the opposite behaviours (e.g., overeating) to those expected. In most cases, criticism is based on a lack of knowledge regarding the causes of obesity—a condition that people often deem to be the person's own fault, due to their lack of willpower, gluttony and laziness [9]. If they are to help the patient control their weight, therefore, significant others should be educated about obesity and how it is treated. In particular, the therapist should inform them that obesity is, in fact, the result of a complex interaction of genetic and environmental factors [10]; it is a chronic condition requiring lasting lifestyle modification [11], and dysfunctional eating and exercising habits are maintained by several biological, environmental, cognitive, emotive and behavioural mechanisms—not by a simple lack of willpower. To better explain this concept, the therapist should show to the significant others the patient's Personal Formulation and inform them that the obstacles to weight loss will be addressed by the treatment through specific procedures. The aim is to engage the significant others in providing active support and help to the patients, avoiding any form of criticism, because this will reduce the chances of success rather than promoting it.

10.1.1 Addressing a Patient's Resistance to the Involvement of Significant Others

It is not uncommon for patients to resist the idea of involving significant others in the sessions, even if the therapist feels that this is indicated. This is often because they are sceptical of their significant others' ability and/or willingness to change their attitudes and behaviours. This happens frequently when family members are critical and hostile towards the treatment, which they see as another failed attempt to lose weight in the making. Some comments by significant others that our patients have reported are of the type: "Why do you bother? It's just a waste of time", "We already know how this will end up…", and "Your willpower is the only thing necessary to eat less and lose weight; why do you need specialist treatment?" In such cases, we discuss with the patient whether this attitude from a significant other may be an obstacle to weight loss. They usually agree that this is the case, and we therefore reiterate the importance of involving them in therapy.

We explain that "losing weight is only a matter of willpower" is a message continuously reinforced by the mass media, even though it is categorically untrue. However, it is common that even patients have the same attitude until they receive scientific information about the real nature of obesity and the obstacles to weight loss. We tell patients that family members, for example, often feel impotent and do not know how to help, and this can lead them to react with anger and detachment to every new weight-loss attempt. We discuss with the patient that in most cases it is useful to explain to their significant others that dysfunctional eating and physical activity habits are not the result of a lack of willpower, but rather several mechanisms that can be addressed successfully via CBT-OB. Moreover, if they consent to the involvement of significant other(s), they will be helped to understand the importance of their role in the treatment outcome, and how they can be of use, which will likely improve both their attitude and the treatment outcomes.

If, despite this discussion, the patient decides not to involve significant other(s), or if the significant other(s) are not willing or able to participate in the therapy, it is important to point out that CBT-OB is in any case an individual treatment and that the patient, with the help of the therapist, will learn several strategies and procedures for addressing the main obstacles to weight loss, including those created by significant others.

10.2 Social Support

Family involvement is not the only form of assistance that the patient can receive from others. Another form is the social support from other people that are not involved in the CBT-OB sessions. The importance of social support in the treatment of obesity has been demonstrated by several studies which show that it is a major determinant of success in weight loss and maintenance [12, 13]. In general, the need for outside help varies from person to person, but social support from friends or other family members can be solicited in several situations. Permanent help may be necessary to change the domestic environment with a view to reducing exposure to eating or sedentary stimuli, for example. Friends and colleagues may also be recruited to help in social occasions in which there will be opportunities to eat, e.g., dinner parties, days out, holidays, etc. A wider support network may also be useful to the patient in the event of crises, for example, when the patient feels at risk of losing control over eating.

10.2.1 Identifying Potential Helpers

If patients agree that it would be helpful for them to receive social support, they should be educated on identifying people who might be of assistance. Ideal characteristics of potential helpers are willingness, availability, and a positive and empathic attitude towards those who suffer from obesity. However, people who have no understanding of obesity and say things like "People with obesity lack control and self-discipline!" should not be involved as potential helpers. It is also not advisable to involve those who, unwittingly or not, sabotage the patient's weight-loss attempt by making comments such as "Dieting makes you sad, why do you bother?" "I've spent all morning cooking this for you, please do not refuse to eat all the food I prepared!", "Oh go on, have a day off!", "Just one won't hurt!", and "Today, I don't want to hear the word diet, didn't we all get together to have fun?"

10.2.2 How, What and When to Ask People Who Can Help

The patient should be educated that the second step in recruiting social support is to ask the helpers they have identified for assistance. To this end the following strategies can be suggested to the patient:

- *Asking for help openly, without fear.* Usually, the best strategy is to take a potential helper aside and explain the problem calmly. If the patient is shy, or fearful of the other person's reaction, they should be asked to think how they would feel if a friend asked them for help. In most cases patients respond that they would be honoured by such a request, which helps them to overcome their timidity.
- *Describing their problems without fear.* The patients should explain to the person the nature of the programme they are following, what their difficulties are, and what type of help they would like to receive.
- *Making specific requests.* Patients should be informed that they may not get the support they need if they do not make specific requests. "Could you help me to stick to my diet?" for example, is too generic, while "Can we take a walk together sometimes?"; "When we have dinner together, do you mind if we go to a restaurant where I can have a low-calorie option?"; and "When we go to lunch with other friends, can you stand up for me if anyone suggests that I should eat everything on my plate?" make it clear precisely what kind of assistance would be appreciated.
- *Using assertive communication.* For example, a patient complained because her partner regularly eats crisps in front of the television; this makes her angry because it threatens to undermine her self-control. Reacting aggressively by saying "Don't do that!" will be unlikely to produce change, but a more assertive statement such as "It would be very helpful for me if you would not eat crisps in front of the television; you know that for me that it takes a great deal of effort not to join you" is more likely to provoke a positive response.
- *Thanking for the help received.* The therapist should also tell the patient that the help of family or friends can only be extended over time if it is reinforced by continually rewarding their efforts. For example, a patient, after having received help from a friend during a party, could say to her: "Thank you so much for the support you gave me by not offering me pastries"; or, in a moment of crisis, a patient comforted by her husband could reinforce his commitment saying: "Thanks for listening to me when I was in crisis; you've been very helpful." Patients are also advised to give a small gift or send a thank-you card to the people who are supporting their weight-loss attempt.

References

1. Kelsey K, Earp JAL, Kirkley BG. Is social support beneficial for dietary change? A review of the literature. Fam Community Health. 1997;20(3):70–82.
2. Okun MA, Ruehlman L, Karoly P, Lutz R, Fairholme C, Schaub R. Social support and social norms: do both contribute to predicting leisure-time exercise? Am J Health Behav. 2003;27(5):493–507.

3. Wing RR, Jeffery RW. Benefits of recruiting participants with friends and increasing social support for weight loss and maintenance. J Consult Clin Psychol. 1999;67(1):132–8.
4. Soubhi H, Potvin L, Paradis G. Family process and parent's leisure time physical activity. Am J Health Behav. 2004;28(3):218–30.
5. van Dam HA, van der Horst FG, Knoops L, Ryckman RM, Crebolder HF, van den Borne BH. Social support in diabetes: a systematic review of controlled intervention studies. Patient Educ Couns. 2005;59(1):1–12. https://doi.org/10.1016/j.pec.2004.11.001.
6. Heitman LK. The influence of social support on cardiovascular health in families. Fam Community Health. 2006;29(2):131–42.
7. Bull S, Eakin E, Reeves M, Kimberly R. Multi-level support for physical activity and healthy eating. J Adv Nurs. 2006;54(5):585–93. https://doi.org/10.1111/j.1365-2648.2006.03861.x.
8. Eyler AE, Wilcox S, Matson-Koffman D, Evenson KR, Sanderson B, Thompson J, et al. Correlates of physical activity among women from diverse racial/ethnic groups. J Womens Health Gend Based Med. 2002;11(3):239–53. https://doi.org/10.1089/152460902753668448.
9. Phul RM. Stigma, discrimination, and obesity. In: Brownell KD, Walsh BT, editors. Eating disorders and obesity: a comprehensive handbook. New York: Guilford Press; 2017. p. 134–9.
10. Reddon H, Gueant JL, Meyre D. The importance of gene-environment interactions in human obesity. Clin Sci (Lond). 2016;130(18):1571–97. https://doi.org/10.1042/cs20160221.
11. Rippe JM, Crossley S, Ringer R. Obesity as a chronic disease: modern medical and lifestyle management. J Am Diet Assoc. 1998;98(10 Suppl 2):S9–15.
12. Wadden TA, West DS, Delahanty L, Jakicic J, Rejeski J, Williamson D, et al. The Look AHEAD study: a description of the lifestyle intervention and the evidence supporting it. Obesity (Silver Spring). 2006;14(5):737–52. https://doi.org/10.1038/oby.2006.84.
13. Perri MG, Limacher MC, Durning PE, Janicke DM, Lutes LD, Bobroff LB, et al. Extended-care programs for weight management in rural communities: the treatment of obesity in underserved rural settings (TOURS) randomized trial. Arch Intern Med. 2008;168(21):2347–54. https://doi.org/10.1001/archinte.168.21.2347.

Adapting CBT-OB for Groups

11

Naturally, in this era of striving towards personalised medicine, it is preferable that patients are treated one-on-one. However, realistically speaking, this is not always feasible, as the high costs of individual treatment may outweigh the financial possibilities of the patient and/or the healthcare provider. It is also important to note that the number of patients with obesity is increasing year on year, and in some areas the demand for treatment significantly outstrips the supply of adequately trained therapists. With this in mind, we have adapted CBT-OB for group delivery, as described below.

11.1 Advantages and Disadvantages of Group CBT-OB

Little data is available to compare the effect on weight loss of group BT-OB versus individual BT-OB, and what information is available is contradictory. One 6 month randomised controlled trial found that group treatment performed better than individual counselling in terms of weight loss, regardless of the individual's preferred method of treatment [1], but another study found no difference between the two ways of delivering the treatment at 12- and 36-month follow-ups [2].

However, the CBT-OB approach for groups presents some advantages with respect to that administered to individual. In particular, treating groups costs less, which lessens the burden on the public healthcare setting and/or makes the treatment accessible to a greater number of people in a private setting. Furthermore, those treated as part of a group may receive social support, as well as a potentially healthy dose of competition [3], which may potentiate the effects of the intervention on weight loss. Moreover, according to the social learning theory, patients can learn from one another via observation, imitation and modelling [4]. In our clinical experience, group treatment can also favour the development of a "group mindset" in participants; they report that members of the group stimulate each other to adopt the mindset and the strategies used by the other group members to address problematic situations outside the group sessions.

R. Dalle Grave et al., *Treating Obesity with Personalized Cognitive Behavioral Therapy*, https://doi.org/10.1007/978-3-319-91497-8_11

Vignette

A group CBT-OB participant, reviewing the strategies she had been using to address some weight-loss obstacles, reported the following experience: "I am handling high-risk situations pretty well because outside the group sessions I often think about Luigi, who parks his car a bit farther away from his workplace in order to have a walk, and also Marco, who on vacation decided to book a hotel in the hills to practice Nordic Walking. I also imagine Elisabeth, who at work dinners sits close to the colleague that eats healthily. These thoughts help me to stay in control and keep my focus on applying the programme's strategies."

Although it undoubtedly brings certain benefits, group treatment also has some potential disadvantages. Besides fewer opportunities to personalise the intervention, there is the risk that some participants can negatively influence the motivation and adherence of other members. For example, the early interruption of the treatment by one participant may be contagious, prompting others to make the same decision. Likewise, a critical or sceptical attitude towards the treatment of a subset of group members may discourage other members from actively working to achieve change.

Another disadvantage of group therapy with respect to individual treatment is the difficulty in addressing some individual problems that may interfere with the treatment, such as marked interpersonal difficulties, mood intolerance, severe low self-esteem or other important psychological problems. Indeed, the patients usually do not feel ready to discuss these private issues in a group, and such problems require a more targeted therapy than group CBT-OB can offer.

Finally, as group CBT-OB is delivered in closed groups, another potential disadvantage is the waiting list, whose duration varies on the basis of the time required to recruit eight to ten participants. It is our experience that a waiting list longer than 3 months is associated with a higher dropout rate in the first part of the treatment, presumably because the patients have lost the motivation necessary to change that they may have had when they attended their first consultation.

11.2 Preparing Patients for Group CBT-OB

If, at the end of the assessment session (see Sect. 3.6), the therapist decides, in agreement with the patient, the option of group treatment, they should participate in two individual sessions with the aim of assessing more in depth if group CBT-OB is suitable for them.

The first part of these preparatory sessions is dedicated to explaining to the patient the organisation, content and rules of group CBT-OB. In particular patients are informed on the following group rules:

- Being punctual. It is important that every group session begins and ends on time. It is also a good idea to get to the session a little early (about 10–15 min

before) in order to acclimatise, relax and prepare the things to be discussed by the group.
- Adopting an active role in the group and considering the treatment a priority.
- Working collaboratively with the therapists and the other group members. In group CBT-OB, the patients and therapists work together as a team to address the obstacles to weight loss and weight maintenance. Together, they agree on specific homework that patients should make the commitment to do between one session and another. These tasks are of paramount importance and should be given absolute priority; it is what patients do between sessions that will determine the success of treatment.
- Assuming the responsibility of not negatively affecting other participants with your behaviour, attitudes and adherence to treatment. In group CBT-OB, patients interact with each other, and this can have positive or negative effects. One of the main tasks of the therapists is to create a positive atmosphere in which patients help each other to address the obstacles to weight loss and weight maintenance. However, it is common that some patients, even involuntarily, may have a negative influence on other patients. Examples of behaviours that tend to adversely affect other participants are as follows: criticising the treatment and therapists, stating that no one will lose weight, not applying the treatment procedures consistently, introducing drugs and alcohol into the group and not maintaining confidentiality outside the group. Constructive criticisms of the treatment are welcome, but they must be conveyed to therapists in private, not in front of other group members.

At the end of the first preparatory session, the therapist asks the patient to fill in a Monitoring Record every day for 7 days. They will not be admitted to the group if they cannot adhere to this procedure, recording all the food eaten each day (without counting calories).

In the second preparatory session, the therapist will review with the patient the number of Monitoring Records they have completed and assess whether they are comfortable with the content, rules and engagement required to participate in the group treatment. If the patient has filled in the Monitoring Record consistently and agrees with the group CBT-OB requirements, they should be put on the waiting list and included in a group as soon as possible.

Our clinical experience suggests that the two preparatory sessions before the group are very effective in reducing dropout and preventing some of the problems described above, such as a critical attitude towards the treatment.

11.3 General Organisation of Group CBT-OB

Like the individual version of the treatment, group CBT-OB lasts 18 months and is structured in two main phases:

- *Phase 1 (weight loss).* This phase is delivered in 16 sessions across 24 weeks, held once a week in the first 8 weeks, and then every 2 weeks.

- *Phase 2 (weight maintenance).* This phase is delivered in 12 sessions across 48 weeks, held every 4 weeks.

The groups are closed and made up of eight to ten participants aged between 20 and 65 years with a BMI ≥30.0. Before each group session, the patients meet with their therapist for few minutes to be weighed and plot their weight graph (see Sect. 4.4). Patients are required not to disclose their weight to other group members. Each session lasts 90 min and is delivered by two therapists (i.e., one clinical psychologist and one dietician), who, in the event of absence, are substituted by another CBT-OB therapist.

To maintain a personalised approach, the group sessions adopt a format similar to that used in CBT-OB for individuals and cover the same material. The session begins by reviewing one Monitoring Record and other homework that participants have chosen to discuss. It then continues by collaboratively setting the agenda, working through the agenda and agreeing on homework tasks. Finally, the session is concluded by summarising what was addressed in the session, repeating the homework assignments and arranging the next appointment.

Except for the first two sessions, in which the therapist describes the use of self-monitoring in real time (see Sect. 4.3), the change in eating (see Sect. 5.3) and strategies for developing an active lifestyle (see Sect. 6.2.1), sessions are dedicated to discussing how to address the weight-loss obstacles that each participant has identified in their Weight-Loss Obstacles Questionnaire (see Appendix D). The therapists write every obstacle identified on a general formulation of weight-loss obstacles on a black- or whiteboard and then invite each participant to include their individual obstacles on their own Personal Formulation (see Sect. 7.3). They should then be asked to consider which strategies and procedure to use to address each obstacle. Homework assignments are collaboratively agreed upon, just as in individual treatment. In addition, the therapists encourage patients to share common experiences, provide support for each other and collectively problem-solve obstacles that they encounter. However, it is advisable that this support occur only during the group sessions, as patients are asked not to contact each other outside the group. A lack of contact between sessions will prevent schisms and potentially unhelpful conversations.

Vignette

During a review of the group's weight-loss obstacles, one patient reported having encountered the following unexpected difficulty. Like every year, the patient had been asked to help install stands for the village fête with some friends. He reported that, buoyed up by the enjoyable atmosphere, he had drunk five beers during the various breaks in proceedings. The patient was disappointed in the way he had handled the situation, especially because he had drunk more than he had planned. At this point the therapist asked the patient why he had been unable to do what he wanted in this situation. The patient responded by saying that if he had continued to work, refusing to take a break and drink with his workmates, he would have appeared to be unsociable. Then the therapist asked whether, put in a similar situation, it would be possible for him to take a break with the others but drink in more moderation, e.g., drinking only one beer on one break and water on the others. The patient commented that this would be possible, but did not resolve the problem of being seen as an unsociable person. The therapist therefore asked the other group participants what they thought about this high-risk situation. One of them said that she frequently encountered similar situations and was still conditioned by them. Another patient admitted that this was a typical difficulty that he had encountered in the past, but had since come to realise that drinking and eating together did not in themselves define the sociability of an occasion, but that the social interactions themselves were more important. The patient also added that in these situations we may needlessly worry too much about what others think of us. Another patient said that these situations can sometimes reveal the excuses that we use to justify our behaviour and give in to our wish to gratify ourselves by drinking or eating. However, the patient who reported the problem said that he did not agree that it was an excuse but rather a question of self-image—others were used to see him as a person who was "game for anything." The therapist brought the discussion to a close by asking the patient whether he would consider his groupmates' suggestions and put his hypothesis to the test in a similar situation—trying to be a sociable person while drinking less. If he agreed, he could try sipping his beer or wine without emptying the glass, so that others would be less likely to fill it up again, and see whether anyone got upset about him being "less sociable." He agreed to try out this experiment and at one of the subsequent meetings reported to the group that in another social situation, a friend of his joked about his weight loss and drinking in moderation, asking him if he was thinking of becoming a fashion model. However, this was offset by others expressing admiration for his ability to moderate his drinking, saying that it was high time that they too began to cut down on alcohol.

The above *Vignette* provides a good example of the potential benefits of group treatment and, in particular, how the experiences and way of thinking of one patient can suggest behavioural changes and promote cognitive change in another. In this context, the group effectively becomes the therapist of the individual. Indeed, the comments of the other group members and the initial patient's willingness to try the experiment provided several lessons for all participants. Firstly, food and drink are not the only components of being sociable. Secondly, it is possible to enjoy social interactions while moderating the intake of food and drink. Thirdly, it is important to pay attention to problematic thoughts that justify excessive eating and drinking, even if this did not seem to be the case in this particular patient.

The weight-maintenance phase of group CBT-OB includes Module 6 (see Chap. 9), in which patients review the changes achieved through weight loss, are educated on weight maintenance, and are involved actively in the decision to begin weight maintenance. The therapists then introduce specific procedures for weight maintenance to the group, i.e., establishing weekly self-weighing and the weight-maintenance target range, adopting eating and physical activity habits to maintain weight, constructing the weight-maintenance mindset, identifying and addressing situations that could lead to weight regain, preventing lapses from becoming relapses and addressing potential weight regain.

In the last part of the weight-maintenance phase, group participants, like individual patients, are encouraged to discontinue real-time self-monitoring of food intake and prepare a personalised weight-maintenance plan (see Sect. 9.8).

11.4 Some Considerations on Group CBT-OB

There is as yet no research upon which to base a definitive conclusion on whether this version of CBT-OB is as effective as CBT-OB delivered individually or even more so. That being said, data from a pilot study seems promising [5]. This cohort study included 67 patients with morbid obesity (BMI kg/m^2 39.84 ± 5.7; 106.76 ± 16.64 kg) treated in seven CBT-OB groups (maximum ten people per group). 76.2% of the patients were able to complete the treatment, and in these patients, there was a substantial and healthy reduction in weight (11.6% in completers and 10.4% at the intention-to-treat analysis), which was largely maintained at 18 months. The treatment was also associated with a significant improvement in cardiovascular risk factors and psychological variables.

It is clear, however, that group treatment is much more difficult to organise than CBT-OB for individuals. Indeed, many patients do not like the idea of addressing their problem with others, and it is difficult to schedule sessions without any interruptions. Mainly, however, the biggest issue is adequate personalisation of sessions. Although we have introduced the specific procedures described in Sect. 11.3 to overcome this issue, it remains problematic for some. For this reason we, on occasion, arrange extra individual sessions with some group participants to address severe interpersonal difficulties that they were experiencing but did not want to discuss in front of the group. Another problem is the heterogeneity of the problems and obstacles reported by the patients, for instance, some participants encounter problems on social occasions, while others have difficulties when they are home alone. That being said, the strong social support engendered by the group setting is helpful to many patients, and both the psychoeducational aspects of CBT-OB and the self-monitoring procedure are ideal for delivery in a group setting and are generally very well received.

References

1. Renjilian DA, Perri MG, Nezu AM, McKelvey WF, Shermer RL, Anton SD. Individual versus group therapy for obesity: effects of matching participants to their treatment preferences. J Consult Clin Psychol. 2001;69(4):717–21.
2. Cresci B, Tesi F, La Ferlita T, Ricca V, Ravaldi C, Rotella CM, et al. Group versus individual cognitive-behavioral treatment for obesity: results after 36 months. Eat Weight Disord. 2007;12(4):147–53.
3. Wadden TA, Butryn ML, Byrne KJ. Efficacy of lifestyle modification for long-term weight control. Obestet Res. 2004;12(Suppl):151s–62s. https://doi.org/10.1038/oby.2004.282.
4. Bandura A. Social learning theory. New York: General Learning Press; 1977.
5. Zini D, Bosco G, Corbelli G, Valenti C, Valerio L, Casini M, et al. Personalized group cognitive behavior therapy (CBT-OB) for morbid obesity: a longitudinal outcome study. Oral presentation at the XI Congresso Nazionale SISDCA "Ricerca, pratica clinica, relazioni internazionali: nuove frontiere nel trattamento dei disturbi dell'alimentazione e dell'obesità," March 8–10 Rome; 2018.

Adapting CBT-OB for Intensive Levels of Care

12

The mainstay of obesity management is outpatient treatment. It is less costly and disruptive than residential or day hospital treatment, and the changes made are more likely to last as patients make them while living in their usual environment. Nevertheless, some patients suffer from severe obesity associated with severe comorbidities, disability and poor quality of life and may therefore require a more intensive version of the treatment administered in specially designed rehabilitation units.

This chapter discusses the association between obesity and disability, the rationale of adopting a rehabilitative perspective for severe obesity and the indications for intensive rehabilitation treatment. It then goes on to describe the rehabilitative intensive treatment developed for patients with disabling obesity at the Department of Eating and Weight Disorders of Villa Garda Hospital (Italy), adopting the principles, strategies and main procedures of CBT-OB.

12.1 Obesity and Disability

Disability is defined as a restriction or lack of ability to perform an activity in any domain of life [1]. Obesity is a significant risk factor for disability and chronic illness, independent of age and physical activity level [2]. It has been estimated that adults with obesity aged between 30 and 49 years lived 5.70 (men) and 5.02 (women) fewer years free from limitations in daily living activities (DLAs) after the age of 50 than their normal-weight counterparts [3].

Obesity in adulthood may lead to disability through one or more of the following biological processes: skeletal stress, protein glycation in connective tissue and atherogenesis [4]. These conditions may result in motor (i.e., joint pain and osteoarthritis), metabolic and cardiorespiratory complications that lead to limitations in DLAs.

Examples of DLAs affected by obesity include walking, taking the stairs, climbing on a stool, getting up from a couch, picking up objects from the ground, putting

R. Dalle Grave et al., *Treating Obesity with Personalized Cognitive Behavioral Therapy*, https://doi.org/10.1007/978-3-319-91497-8_12

on shoes, bathing and showering, dressing, personal hygiene, work activities (due to premature fatigue), postural pain, frequent absences from work or school and inability to perform some tasks. The physical functions affected by disability associated with severe obesity predominantly involve the lower limbs (i.e., strength and maintaining balance), although the function of upper limbs (i.e., strength and manual skills) can also be compromised [4]. The impact of obesity on disability is particularly severe among the elderly (i.e., >65 years of age) because sarcopenia—the physiological decline in lean mass—interacts negatively with the effects of obesity in this age range [5].

Obesity also has negative impacts on psychological wellbeing and interpersonal relationships and is associated with an increased risk of clinical depression, anxiety, low self-esteem, negative body image, pathological eating, substance misuse and suicidal thoughts and behaviours [6]. Since some of these outcomes persist after accounting for BMI, age of obesity onset, gender and age, many negative psychological consequences seem to derive from stigmatising experiences rather than obesity per se [6].

The Italian Society of Obesity (SIO) has recently proposed and validated—in a multicentre study conducted in 16 Italian hospitals—the Obesity-Related Disability Test (Test SIO Disabilità Obesità Correlata, TSD-OC) [7]. This test comprises 36 items divided into seven sections (pain, stiffness, DLAs and indoor mobility, housework, outdoor activities, occupational activities and social life). Responses are significantly correlated with measures of functional (i.e., 6-min walk test and handgrip strength) and health-related quality of life (i.e., the 36-item Short Form Health Survey). On the Obesity-Related Disability Test, the degree of disability of the subject is evaluated by comparing the score obtained with the maximum possible score (360 pts). A person who has a global score greater than 33% of the total or a score of 8/10 on any of the individual items is considered to suffer from disabling obesity.

12.2 Rationale for Adopting a Rehabilitative Perspective

The cycle between obesity, physical and psychosocial complications, disability and weight gain represents a considerable social and economic burden on national health systems worldwide, as a rehabilitative therapeutic perspective is required for effective treatment [8]. Unfortunately, people with disabling obesity tend to have difficulties gaining admission to standard rehabilitation units, which are in most cases structurally and technologically inadequate for the treatment of pathological conditions in such patients, being designed predominantly for individuals of normal weight.

To address this issue in Italy, some rehabilitation units have been specially established to treat patients with disabling obesity, and a consensus endorsed by SIO and the Italian Society of Eating Disorders (SISDCA) has laid out the standards applicable to units for the metabolic, nutritional and psychological rehabilitation of patients with severe obesity [9]. Briefly, this report states that any such rehabilitative treatment programme should encompass nutritional intervention, functional rehabilitation, physical reconditioning, psychoeducational and psychotherapeutic interventions and rehabilitation nursing, combined in a multidimensional interdisciplinary approach [9].

12.3 Indications for Intensive Rehabilitation Treatment

Intensive residential or day hospital rehabilitation should be incorporated into the obesity care network and should be taken into consideration when [9]:

- The severity of medical and/or psychiatric comorbidities of obesity is high.
- The obesity has a strong impact on the patient's disability and quality of life.
- Numerous interventions are required to treat the patient, and it would be advisable (for both clinical and financial reasons) to administer them over a relatively short period, as part of a coordinated project (case management).
- Less intensive routes (previous outpatient and/or day hospital treatment) have not yielded the hoped-for results, and the risk to the health of the patient is increasing.

In our unit, the appropriate setting for treating patients with obesity is assessed by means of the Comprehensive Appropriateness Scale for the Care of Obesity in Rehabilitation (CASCO-R). This was developed by a panel of experts under the aegis of the SIO-SISDCA consensus [10] and is designed to be completed by a physician during the patient's initial assessment. It consists of evaluating the following four criteria, each via a dedicated section (Fig. 12.1):

1. BMI and waist circumference
2. Comorbidities associated with obesity (type 2 diabetes; dyslipidaemia; cardiovascular diseases; respiratory, gastrointestinal, skeletal and genital–urinary tract diseases; pro-inflammatory and pro-coagulative status; malnutrition)
3. Risk factors potentially increasing obesity-related morbidity (family history, age, lifestyle habits such as smoking and sedentary lifestyle, major disturbances in eating behaviour, other clinically significant psychopathological disorders)
4. Previous unsuccessful hospitalisations for nutritional–metabolic rehabilitation (this section assigns negative scores after one or more previous hospitalisations in metabolic and nutritional rehabilitation units)

A significant correlation was found between the CASCO-R scale score, overall workload and adverse clinical events. Moreover, the CASCO-R scale demonstrated excellent performance in terms of internal validity and test–retest analysis. Three global score cut-offs have been proposed: >25 for intensive residential rehabilitation, 20–25 for day hospital treatment and <20 for outpatient treatment [10].

Intensive rehabilitation treatment may be also indicated for a subgroup of patients with severe obesity and several complications scheduled for bariatric surgery. This

Patient name			Date	
			Attributable score	Obtained score
Obesity degree And related risk for cardiovascular and metabolic disorders		BMI ≤ 40 kg/m²	8	
		BMI 35-39.9 kg/m²	6	
		BMI 30-34.9 kg/m²	4	
		Waist circumference > 102 cm ♂; 88 cm ♀	2	
Comorbidity	Dyslipidemia	LDL-cholesterol ≥ 130 mg/dl or antidyslipidemic medications	4	
		HDL-cholesterol ≤ 40 mg/dl ♂; 50 mg/dl ♀	2	
		Triglyceride > 150 mg/dl or antidyslipidemic medications	1	
	Impaired glucose metabolism	IFG (fasting blood glucose 110-125 mg/dl) or hyperinsulinemia (insulin > 25 mcU/ml or > 80 mcU/ml on the 75-g OGTT between 60' and 120' or with a peak > 90') or HOMA (Glic * Ins/405) > 2.77	2	
		IGT (2 h glucose levels of 140 to 199 mg/dl on the 75-g OGTT)	4	
		T2DM (fasting plasma glucose ≥ 126 mg/dl) or 2 h glucose levels ≥ 200 mg/dl on the 75-g OGTT) or antidiabetic medications	6	
	Cardiovascular system	Hypertension (SBP > 130 mmHg or DBP > 85 mmHg or antihypertensive medications)	3	
		Atherosclerosis (ischemic cardiomyopathy, stroke, …)	4	
		NYHA: class III (marked limitation in activity due to symptoms, even during less-than-ordinary activity) or IV (severe limitations; symptoms even while at rest)	4	
		Asymptomatic left ventricular hypertrophy	3	
	Respiratory system	OSAS, restrictive respiratory failure	4	
		Dyspnea, Epworth scale > 10	2	
	Skeletal system	Osteoarthritis (hip, knees, spine)	3	
	Genitourinary system	Gynecological problems (dysmenorrhea, PCOS)	2	
		Impaired sexual function	2	
		Urinary incontinence	2	
	Gastrointestinal tract	NAFLD, biliary calculi	1	
	Proinflammatory status	C-reactive protein > 10 mg/l	3	
	Procoagulant status	Fibrinogen > 450 mg/dl	3	
Risk factors that contribute to increase the obesity-related comorbidity	Family diseases	Early cardiovascular diseases (myocardial infarction, stroke, sudden death before age 65 in ♀ relatives or before age 55 in ♂ relatives)	4	
	Age	≥ 45 years ♂; 55 years ♀ (or premature menopause without hormonal replacement treatment)	2	
	Life habits	Sedentary lifestyle (< 10 METs/week)	1	
		Smoking > 10 cigarettes/day	1	
	Behaviour	Psychic alterations (depression, anxiety)	2	
		Eating disorders: prandial hyperfagia, grazing, emotional eating, night eating	3	
		Eating disorders: bulimia nervosa, BED	4	
	Anamnesis	Failure of > 3 out-patient treatments for weight loss	2	
	Malnutrition (undernutrition)	Hb < 12 g/dl ♀, 13 g/dl ♂; albuminemia < 35 g/l; total cholesterol < 150 mg/dl (without antidyslipidemic medications); arm circumference < 22 cm; calf circumference < 31 cm	4	
Previous in-patient rehabilitation treatments		First return (weight gain > 50% of that lost during the previous admission)	-5	
		Following returns (weight gain > 50% of that lost during the previous admission)	-10	
a. > 25: in-patient rehabilitation b. 20-25: intensive out-patient rehabilitation c. < 20: out-patient treatment			**TOT**	

Fig. 12.1 CASCO-R. Comprehensive Appropriateness Scale for the Care of Obesity in Rehabilitation. From Donini LM, Dalle Grave R, Di Flaviano E, Gentile MG, Mezzani B, Pandolfo Mayme M, Brunani A, Rovera G, Santini F, Lenzi A, Cuzzolaro M (2014) Assessing the appropriateness of the level of care for morbidly obese subjects: validation of the CASCO-R scale. Ann Ig 26 (3):195–204. Reprinted with permission of Società Editrice Universo – Roma

should reduce the risks associated with the operation and/or the postsurgical period in patients who are having difficulty implementing the lifestyle modifications necessary to achieve adequate weight loss. It is also indicated in pre-surgical patients with persistent weight-related disabilities and/or the onset or recurrence of eating disorder, which may compromise the success of surgical intervention.

Vignette

The patient, a 60-year-old woman with a BMI of 52.0, had steadily gained weight from the age of 20. At the age of 55, she was given surgical knee replacement due to severe arthritis. However, this failed to resolve the knee pain and left her reliant on a walking stick to get around. She also suffered from type 2 diabetes, hypertension, obstructive sleep apnoea (being treated with C-PAP) and severe lower limb oedema. She reported not being able to climb the stairs or put on shoes and having extreme difficulties in maintaining adequate personal hygiene, dressing and doing housework. Due to fatigue and postural pain, she was forced to stop work (as a shop assistant) at the age of 55, and since then her weight had increased by 25 kg due to the progressively reduction in her mobility and worsening eating habits (characterised by frequent snacking during the day). She scored 55% on the Obesity-Related Disability Test, confirming the presence of disabling obesity, and 28 on the CASCO-R, indicating the appropriateness of residential rehabilitation.

12.4 Intensive CBT-OB-Based Rehabilitation Treatment

Rehabilitative CBT-OB has been developed at the Department of Eating and Weight Disorders of Villa Garda Hospital (Italy) and combines a rehabilitative approach with intensive CBT-OB [11].

12.4.1 The Unit

Intensive rehabilitation treatment based on CBT-OB should be provided in a specialised unit for the treatment of disabling obesity. The patients' rooms should have a private bathroom, and wardrobes, desks and beds adapted for people with severe obesity (Fig. 12.2). The unit should also include a nurses' office with a high-capacity scale with a large platform for private weighing, as well as rooms for medical offices, a dining room with a kitchen for cooking, rooms for individual and group CBT-OB sessions, a suitably equipped gym for physical activity and a room for recreational activities. The unit should be open, so that patients are exposed to the environmental eating triggers that they will encounter after discharge.

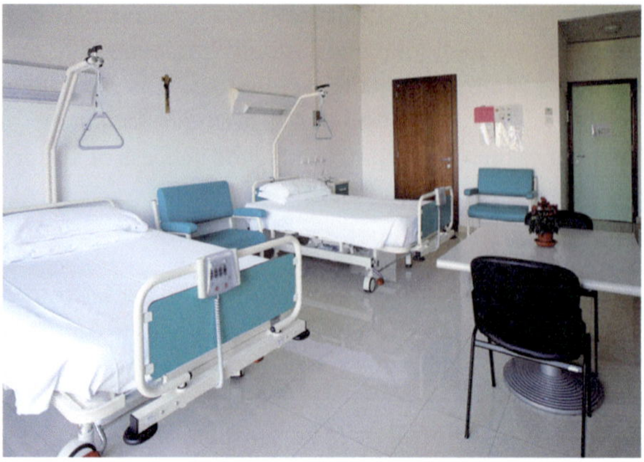

Fig. 12.2 A room with beds for patients with disabling obesity

12.4.2 The Non-eclectic Multidisciplinary Team

The organisation of intensive rehabilitative units makes a multidisciplinary team essential for treatment delivery in the vast majority of cases. However, a team approach presents both advantages and disadvantages. The main advantage is that the team includes clinicians with various areas of expertise, which may facilitate the management of complicated patients with severe comorbidities and disability—the typical subgroup of patients with obesity admitted to rehabilitation units.

The disadvantages may be divided in two main categories. First, treatment involving multiple therapists (e.g., physicians, psychiatrists, psychologists, dieticians and physiotherapists) encourages patients to partition their problems and to talk about specific topics with specific people. There is a risk, therefore, that—without proper mediation—no one therapist is party to the entire clinical picture. This is a problem that does not occur with outpatient CBT-OB, where just one therapist (or two when the treatment is delivered in a group) is responsible for each patient's care. Furthermore, in most treatments that manage disabling obesity, an "eclectic" approach is adopted, incorporating a wide variety of procedures, including rehabilitative, medical, psychiatric, psychological, nursing and social interventions based on different and often conflicting theories. For example, the physician and the psychiatrist are likely to follow a biomedical approach—prescribing drugs to treat the medical and psychiatric complications associated with obesity, respectively; the psychologist may apply some forms of generic CBT; and the dietician and the physiotherapist may give the patient advice on diet and physical activity, respectively, using a traditional prescriptive approach. In other words, each member of an eclectic treatment team adopts the theory and practice dictated by their area of expertise, pursuing therapeutic goals related to their own professional role rather than those of the team as a whole (and therefore the patient).

While each of these approaches undoubtedly has it merits, and will benefit the patient to a certain extent, their co-administration inevitably entails some significant drawbacks:

- It facilitates the delivery of contradictory information to patients about obesity and the procedures and strategies required to address it. This may create confusion in patients about which problems to address, when and how and may thereby compromise the effectiveness of the individual treatments themselves.
- Therapeutic boundaries are unclear. Therapists may, unwittingly or otherwise, cross over into the territory of another team member, generating further confusion in the patient. For example, a dietician, frustrated by the patient's difficulties adhering to their meal plan, may give patients an untrained psychological interpretation of their resistance, thereby effectively taking on the role of the psychologist.
- It increases the risk of conflicts among team members, who likely have different beliefs about the best way to treat obesity and the issues to address with patients.
- It makes it difficult to produce substantial improvements in treatment. Without a shared theory, it is almost impossible to understand which are the active and inactive elements of a treatment approach.

As the involvement of more than one therapist is inevitable in intensive rehabilitative settings, CBT-OB has been designed to ensure a unified, rather than eclectic, multidisciplinary approach. To guarantee that all members of the team are cognisant of the full clinical picture, and to prevent conflicting advice being given to patients, the following three main strategies are put into practice:

1. All therapists involved in treating patients with disabling obesity (i.e., physicians, psychiatrists, psychologists, dieticians, physiotherapists and nurses) receive extensive training in CBT-OB before joining the team. This ensures that while the therapists maintain their specific professional roles, they all share the same philosophy (cognitive behavioural theory and treatment) and therefore use a similar language with patients.
2. Therapeutic roles are well defined and coordinated within the team. Thus, the dietician is primarily concerned with addressing modification of eating habits and weight, the psychologist conducts individual and group CBT-OB sessions, the physician oversees the medical health of the patients and the prescription of any medication, the physiotherapist manages the physical activity program, and the nurse supervises the administration of medication and assists patients in weighing and managing everyday difficulties.
3. A review meeting (round table) attended by the patient and all their therapists is held on a weekly basis. At this meeting, the patient's progress is assessed, and the various elements of the treatment and their relationship to one another are discussed. This allows all team members to form a complete picture of the patient's eating problem, and gives the patient a sense of empowerment, at the same time obviating the risk of mixed messages arising.

Table 12.1 Practical advice on building a CBT-OB clinical team

1. Select, if possible, open-minded therapists who like to work in teams and follow a manual-based treatment. They should not be committed to other theories and therapeutic practices, because strong alternative influences may be dangerous, causing a therapist to deviate too far from CBT-OB guidelines
2. Train all therapists (physicians, psychologists, dieticians, physiotherapists and nurses) in CBT-OB and the team approach before they start to see patients. Neither universities nor psychotherapy schools (even CBT-based) tend to prepare therapists in either intensive CBT-OB or teamwork
3. Monitor therapist adherence and consistency by adopting the following procedures: • Providing the therapists with a written treatment protocol to implement • Planning a weekly peer-supervised meeting between therapists to discuss clinical work, freely and at length • Asking the therapists to record individual sessions and encouraging them to listen to selected recordings of each other's treatment sessions • Asking the therapists to give evidence of the topics covered in each session, which should be included in the medical records • Introducing new procedures and strategies only when mutually agreed upon • Providing the following procedures to improve the team approach: – Maintaining the highest standard of professional skill in the team, with regular group updates on obesity literature – Pooling knowledge gained with all team members – Helping other team members to resolve any problems implementing CBT-OB – Never criticising other team members (especially in the presence of the patient or other team members) – Organising a weekly team meeting to set out the professional tasks of each member in detail, to address any difficulties raised by implementation of the treatment and to integrate new strategies and procedures

The potential advantages of a non-eclectic CBT-OB team are that patients have the opportunity to benefit from a theory-based treatment, even at intensive levels of care, and the treatment itself can be continually refined and adjusted to suit the individual. Moreover, it facilitates the construction of a collaborative therapeutic relationship with the patient, who is reassured by the support received from different professionals on several fronts. In this way patients can benefit from being treated as a whole person by means of a coherent, non-contradictory approach. Last but not the least, a common line of attack unites the team and facilitates evaluation of the strengths and limitations of the treatment itself—something that is invaluable from a research perspective and can ultimately only lead to improvement in therapeutic strategies. Table 12.1 gives some practical advice on how to put together a CBT-OB clinical team.

12.4.3 The Patient's Role in Intensive CBT-OB

Like standard outpatient CBT-OB, intensive CBT-OB adopts a collaborative approach, encouraging the patients to play an active role in their own treatment. They are required to put the maximum effort in applying the CBT-OB procedures and to do homework between sessions. They are also asked to be punctual and to arrive at each therapy session (individual and group CBT-OB sessions, meals, weekly review meetings, physical exercise sessions) 10–15 min early so that they can be adequately prepared. Patients should make participation in all therapy sessions a priority and consider the impact of their behaviour—in intensive rehabilitative settings, it is easy for patients to affect each other positively or negatively, so they are encouraged to do their best to create a positive atmosphere, in which they can help each other to address their obesity. Nonetheless, some patients, even involuntarily, may have a negative influence on other patients. Examples of behaviours that tend to adversely affect other patients are the following:

- Criticising the treatment and therapists
- Openly stating their belief that no one can maintain the weight lost in the long term
- Failing to commit in applying the treatment's procedures
- Introducing food and alcohol into the unit
- Talking about food, weight and body shape

Patients are told that in order to be admitted to the intensive CBT-OB unit, they will need to take the responsibility of not influencing the adherence of other patients by exhibiting negative behaviours and attitudes. Constructive criticism of the treatment is, of course, welcome, but comments and suggestions should be communicated to the therapists in private—not in front of the other patients. We also discourage patients from talking to other patients about food, weight and shape.

12.4.4 Assessment

The assessment of patients with disabling obesity admitted to intensive CBT-OB includes the following procedures:

- *Medical assessment.* The physician conducts a physical examination and takes down an accurate obesity-focused history (see Sect. 3.2) to clarify and establish the specific diagnostic and therapeutic needs of the patient not covered in the diagnostic workup (which should be performed as described in Sect. 3.7.2).
- *Psychological assessment.* The clinical psychologist conducts a psychological evaluation, assessing eating disorder psychopathology by means of the Eating Disorder Examination interview (EDE 17.0D) [12, 13], general psychopathology with Brief Symptom Inventory (BSI) [14], obesity-related quality of life using the ORWELL-97 questionnaire [15] and scores on the SIO Obesity-Related Disability Test [7].
- *Dietetic assessment.* The dietician takes an exhaustive dietary history of the patient using a structured interview to assess usual food and/or nutrient intake over the last year.

- *Physical fitness assessment*. The physiotherapist uses the tests described in Sect. 6.1.2 to assess muscle strength, aerobic capacity, flexibility and balance, with the aim of planning an individualised fitness rehabilitation program.
- *Body composition assessment*. In a well-equipped unit, this will include bioelectrical impedance analysis (BIA) and dual-energy X-ray absorptiometry (DEXA), as well as standard measurement of weight, height and waist circumference. Both BIA and DEXA provide an estimate of body composition, in particular the amount of body fat, and enable the detection of sarcopenia associated with obesity.
- *Energy expenditure assessment*. This is conducted via indirect calorimetry to assess the basal metabolic rate and by means of metabolic Holter monitoring of the type and intensity of physical activity performed by the patient during the day.

12.4.5 Individual Rehabilitation Plan

The above assessment should be used to design a personal rehabilitation plan which takes into account the individual patient's needs and recovery potential, as well as their preferences and the resources available. The plan should be designed to meet not only the patient's medical and psychological needs but also improve their overall quality of life. As we have seen in the preceding chapters, a patient's expectations will be a key factor in determining outcomes and should therefore be thoroughly explored. The patient should be given a full description of the goals of the programme, the indicators used to assess its effectiveness, the interventions that they will be prescribed and the operators responsible for each. During implementation of their rehabilitation plan, regular monitoring should be conducted to enable "mid-course correction", i.e., modification and adaptation of the plan to take into account any changes and emerging needs. At the end of the treatment programme, assessment should be performed as a matter of course, to evaluate the extent to which the individual CBT-OB rehabilitation plan achieved its stated goals. An example individual CBT-OB rehabilitation plan is provided in Table 12.2.

12.4.6 Specific Intervention Areas

12.4.6.1 Nutritional Interventions

The nutritional programme is designed to produce a 500–1000 kcal energy deficit per day to achieve a variable weight loss of about 0.5–1 kg a week. As in outpatient CBT-OB (see Sect. 5.3), this energy deficit is calculated by subtracting 250–500 kcal from the patient's basal metabolic rate (as measured by indirect calorimetry), adjusting the caloric deficit according to the individual's physical activity level.

A low-energy meal plan is a fundamental part of the programme. It is based on a Mediterranean-style low-glycaemic-index diet composed of about 25% protein, 45% carbohydrates and 30% fats [16]. A high level of dietary protein has been adopted because there is evidence that this could help prevent and treat obesity,

Table 12.2 Example of an individual CBT-OB rehabilitation plan

• Global outcomes (i.e., expected long-term outcome): – Achieving healthy weight loss (i.e., a weight loss of at least 10%) – Reducing the cardiovascular risk – Reducing obesity-related disabilities – Achieving a satisfactory quality of life – Developing a lifestyle and mindset conducive to long-term weight maintenance
• Functional outcomes (i.e., expected outcomes at the end of the intensive CBT-OB-based rehabilitation treatment, taking into account the complete set of parameters covered by all interventions delivered): – Learning the cognitive behavioural skills for long-term weight control – Starting the weight-loss process – Starting to manage cardiovascular risk and the complications associated with obesity – Improving cardiovascular fitness – Improving obesity-related disabilities
• Specific outcomes (i.e., outcomes at the end of intensive CBT-OB-based rehabilitation treatment related to smaller or more discrete parameter sets, such as recovering a particular function): – Achieving a weight loss of at least 3% – Increasing knowledge about obesity and acquiring cognitive behavioural weight-management skills (achieving at least a 10% increase in the score on an in-house "test" of knowledge on obesity and CBT-OB procedures) – Improving cardiovascular fitness (achieving at least a 10% increase in distance on the 6-min walking test) – Reducing obesity-related disabilities (achieving at least a 10% reduction in Obesity-Related Disability Test score)
• Specific intervention areas: – Nutrition Goal: achieving at least a 3% weight loss Procedures: 1200 kcal meal plan (25% proteins, 45% carbohydrates, 30% fats) Operators: dieticians – Physical rehabilitation Goal: achieving at least a 10% increase in distance to 6-min walking test Procedures: calisthenics sessions 45 min twice a week, gradual increase in daily step count to reach at least at 7500 by the end of the treatment Operators: physiotherapists – Cognitive behavioural Goal: achieving at least a 10% increase in the score on a questionnaire designed to "test" the patient's knowledge of obesity and CBT-OB procedures Procedures: 12 group cognitive behavioural sessions (90 min each) Operators: psychologists – Medical Goal: normalising blood sugar and blood pressure Procedures: adjusting and/or changing the diabetes and blood pressure drugs Operators: physicians

metabolic syndrome, type 2 diabetes [16] and sarcopenia [17]. Moreover, better weight maintenance has been observed in participants of a large randomised controlled trial who consumed a high-protein, low-glycaemic-index diet with moderate fat content ad libitum [18] and in subjects who followed a Mediterranean diet as opposed to a low-fat diet [19].

We do not routinely recommend very-low-energy diets (VLEDs; 200–800 kcal/day) because there are questions surrounding the safety of an energy intake of under 800 kcal [16]. Moreover, VLEDs are not educational and do not facilitate the gradual modification of eating habits, nutritional knowledge and skills that seems to be required for long-term weight maintenance [16].

Patients are trained to count their daily calorie intake, to use the Monitoring Record, both in real-time, and to plan when, what and where to eat in the weeks after discharge.

12.4.6.2 Physical Rehabilitation

The physical rehabilitation programme should adopt the general strategies and procedures of outpatient CBT-OB but adapted for disabling obesity and personalised on the basis of the patient's baseline fitness.

To this end, at admission, the patient is provided with a pedometer with a view to obtaining a baseline daily step count, and the physiotherapist should assess their performance in the following tests:

- Six-minute walk test—to evaluate functional exercise capacity
- Handgrip test—to measure isometric muscle strength
- Sit-to-stand and up-and-go times—to assess mobility and static and dynamic balance
- Functional reach test—to assess flexibility

After this assessment, the patient should be started on a personalised motor/functional rehabilitation programme that includes the following two components:

- *Lifestyle activity.* Patients are encouraged to cut down on sedentary activities (e.g., watch less TV, sit for less time during the day, etc.) and gradually increasing the number of their daily steps from baseline (e.g., 2500 at baseline; 5000 at week 1; 7500 at week 2; and 10,000 at week 3).
- *Calisthenics.* Patients should participate twice a week in 45-min sessions designed to address the fitness issues that emerged in baseline functional tests. Exercises to improve flexibility, balance and lower limb strength should be included.

Patients are trained to calculate their daily energy expenditure, reporting the number of daily steps, the relative consumption of kcal, the type and duration of formal exercise performed, the amount of kcal consumed in this activity, the basal metabolic rate and the diet-induced thermogenesis in their Monitoring Record.

Since it is fundamental to continue to adopt an active lifestyle after the conclusion of the intensive CBT-OB-based rehabilitation treatment, patients are encouraged to adopt a level of physical activity that is compatible with their work commitments during the treatment, so that their regime will be easily transferable to their daily life in the real world. Finally, before discharge patients should complete an exercise schedule comparing what they used to do in the rehabilitation programme and what they will do now (see Table 12.3).

Table 12.3 An example exercise schedule

Time	What I used to do	Time	What I will do now
6:00		6:00	
7:00	Wake up	7:00	Wake up and take breakfast at home
8:00	Take the bus to work. Breakfast at the bar	8:00	Take the bus to work and get off a stop before
9:00	Start working	9:00	Start work
10:00		10:00	Go up and down the stairs
11:00		11:00	Go up and down the stairs
12:00		12:00	
13:00	Lunch at the office bar	13:00	Lunch in a bar or restaurant 1 km away from the office
14:00	Back to work	14:00	Back to work
15:00		15:00	
16:00		16:00	Go up and down the stairs
17:00		17:00	
18:00	Finish work. Get the bus home	18:00	Finish work. Get the bus home
19:00	Lie down on the couch	19:00	Take the dog for a 30-min walk
20:00	Dinner	20:00	Dinner
21:00		21:00	
22:00	Go to bed	22:00	Go to bed
23:00		23:00	

12.4.6.3 Cognitive Behavioural Interventions

The cognitive behavioural programme is delivered by the psychologist trained extensively in CBT-OB in 12 closed-group sessions of eight participants. Each session lasts 90 min and has the following structure (see also Chap. 11 on how to conduct group CBT-OB): (1) reviewing the homework, (2) setting and working through the agenda and (3) bringing the session to a close. The groups cover psychoeducation on obesity (i.e., obesity has multifactorial causes, is a chronic condition and requires a persistent lifestyle modification and the development of a weight-control mindset to manage it), CBT-OB procedures, behavioural exercises and discussions on how to address weight-loss obstacles. Two group sessions can be held with significant others if indicated and agreed to. Individual CBT-OB sessions can be offered to patients with BED and psychiatric comorbidities associated with obesity.

The patients are trained to use the following CBT-OB procedures (see Chaps. 3, 4, 5 and 6 for details):

- Using the Monitoring Record to plan when, what and where to eat and to record in real time
- Eating consciously (eating slowly; appreciating the sight, smell and taste of food; using the Monitoring Record in real-time; resisting the impulse to deviate from the meal plan)
- Weekly weighing (interpreting the weight change every 4 weeks, not from a single reading)

- Constructing a Personal Formulation (including antecedent food and nonfood stimuli, positive consequences and problematic thoughts hindering weight loss)
- Addressing antecedent food stimuli (e.g., the presence of abundant quantities of food in the environment and social occasions)
- Addressing antecedent nonfood stimuli (e.g., events, changes in mood, impulses to eat, places and times of day)
- Addressing problematic thoughts (i.e., thoughts that hinder adherence to the lifestyle changes needed to lose weight)
- Addressing the positive consequences of food intake (e.g., gratification or elimination of aversive states through food)
- Planning the return home (1-week meal planning, physical activity planning, reducing food stimuli in the home, identifying and avoiding the dysfunctional eating and physical activity that characterised pretreatment habits)

Patients should also be encouraged to practice the following behavioural exercises with the aim of changing some cognitive mechanisms that may be hindering weight loss:

- Calorie counting (energy intake and energy expenditure). Patients should be trained and practice calorie counting, reading food labels, estimating the calorie content of food of uncertain composition (e.g., restaurant dishes) and estimating the amount of calories burned through daily steps and physical activity (using the MET).
- Interpreting the weight-loss graph. Patients should be trained to interpret their weight-loss graph accurately on a weekly basis (see Sect. 4.4).
- Eating slowly. Patients are instructed to record the time taken to consume their meals and to increase it gradually.
- Leaving something on the plate. As part of the rehabilitation programme, two meals a week feature large portions, and the patients are asked to leave something on the plate.
- Addressing a buffet. One meal a week is organised as a buffet, so the patients can practice taking only the food that is included in their meal plan.
- Practicing eating out. Once a week the patients eat in a restaurant outside the unit and should order only the food that they have planned to eat.

As part of the intensive CBT-OB-based rehabilitation treatment, significant others (i.e., the people who can influence the patients' eating) may participate with the patients in two group sessions to discuss how to create a home environment with low exposure to food stimuli. In this way the involvement of significant others can facilitate the patients' adherence to the weight-loss meal plan. Using slides, the psychologist uses the first group session to explain the behavioural chain involving food stimuli (i.e., buying food, storing food, cooking, serving, eating and after meals). The psychologist asks each family group to think about, write down and tell the other group members which stimuli they can reduce in their home environment at various points in the behavioural chain. In the next joint group session, the changes implemented by the significant others to change the home environment are reviewed and discussed.

12.4.6.4 Medical Interventions

The assessment and pharmacological treatment of medical complications associated with disabling obesity must be managed by a trained physician in CBT-OB. Since several drugs are associated with weight gain (see Sect. 3.2), particular attention needs to be paid to find substitutes with a weight-neutral or weight-loss-promoting effect.

12.4.7 Bringing Intensive CBT-OB to a Close

Just as it is important to start well, it is crucial to bring the intensive CBT-OB-based rehabilitation treatment to a satisfactory close. With this in mind, the goal of the last phase of the treatment is to prepare patients to return home, continuing the weight-loss phase begun in the intensive rehabilitation setting and minimising the risk of relapse.

First of all, patients are informed that they have acquired new eating and physical activity habits that will permit them to lose weight at home too and that the tendency to adopt some apparently automatic and uncontrollable dysfunctional eating habits (e.g., eating desserts or grazing) they had before the admission should no longer be a problem due to the process of deconditioning that occurred during their intensive treatment (i.e., the patients did not eat desserts for 21 days and stopped constant snacking). However, the therapist should emphasise to the patients that a habit, once learned, never entirely disappears. For this reason, they are recommended to persist with the new habits learned during intensive treatment and to pay close attention to the early signs of their old eating habits reappearing. Patients are also educated that the risk of relapse is facilitated by exposure to multiple environmental stimuli (i.e., family environment, work and social occasions) not present in the intensive rehabilitation unit and by the transition from intensive to less intensive settings of care.

The final procedure is to assist the patients in preparing a written plan of action for the period after the intensive CBT-OB-based rehabilitation treatment that should include the following elements:

- Tools to use at home (e.g., Monitoring Record, weight-loss graph, pedometer, Personal Formulation, Weight-Loss Obstacles Questionnaire)
- Weighing (e.g., once a week)
- Good eating habits (e.g., eating regularly, meal planning (1200–1500 kcal/day), real-time monitoring, eating consciously)
- Good physical activity habits (e.g., 10,000 steps a day, calisthenics twice a week)
- Weight-loss mindset (e.g., adopting a mindset oriented to achieving healthy weight loss and its associated physical and psychological advantages and to tolerate hunger and cravings for highly palatable foods)

- Procedures to reduce the risk of relapse (e.g., identifying and addressing high-risk weight-regain situations, addressing weight regain—see Sects. 9.5.5, 9.5.6 and 9.5.7, respectively)
- Outpatient treatment (preferably post-intensive outpatient CBT-OB).

12.5 Post-intensive Outpatient CBT-OB

Exposure to numerous dietary environmental stimuli and everyday life stresses after discharge typically makes it difficult to adhere to the lifestyle changes initiated during intensive CBT-OB-based rehabilitation treatment. For this reason, patients are advised to continue their treatment by attending standard outpatient CBT-OB, as described in Fig. 2.1. In this way, the patients can continue to practice the weight-loss procedures learned during the initial intensive phase of treatment and address their individual obstacles to weight loss via the CBT-OB procedures in Module 4.

Vignette

The patient, a 57-year-old man with a BMI of 46.7 and a CASCO-R score of 28, was admitted to the intensive CBT-OB-based rehabilitation unit after the failure of several specialist outpatient treatments for obesity. The patient had disabling obesity associated with type 2 diabetes, high blood LDL cholesterol (HDL), high triglycerides, obstructive sleep apnoea (but could not tolerate C-PAP), hypertension and atrial fibrillation (resistant to two electrical cardioversions). To manage these complications associated with obesity, he was being prescribed eight drugs, but his quality of life was poor nevertheless. Indeed, he had a score of 70 on the ORWELL-97 questionnaire, corresponding to the 75th percentile of the population—considered indicative of a clinically significant impairment in quality of life—and disability score of 45% on the Obesity-Related Disability Test. In particular he scored highly on pain, DLA (in particular walking and taking the stairs), activities out of the home, occupational activities and social life subscales. He also reported several episodes of falling asleep during the day.

The patient was actively engaged in the intensive CBT-OB-based rehabilitation treatment, which included, in addition to group CBT-OB sessions, a nutritional programme with a limit of 1500 kcal (indirect calorimetry indicated he had a basal metabolic rate of 2000 kcal) associated with a programme of gradual physical rehabilitation beginning with 3500 steps/day. At the end of the 21 days of treatment, he had lost about 5% of his initial body weight (7 kg); he was walking 6000 steps/day and showed improvements in the 6-min walk test (from 380 to 500 m) and the ORWELL-97 questionnaire score (from 70 to 48). He also reported sleeping better and feeling less tired during the day.

After discharge, the patient signed up for outpatient CBT-OB and achieved a weight loss of 20% (about 26 kg) after 24 weeks. He maintained this weight loss during the 48 weeks of the weight-maintenance phase and at the last assessment reported a dramatic improvement in his quality of life (ORWELL-97 questionnaire score 20) and no more sleep apnoea. He no longer felt tired or fell asleep during the day, and his metabolic markers were within the normal range, despite the number and amount of medicines he was taking having been reduced.

References

1. World Health Organization. International classification of impairments, disabilities, and handicaps. Geneva: World Health Organization; 1980.
2. Visser M, Langlois J, Guralnik JM, Cauley JA, Kronmal RA, Robbins J, et al. High body fatness, but not low fat-free mass, predicts disability in older men and women: the Cardiovascular Health Study. Am J Clin Nutr. 1998;68(3):584–90.
3. Peeters A, Bonneux L, Nusselder WJ, De Laet C, Barendregt JJ. Adult obesity and the burden of disability throughout life. Obes Res. 2004;12(7):1145–51. https://doi.org/10.1038/oby.2004.143.
4. Ferraro KF, Su YP, Gretebeck RJ, Black DR, Badylak SF. Body mass index and disability in adulthood: a 20-year panel study. Am J Public Health. 2002;92(5):834–40.
5. Zamboni M, Mazzali G, Fantin F, Rossi A, Di Francesco V. Sarcopenic obesity: a new category of obesity in the elderly. Nutr Metab Cardiovasc Dis. 2008;18(5):388–95. https://doi.org/10.1016/j.numecd.2007.10.002.
6. Devlin MJ. Binge eating disorder. In: Brownell KD, Walsh BT, editors. Eating disorders and obesity: a comprehensive handbook. New York: Guilford Press; 2017. p. 192–7.
7. Donini LM, Brunani A, Sirtori A, Savina C, Tempera S, Cuzzolaro M, et al. Assessing disability in morbidly obese individuals: the Italian Society of Obesity test for obesity-related disabilities. Disabil Rehabil. 2011;33(25–26):2509–18. https://doi.org/10.3109/09638288.2011.575529.
8. Capodaglio P, Donini LM, Petroni ML, Brunani A, Dalle Grave R, Di Flaviano CE, et al. Rehabilitation in obesity with comorbidities: a consensus document from experts of the Italian Society of Physical and Rehabilitation Medicine (SIMFER), the Italian Society of Obesity (SIO) and the Italian Society of Eating Disorders (SISDCA). Eat Weight Disord. 2014;19(3):383–6. https://doi.org/10.1007/s40519-014-0121-8.
9. Donini LM, Cuzzolaro M, Spera G, Badiali M, Basso N, Bollea MR, et al. Obesity and eating disorders. Indications for the different levels of care. An Italian Expert Consensus Document. Eat Weight Disord. 2010;15(1–2 Suppl):1–31.
10. Donini LM, Dalle Grave R, Di Flaviano E, Gentile MG, Mezzani B, Pandolfo Mayme M, et al. Assessing the appropriateness of the level of care for morbidly obese subjects: validation of the CASCO-R scale. Ann Ig. 2014;26(3):195–204. https://doi.org/10.7416/ai.2014.1977.
11. Dalle Grave R, Sartirana M, El Ghoch M, Calugi S. Personalized multistep cognitive behavioral therapy for obesity. Diabetes Metab Syndr Obes. 2017;10:195–206. https://doi.org/10.2147/DMSO.S139496.
12. Calugi S, Ricca V, Castellini G, Lo Sauro C, Ruocco A, Chignola E, et al. The eating disorder examination: reliability and validity of the Italian version. Eat Weight Disord. 2015;20(4):505–11. https://doi.org/10.1007/s40519-015-0191-2.

13. Fairburn CG, Cooper Z, O'Connor M. Eating disorder examination (EDE 16.0D). In: Fairburn CG, editor. Cognitive behavior therapy and eating disorders. New York: Guilford Press; 2008. p. 265–308.
14. Derogatis LR, Spencer PM. The brief symptom inventory: administration, scoring and procedures manual. Baltimore: Clinical Psychometric Research; 1982.
15. Mannucci E, Ricca V, Barciulli E, Di Bernardo M, Travaglini R, Cabras PL, et al. Quality of life and overweight: the obesity related well-being (Orwell 97) questionnaire. Addict Behav. 1999;24(3):345–57.
16. Astrup A, Brand-Miller J. Macronutrient composition and obesity treatment. In: Brownell KD, Walsh BT, editors. Eating disorders and obesity: a comprehensive handbook. 3rd ed. New York: Guilford Press; 2017. p. 480–7.
17. Sammarco R, Marra M, Di Guglielmo ML, Naccarato M, Contaldo F, Poggiogalle E, et al. Evaluation of hypocaloric diet with protein supplementation in middle-aged sarcopenic obese women: a pilot study. Obes Facts. 2017;10(3):160–7. https://doi.org/10.1159/000468153.
18. Larsen TM, Dalskov SM, van Baak M, Jebb SA, Papadaki A, Pfeiffer AF, et al. Diets with high or low protein content and glycemic index for weight-loss maintenance. N Engl J Med. 2010;363(22):2102–13. https://doi.org/10.1056/NEJMoa1007137.
19. Schwarzfuchs D, Golan R, Shai I. Four-year follow-up after two-year dietary interventions. N Engl J Med. 2012;367(14):1373–4. https://doi.org/10.1056/NEJMc1204792.

Adaptating CBT-OB for Binge-Eating Disorder

13

The diagnostic concept of binge-eating disorder (BED) was first described in 1959 by the American psychiatrist and researcher Albert Stunkard to illustrate the characteristics of a subgroup of patients with obesity and recurrent episodes of uncontrolled overeating [1]. However, it was not identified as a distinct eating disorder until the second half of the 1980s, when several studies on the prevalence of bulimia nervosa in the population showed a large subgroup of individuals who did not use compensatory behaviours after binge-eating episodes. At the same time, it was noted that about a quarter of individuals requiring treatment for obesity reported recurring episodes of binge eating but did not suffer from bulimia nervosa. Subsequent studies have confirmed that BED has distinctive clinical features that set it apart from bulimia nervosa and obesity [2], but it was not until 2013 that the disorder was recognised as a distinct diagnostic category by the *Diagnostic and Statistical Manual of Mental Disorders* (DSM-5) [3].

13.1 Diagnostic Criteria

According to the DSM-5, a person suffers BED if they meet the following diagnostic criteria [3]:

- Recurrent episodes of binge eating. An episode of binge eating is characterised by both of the following:
  - Eating, in a discrete period of time (e.g., within any <2-h period), an amount of food that is definitively larger than most individuals would eat in a similar period of time under similar circumstances
  - A sense of lack of control over eating during the episodes (e.g., a feeling that one cannot stop eating or control what and how much one is eating)

R. Dalle Grave et al., *Treating Obesity with Personalized Cognitive Behavioral Therapy*, https://doi.org/10.1007/978-3-319-91497-8_13

- The binge-eating episodes are associated with three (or more) of the following:
  - Eating much more quickly than normal
  - Eating until feeling uncomfortably full
  - Eating large amounts of food when not feeling physically hungry
  - Eating alone because of feeling embarrassed by how much one is eating
  - Feeling disgusted with oneself, depressed or very guilty afterwards
- Marked distress regarding binge eating is present.
- Binge eating occurs, on average, at least once a week for 3 months.
- The binge eating is not associated with the recurrent use of inappropriate compensatory behaviours (as in bulimia nervosa) and does not occur exclusively during the course of bulimia nervosa or anorexia nervosa.

13.2 Clinical Features

The core feature of BED is the recurrent episodes of binge eating. However, in contrast to bulimia nervosa, and indeed anorexia nervosa, extreme weight-control behaviours (e.g., purging or extreme and rigid dietary restraint) are absent. In individuals with BED, binge-eating episodes occur against the background of a general tendency to overeat rather than dietary restraint (as typically seen in bulimia nervosa) [4], which explains the strong association of the disorder with obesity.

Another consistent finding is that individuals with BED, compared with those of similar weight without BED, report a higher rate of current and lifetime psychopathology (see Sect. 13.4) and more frequent dieting and weight fluctuations [5]. Indeed, it is common for individuals with BED to report periods of binge eating, during which their weight increases, alternating with other periods of dieting, which determine a transitory weight loss [5].

Overvaluation of shape and weight (i.e., the undue influence of shape or body weight on self-evaluation)—a core criterion of anorexia nervosa and bulimia nervosa—is not a diagnostic criterion for BED in DSM-5, but is present in about 50% in patients with BED [6]. Overvaluation of shape or weight is not associated with BMI (i.e., it does not simply reflect distress with excess weight), but has been linked to a greater severity of eating-related psychopathology and psychological distress, and has reliably demonstrated negative prognostic significance [6]. Moreover, a subgroup of patients with BED and a previous history of anorexia nervosa and/or bulimia nervosa seem to respond less well to treatment [7].

When BED is severe and characterised by daily binge-eating episodes, it impairs quality of life, and individuals may miss work, school or other social activities and place a great burden on healthcare systems [8]. In most cases, sufferers try to control their eating by themselves, but only succeed for a short period of time, and many patients request treatment for their excess weight—not the eating disorder itself.

13.3 Epidemiology, Course and Outcome

The lifetime prevalence of BED in the community, estimated by the National Comorbidity Survey Replication, is around 3.5% among women and 2.0% among men [9]. While about half of individuals with BED in community studies have a condition of overweight or obesity, most of the studies on clinical samples have been conducted in such patients [5]. It is estimated that about 7.5% of patients seeking treatment for obesity suffer from BED [10], which is reported in 15.7% of those assessed for bariatric surgery [11].

Little data is available about the natural course of BED among adults in the community, although an association between binge eating and obesity has been observed. BED also seems to increase the risk of developing overweight and obesity, a finding confirmed by a longitudinal study on adolescents that found that BED is associated with an increased risk of obesity and depression [12].

Patients typically report long histories of binge eating, with an increase in frequency in times of stress, but many also report long periods free from this behaviour. Indeed, findings from short-term natural history studies and clinical trials indicate that BED is characterised by high remission rates [13], even with minimal intervention or placebo [5]. That being said, whether this outcome represents a stable remission is not yet known.

13.4 Coexisting Psychological and Medical Comorbidities

Individuals with BED often report low self-esteem, depressive features and mood intolerance, while the most frequently seen personality traits and coexisting psychiatric disorders diagnosed in individuals with BED include impulsive traits, mood disorders, anxiety disorders and substance use disorders [14]. These associations persist even when the weight status is controlled, indicating that they are specific to binge eating and not the severity of obesity [5].

The association between BED—independent of weight—and medical complications is less clear. Studies controlling for weight showed that individuals with BED report higher rates of new diagnoses of metabolic syndrome components, including dyslipidaemia, impaired glucose levels and type 2 diabetes [15]. Indeed, individuals with BED often have an unhealthy lifestyle characterised by daily smoking, low exercise frequency, poor nutrition—as binge-eating episodes usually involve foods that are high in fat, sugar and/or salt but low in vitamins and minerals—and alcohol misuse. This explains why they present both the typical complications associated with obesity (e.g., metabolic syndrome, type 2 diabetes) and also several that are independent of the excess weight but related to their unhealthy lifestyle, such as irritable bowel syndrome; alcohol and smoking complications; neck, shoulder and lower back pain; and chronic muscle pain [16].

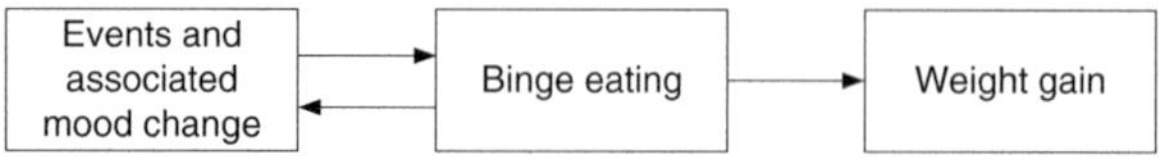

Fig. 13.1 The principal maintenance mechanisms of binge eating in individuals with binge-eating disorder without overvaluation of shape or weight

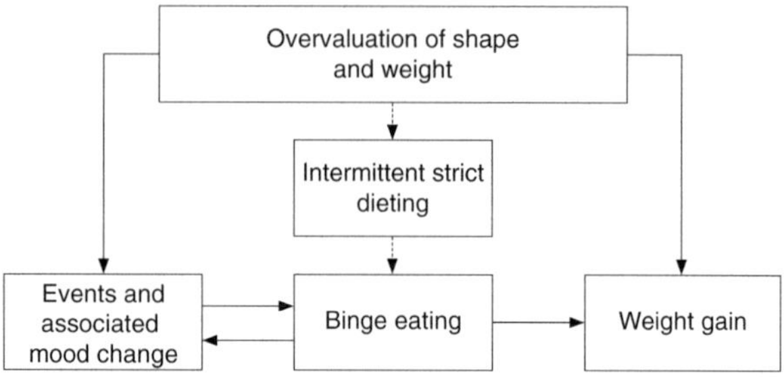

Fig. 13.2 The principal maintenance mechanisms of binge eating in individuals with binge-eating disorder and overvaluation of shape or weight

13.5 Mechanisms Maintaining Binge Eating

The psychopathology underlying and maintaining episodes of binge eating is very heterogeneous. However, according to cognitive behavioural theory, individuals with BED can be divided into two subtypes based on the presence or absence of overvaluation of shape and weight [6].

In individuals without the overvaluation of shape and weight (about 50% of those with BED), binge-eating episodes are triggered and maintained principally by events and associated mood changes (Fig. 13.1). In these individuals, binge eating may help them to cope with negative events or adverse moods by distracting them from troubling thoughts and via direct modulation of mood (it dampens down intense mood states). In other individuals, binge eating may be used as a form of gratification [17]. However, as there is the tendency to interpret binge eating as the result of poor self-control, after a brief period of mood improvement, individuals with BED tend to feel disgusted with themselves, depressed or very guilty, and these negative moods can trigger a new episode of binge eating.

In individuals who do overvalue shape and weight, binge eating is maintained by three principal mechanisms that interact with each other (Fig. 13.2): (1) the perceived or real weight in excess and/or the overvaluation of shape and weight generates negative moods (which may also be brought on by events not related to body image) that are mitigated by binge eating; (2) by producing weight gain, binge eating intensifies the overvaluation of shape and weight; and (3) the overvaluation of shape and weight leads them to adopt a strict but intermittent diet—often characterised by rigid and extreme dietary rules (i.e., multiple, demanding and specific dietary rules that must be adhered to at all costs). The attempt to limit the amount of food eaten may be successful for a certain period of time and even produce a significant amount of weight loss. However, there is the tendency for any minor infraction of their over-strict dietary rules to produce an extremely negative reaction—as evidence of a lack of self-control [17]. Patients tend to respond to rule-breaking by abandoning dietary restraint and succumb to the urge to eat (intensified by the cognitive dietary restraint and the often associated caloric restriction). The result is an episode of binge eating, which in turn intensifies the overvaluation of shape or weight [17].

13.6 Treatment: The Problem of Weight Loss

Both CBT for eating disorders and interpersonal psychotherapy (IPT) are the interventions for BED with the most empirical support. Both treatments produce short- and long-term reductions in binge eating (>50% remission rates throughout 48-month follow-up) and associated psychopathology, but they do not produce weight loss [18]. Promising results have also been reported for guided self-help based on CBT, with about 46% of patients achieving remission from BED, but this treatment too does not produce weight loss [18]. Nonetheless, the 2017 National Institute for Health and Care Excellence (NICE) guidelines "Eating disorders: recognition and treatment" recommends guided self-help programmes based on CBT for adults with BED. If this is unacceptable, contraindicated or ineffective after 4 weeks, the guidelines recommend offering group or individual CBT for eating disorders [19]. The NICE guidelines also advise explaining to individuals with BED that "psychological treatments aimed at treating binge eating have a limited effect on body weight, and that weight loss is not a therapy target in itself" [19].

In order to provide an "all-round" treatment option for individuals with BED and obesity, weight-loss programmes based on BT-OB and bariatric surgery have been introduced. However, available data suggest that BT-OB is not as effective as CBT or IPT in reducing the frequency of binge-eating episodes. Furthermore, although BT-OB produces a greater short-term weight loss, at 2-year follow-up, the weight loss is no longer significantly different to that achieved through IPT or guided self-help CBT [20].

The presence of BED also seems to predict a lesser weight loss and a higher weight regain in patients treated with bariatric surgery, especially in the subgroup of individuals in whom there is a recurrence of the loss of control over eating. Although these episodes are not usually associated with the intake of a large amount of food—due to the limitations imposed by surgical gastric restriction—they will inevitably lead to regain if they are recurrent throughout the day [5].

Finally, some studies have tested different drugs for BED, revealing that several medications are superior to placebo for reducing binge eating over the short term [21]. However, except for topiramate—which significantly reduces both binge eating and weight over the short term—tested drugs have yielded minimal weight loss. In 2015, the Food and Drug Administration approved lisdexamfetamine dimesylate (LDX) on the basis of some studies showing its short-term superiority to placebo for reducing binge eating after 12 weeks of treatment (about 40% remission on LDX vs. 21% on placebo) [21]. However, LDX is a stimulant, and its use is restricted as it is not indicated for weight loss or obesity; it also bears a "black box" warning due to its high potential for abuse/dependence.

Almost no data exists regarding the longer-term effects of pharmacotherapy for BED, although treatment with fluoxetine was shown not to be as effective as CBT over time. Moreover, the addition of medication to CBT does not enhance outcomes in either the short or the long term. Hence the NICE guidelines recommend not offering medication as the sole treatment for BED [19].

Interestingly, the research into BED treatments has revealed two potentially useful outcome predictors [18]. The first is that patients with overvaluation of shape and weight tend to show less overall improvement across treatments over time than those without and benefit less from medication than from CBT. The second is that patients who display a rapid response to treatment (defined as a 70% or greater reduction in binge eating by week four) are more likely to remit than those with no rapid response when treated with BT-OB or medications, while this effect is less evident in those treated with CBT.

In conclusion, it appears that, while patients with BED seem to respond quite well to psychological interventions, especially guided self-help CBT, these are limited by the fact that none produce significant weight loss. BT-OB and pharmacological approaches have also failed in this regard, indicating the need to develop new treatments able to produce both remission from BED and a healthy weight loss in patients with concomitant obesity. With this in mind, we have developed a version of CBT-OB specially adapted for BED.

13.7 CBT-OB for BED

CBT-OB has been adapted for BED specifically to address both the heterogeneous and multiple mechanisms that can operate in individuals with this disorder and weight loss, if not contraindicated, in those with associated obesity. The treatment integrates CBT-E, a treatment designed to address the maintenance mechanisms of binge eating—recommended for all eating disorders and ages by the recent NICE guidelines [19]—with the weight-loss CBT-OB described in this book.

CBT-E is a personalised transdiagnostic treatment for eating disorder psychopathology rather than for a particular eating disorder diagnosis [17]. It was originally designed as an individual treatment for adult outpatients, but has subsequently been adapted for use with younger patients [22] and for more intensive use in outpatient, day hospital and residential settings [23]. The treatment is guided by a personalised formulation of the patient's eating disorder, constructed at the beginning of treatment and revised as necessary as the treatment progresses. The strategies and procedures used in CBT-E address the expressions of the eating disorder psychopathology (i.e., binge-eating episodes) and specifically target and disrupt the mechanisms maintaining it. The main strategy is encouraging patients to make changes in the way they behave and then helping them to understand and reflect on the effects and implications of these changes. In this way, they learn to decentre from their eating problems and eventually to identify their eating disorder mindset and learn to control and manipulate it.

With patients who are normal weight, CBT-E has four stages and involves an initial assessment appointment followed by 20 50-min treatment sessions over 20 weeks [17]. The treatment can be delivered in two versions: a "focused" version that exclusively addresses the core processes maintaining the eating disorder psychopathology and a "broad" version that also addresses one or more of the three additional hypothesised maintenance processes (i.e., clinical perfectionism, core low self-esteem and marked interpersonal difficulties). Both versions are transdiagnostic in scope, with the first stages of each being identical; the treatment diverges in the later stages based on the patient's psyhcopatology and clinical presentation.

In our CBT-OB programme, patients with BED and obesity start their treatment with Stage 1 of CBT-E. After 4 weeks, during Stage 2, the decision is made whether to continue with CBT-E or to shift over to standard CBT-OB. The outcome of this decision will depend upon an individual patient's response to treatment and whether or not their psychopathology features overvaluation of shape and weight. The patient's opinion should, of course, be sought, but CBT-OB is generally started if the patient presents a remission from binge eating and does not report the overvaluation of shape and weight. Otherwise, the treatment continues with Stage 3 of CBT-E, which includes specific modules to address the mechanisms that are maintaining the patient's binge eating. After completing Stage 4 of CBT-E, CBT-OB can be started if the patient has achieved remission from binge eating and does not report the overvaluation of shape and weight at the post-treatment review session, held 20 weeks after the end of CBT-E (see Fig. 13.3).

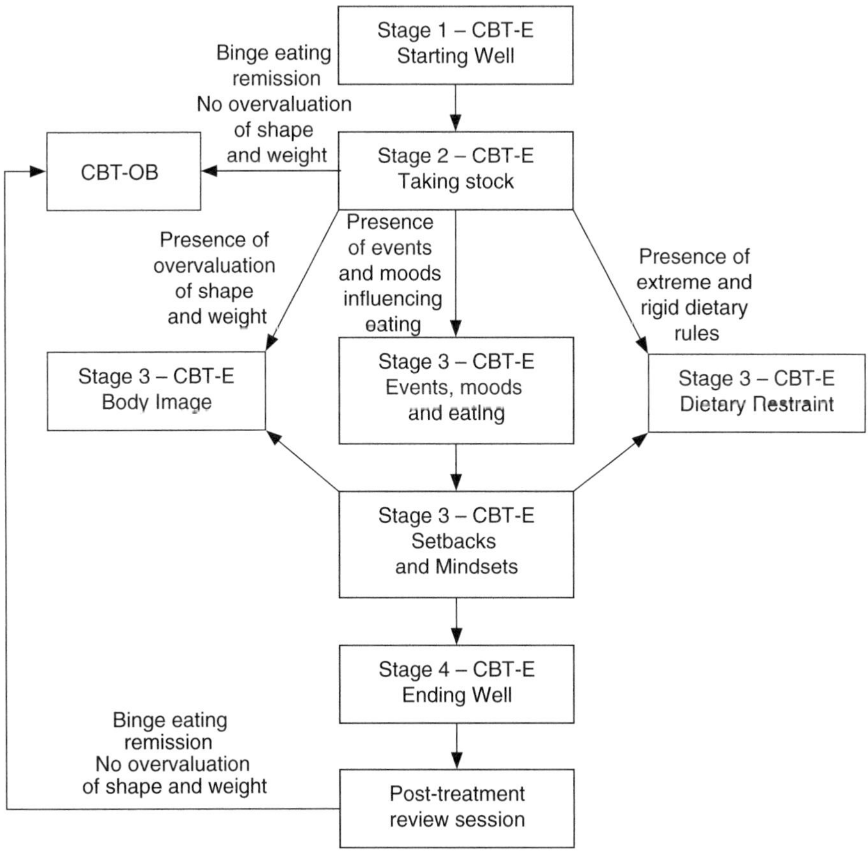

Fig. 13.3 The CBT-E/CBT-OB map for binge-eating disorder

This stepped-care approach was developed because in our clinical setting we observed that a large subgroup of patients with BED without overvaluation of shape and weight achieve complete remission from binge eating after just a few sessions, thanks to real-time self-monitoring, in-session weighing and regular eating procedures. These patients therefore do not require a full course of CBT-E treatment and after 5 or 6 weeks will be ready to start addressing weight loss via CBT-OB. However, a subgroup of patients—with severe BED psychopathology, often associated with the overvaluation of shape and weight—do not respond so rapidly to the treatment and require the full course of CBT-E to achieve remission from BED. These patients run a high risk of relapse, and we suggest that they start CBT-OB only if their remission from binge eating lasts until the post-treatment review conducted 20 weeks after the end of CBT-E.

13.7.1 Involving Patients in the Decision to Address Binge Eating First

The therapist should always assess for the presence of BED in patients seeking treatment for obesity, as about 10% of this population suffer from this eating disorder. They should therefore be asked whether or not they have had episodes of overeating or loss of control over eating over the past 4 weeks. The therapist should explain to patients that "overeating" means eating what most people would regard as an unusually large amount of food within any 2-h period, while "loss of control over eating" means having the feeling of not being able to stop eating or control what or how much is being eaten. If patients report episodes of overeating associated with the loss of control over eating, the therapist should ask, on average, how often they ate in this way in the last 3 months. Additional questions to confirm the diagnosis of BED are asking the patients if these episodes have been associated with eating much more than normal, if they ate until feeling uncomfortably full, if they ate a lot even when not feeling physically hungry and/or if they did this alone due to feelings of embarrassment about how much they were eating. Patients should also be asked if they felt disgusted with themselves, depressed or very guilty after these episodes. Finally, for an accurate diagnosis of BED, the therapist must exclude the presence of bulimia nervosa or anorexia nervosa and ensure that patients do not make recurrent use of inappropriate compensatory behaviours (as in bulimia nervosa). It is advisable to use the EDE 17.0D interview [24, 25], which not only aids in the differential diagnosis but also enables thorough assessment of the patient's core eating disorder psychopathology (i.e., overvaluation of shape and weight) and behavioural symptoms (i.e., binge eating, self-induced vomiting, laxative and diuretic misuse, excessive exercising and dietary restraint) over the preceding 28 days and in the past 3 months.

Once a diagnosis of BED has been made, the therapist should explain to the patient the rationale behind addressing the eating disorder before weight loss. The first step is to collaboratively create a provisional version of the patient's Personal Formulation (see Figs. 13.1 and 13.2), emphasising the role of both the principal mechanisms maintaining binge eating and their role in promoting weight gain and hindering weight loss. It is also useful to review any previous weight-loss attempt failures, focusing the patient's attention on the role played by binge-eating episodes in favouring their negative outcomes. The therapist should also say to the patients that trying to lose weight without first addressing the binge-eating episodes and the mechanisms that maintain them would be like trying to build a house without first laying the foundations.

Patients should be informed that in most cases weight-loss treatment (CBT-OB) can be started after 5–6 weeks, and in a minority of cases after 40 weeks, when a persistent remission from binge-eating episodes has occurred and their self-evaluation schema does not rely excessively on their shape and weight. Patients should also be told that the treatment used to address binge eating (CBT-E) has been shown by several studies to be very effective in treating BED. The therapist should briefly describe CBT-E, underlining the following points:

- CBT-E is a one-to-one treatment that is primarily focused on what makes it difficult to stop binge eating.
- The treatment is tailored specifically to tackle binge eating and the needs of the individual. Both patient and therapist will become experts on the individual's eating issues and what is driving them.
- CBT-E has four stages: Stage 1 lasts 4 weeks and includes twice-weekly sessions; Stage 2 is a progress review that lasts one or two sessions; Stage 3 focuses on addressing the main mechanisms driving binge eating and features eight weekly sessions; and Stage 4 aims to minimise the risk of relapse over 20 weeks, ensuring progress is maintained at sessions held every 2 weeks. If after Stage 2 there is stable remission from binge-eating episodes and no significant problems with body image, CBT-E can be interrupted and weight-loss CBT-OB can be started. In all the other cases, the full CBT-E should be completed, and CBT-OB can start at the post-treatment review—conducted 20 weeks after the end of CBT-E—if there is a lasting remission from binge eating and no significant problems with body image.
- It is crucial to have as few breaks in the treatment as possible. This is because it is important to establish "momentum"—working together from session to session to break the binge-eating cycle. Breaks in treatment are very disruptive as momentum is lost. It is especially important that there are no breaks in the first 6 weeks and no longer than 2-week breaks thereafter. This needs to be taken into account when deciding when to start treatment.
- Each appointment lasts 50 min and should start and finish on time.
- The patient and therapist will work together as a team to overcome the binge-eating problem and agree on specific homework tasks to be done between sessions. These tasks are very important and should be given priority. What the patient does between sessions has the greatest influence on the treatment outcomes.
- The treatment will be hard, but it will be worth it. The more effort the patient puts in, the greater the benefits.

The final step in helping the patient to decide to address binge eating first is to discuss with them the pros and cons of delaying weight loss in favour of tackling binge eating. In our clinical experience, this leads to most patients deciding to start CBT-E, because they realise that without addressing binge eating the probability of weight-loss success is low. If patients are ambivalent about our proposal, we ask them to take some days off to decide and to write the pros and cons in a table to be discussed in the next assessment session.

13.7.2 Addressing Questions and Concerns About Postponing Weight Loss

The therapist should always ask the patient to raise any questions or concerns they may have about the proposal to postpone weight loss and to address binge eating first. Some examples are listed below, together with the appropriate responses from the therapist.

- *PATIENT*: "If I stop binge eating, will I lose weight?"
- *THERAPIST*: "It is difficult to predict if you will lose weight or not. In most cases there is little or no change in weight, although sometimes it does occur. Nevertheless, I suggest that you focus all your efforts on addressing the mechanisms that are maintaining your binge-eating episodes. We will deal with weight loss once you have control of your eating."

- *PATIENT*: "It is difficult for me to accept not trying to lose weight now because I need to lose weight for medical reasons—I need to get my diabetes under control."
- *THERAPIST*: "I understand, and I know that you need to lose weight for medical reasons. However, if you stop binge eating and establish a pattern of regular eating and an active lifestyle—which CBT-E will help you to do—your blood sugar control will improve, and then we will address weight loss with more chance of success."

- *PATIENT*: "I am disgusted with my body. I need to lose weight so I can start feeling good about myself."
- *THERAPIST*: "Your negative body image is an important issue that we will address in the treatment. However, I suggest that now you concentrate your efforts on regaining control over your eating. In my experience, interruption of binge eating improves self-confidence, and is a necessary condition for addressing both negative body image and weight loss successfully."

- *PATIENT*: "I really do not know how to stop binging. It cannot resist eating. I have no control whatsoever."
- *THERAPIST*: "As I showed you in this diagram (the BED Formulation), your binge eating seems to be maintained by certain events and associated negative emotions, and it is more common when you skip lunch. Stopping binge eating does not depend on willpower, but on the interruption of these maintenance mechanisms."

13.7.3 CBT-E Stage 1

In this and the following sections, we report a brief description of the four stages of CBT-E, as applied to patients with BED. A detailed description of the treatment can be found in the complete treatment guide [17].

The aims of CBT-E Stage 1 are to engage the patient in treatment and change. Appointments are held twice weekly for 4 weeks and involve the following:

- Jointly creating with the patient a personalised formulation of the processes maintaining the binge eating (see Figs. 13.1 and 13.2).
- Establishing real-time self-monitoring of eating and other relevant thoughts and behaviours, by writing them down when they occur on a specific Monitoring Record (which can be downloaded at: http://www.credo-oxford.com/4.4.html).
- Education on body weight regulation and fluctuations (a procedure also adopted by CBT-OB, see Sect. 4.4).
- Introducing and establishing weekly in-session weighing and practising interpreting and coping with weight fluctuations (a procedure also adopted by CBT-OB, see Sects. 4.4 and 5.1).
- Introducing and adhering to a pattern of regular eating, with planned meals and snacks. Patients are encouraged to take three planned meals each day plus two or three planned snacks and not to eat in the intervals. This ensures that there is rarely an interval greater than 4 h between eating. Two principal strategies can be taught by the therapist and employed by the patient to help the patient resist eating between meals. These comprise two lists of distractive tasks, which can be drawn up beforehand and referred to by the patient when they feel tempted to eat. These tasks, or behaviours, should be loosely grouped under the headings: "Things to Do" and "Things to Say". Examples of the former should be activities that are incompatible with eating and therefore distract from the urge to binge (e.g., taking a bath, doing a crossword) or those that reduce the risk of eating (e.g., going to a place where food is inaccessible). The latter group, "Things to Say" (to oneself), comprises external vocalisations of statements reiterating, for example, that the urge to eat is a temporary phenomenon that can be tolerated and overcome. During meals, on the other hand, patients are free to eat whatever they wish, with the sole condition that the meals and snacks not be followed by purging. The regular eating pattern should be the priority of the day and must therefore take precedence over other activities. That being said, mealtimes may be adjusted each day to suit the patient's commitments.
- Developing an active lifestyle. This follows the procedures of CBT-OB Module 3 and is introduced in the second week of our adaptation of CBT-E for BED.
- Involving significant others if they will facilitate treatment.

13.7.4 CBT-E Stage 2

This stage involves one or two appointments, a week apart, that feature the following elements:

- Collaborative review of progress and compliance with treatment
- Identifying barriers to change—both general (e.g., work pressures) and specific features of the eating disorder itself (e.g., the presence of events and moods influencing eating, overvaluation of shape and weight, dietary restraint) or external maintenance mechanisms (i.e., clinical perfectionism, core low self-esteem, interpersonal difficulties) that maintain binge eating
- Modifying the initial formulation as needed in order to plan Stage 3
- Deciding to continue with the CBT-E (the focused or broad version) or to shift to CBT-OB

As described above, CBT-OB is initiated if patients present a stable remission from binge-eating episodes (e.g., in the last week) and show no overvaluation of shape and weight. This core eating disorder psychopathology can be assessed by the following questions derived from EDE 17 0.D interview [25]:

- "Over the past four weeks has your weight (the number on the scale) been important in influencing how you feel about (judge, think, evaluate) yourself as a person?"
- "... If you imagine the things which influence how you feel about (judge, think, evaluate) yourself, such as your performance at work, being a parent, your marriage, how you get on with other people, and put these things in order of importance, where does your weight fit in? What about your shape? How has it compared in importance with your weight in influencing how you feel about yourself?"
- "If, over the past four weeks, your weight had changed in any way, would this have affected how you felt about yourself? Did you have a negative emotional reaction? If Yes, how long did it last?"

If, from these questions, it emerges that shape and weight are among the most important things used by patients to evaluate themselves, and they have an intense and longstanding negative reaction when their weight increases, overvaluation of shape or weight is confirmed. If a patient reports residual binge eating and/or overvaluation of shape or weight, it is advisable to postpone the start of CBT-OB and continue with CBT-E Stage 3.

Vignette

The patient, a 32-year-old woman with a BMI of 32.0, had had a progressive increase in body weight from the age of 25, after her first and only pregnancy. At the age of 27 years she made her first weight loss attempt, implementing a strict low-carbohydrate diet, and lost about 15 kg, which she only managed to maintain for a few months. Afterwards she made several other weight-loss attempts, but without success. At the age of 31 she divorced from her husband and started to experience binge-eating episodes, especially at the weekends when her son was with her ex-husband, which made her feel lonely and sad. To compensate for overeating, she tried to diet during the week by eliminating carbohydrates, but after a few weeks she started to have recurrent episodes of binge eating in the evening after putting her son to bed. During these episodes she started by eating large amounts of "healthy foods"—such as a box of almonds or walnuts or dried berries—but then these were supplanted by junk food such as crisps, cookies and sweets. She ate these things very rapidly, when no one else was around, until she felt uncomfortably full. She also felt very guilty afterwards. After a few months, she also started to eat large amounts of food at some mealtimes. She gave up checking her weight, and in about 1 year she had gained about 15 kg.

At the assessment interview, she reported feeling very distressed about her eating behaviour and that her goal was to lose 30 kg to improve her self-esteem and make her feel more confident in interpersonal relationships. The therapist, after having confirmed the diagnosis of BED, explained to the patient the rationale behind addressing binge eating first and then weight loss. Together they drew a provisional Personal Formulation including the main mechanisms maintaining her binge eating (i.e., the negative emotions associated with the divorce and the sense of loneliness and the strict diet that she intermittently adopted in the attempt to compensate for the excess of food she ate during the binge episodes). They then reviewed the failure of the patient's attempts to lose weight in the last year and their association with the increased frequency of binge-eating episodes. The therapist explained that it would only make sense to start the weight-loss treatment after the problem of binge eating had been resolved. Finally, the therapist explained the nature of CBT-E and discussed with the patient the pros and cons of this proposal. Although initially ambivalent about the idea of postponing weight loss, the patient agreed to start CBT-E to address the binge eating first.

The patient was very engaged in the treatment from the beginning, applying with commitment the CBT-E Stage 1 procedures (i.e., self-monitoring in real time, weekly weighing and regular eating). After 1 week of regular eating, she stopped having episodes of binge eating and at Stage 2 was in remission from BED, displaying no overvaluation of shape and weight. She was therefore started on CBT-OB, and at the end of the programme, she had lost and maintained a weight loss of about 15 kg and was very satisfied with results achieved.

13.7.5 CBT-E Stage 3

The aim of this stage is to address the key mechanisms that are maintaining the patient's binge eating. There are eight weekly appointments and four modules in the focused version of CBT-E (the broad version includes also adjunctive modules to address one or more external maintaining mechanisms):

- *Events, Mood and Eating Module*. This is the Module most commonly used in patients with BED. It includes the following procedures: (1) using proactive problem-solving skills to tackle events triggering binge eating and (2) developing skills to accept and modulate intense moods without binge eating.
- *Body Image Module*. This is used in patients who display overvaluation of shape and weight. It includes the following procedures: (1) providing education about this overvaluation and its consequences, (2) developing previously marginalised domains of self-evaluation, (3) reducing unhelpful body checking and avoidance, (4) relabelling unhelpful thoughts or feelings such as "feeling fat" and (5) exploring the origins of the overvaluation.
- *Dietary Restraint Module*. This is used in patients who adopt extreme and rigid dietary rules between episodes of binge eating. It includes procedures for changing inflexible dietary rules into flexible guidelines and introducing previously avoided food.
- *Setbacks and Mindsets Module*. This is implemented towards the end of Stage 3 and includes procedures for learning to identify setbacks and control the eating disorder mindset.

13.7.6 CBT-E Stage 4

The aims of the final stage of CBT-E are to ensure that the progress made in treatment is maintained and that the risk of relapse is minimised. There are three appointments, each 2 weeks apart, which cover the following:

- Addressing concerns about ending treatment
- Devising a short-term plan to continue to implement changes made in treatment (e.g., reducing body checking, introducing other avoided foods, eating more flexibly, maintaining involvement in new activities) until the post-treatment review session
- Phasing out treatment procedures, in particular self-monitoring and in-session weighing
- Education about realistic expectations and identifying and addressing setbacks
- Devising a long-term plan to prevent relapse, cope with setbacks and minimise their occurrence

Finally, there is a post-treatment review session, 20 weeks after the penultimate appointment, to review progress and to revise, if necessary, the long-term maintenance plan. Patients who are in remission from binge eating and do not display overvaluation of shape or weight can be offered CBT-OB to address weight loss at this point.

References

1. Stunkard AJ. Eating patterns and obesity. Psychiatry Q. 1959;33:284–95.
2. Wonderlich SA, Gordon KH, Mitchell JE, Crosby RD, Engel SG. The validity and clinical utility of binge eating disorder. Int J Eat Disord. 2009;42(8):687–705. https://doi.org/10.1002/eat.20719.
3. American Psychiatric Association. Diagnostic and statistical manual of mental disorders (DSM-5). 5th ed. Washington, DC: American Psychiatric Association; 2013.
4. Engel SG, Kahler KA, Lystad CM, Crosby RD, Simonich HK, Wonderlich SA, et al. Eating behavior in obese BED, obese non-BED, and non-obese control participants: a naturalistic study. Behav Res Ther. 2009;47(10):897–900. https://doi.org/10.1016/j.brat.2009.06.018.
5. Devlin MJ. Binge eating disorder. In: Brownell KD, Walsh BT, editors. Eating disorders and obesity: a comprehensive handbook. New York: Guilford Press; 2017. p. 192–7.
6. Grilo CM. Why no cognitive body image feature such as overvaluation of shape/weight in the binge eating disorder diagnosis? Int J Eat Disord. 2013;46(3):208–11. https://doi.org/10.1002/eat.22082.
7. Utzinger LM, Mitchell JE, Cao L, Crosby RD, Crow SJ, Wonderlich SA, et al. Clinical utility of subtyping binge eating disorder by history of anorexia or bulimia nervosa in a treatment sample. Int J Eat Disord. 2015;48(6):785–9. https://doi.org/10.1002/eat.22422.
8. Agh T, Kovacs G, Supina D, Pawaskar M, Herman BK, Voko Z, et al. A systematic review of the health-related quality of life and economic burdens of anorexia nervosa, bulimia nervosa, and binge eating disorder. Eat Weight Disord. 2016;21(3):353–64. https://doi.org/10.1007/s40519-016-0264-x.
9. Hudson JI, Hiripi E, Pope HG Jr, Kessler RC. The prevalence and correlates of eating disorders in the National Comorbidity Survey Replication. Biol Psychiatry. 2007;61(3):348–58. https://doi.org/10.1016/j.biopsych.2006.03.040.
10. Ricca V, Mannucci E, Moretti S, Di Bernardo M, Zucchi T, Cabras PL, et al. Screening for binge eating disorder in obese outpatients. Compr Psychiatry. 2000;41(2):111–5.
11. Mitchell JE, King WC, Courcoulas A, Dakin G, Elder K, Engel S, et al. Eating behavior and eating disorders in adults before bariatric surgery. Int J Eat Disord. 2015;48(2):215–22. https://doi.org/10.1002/eat.22275.
12. Field AE, Sonneville KR, Micali N, Crosby RD, Swanson SA, Laird NM, et al. Prospective association of common eating disorders and adverse outcomes. Pediatrics. 2012;130(2):e289–95. https://doi.org/10.1542/peds.2011-3663.
13. Fairburn CG, Cooper Z, Doll HA, Norman P, O'Connor M. The natural course of bulimia nervosa and binge eating disorder in young women. Arch Gen Psychiatry. 2000;57(7):659–65.
14. Treasure J, Claudino AM, Zucker N. Eating disorders. Lancet. 2010;375(9714):583–93. https://doi.org/10.1016/s0140-6736(09)61748-7.
15. Mitchell JE, King WC, Pories W, Wolfe B, Flum DR, Spaniolas K, et al. Binge eating disorder and medical comorbidities in bariatric surgery candidates. Int J Eat Disord. 2015;48(5):471–6. https://doi.org/10.1002/eat.22389.
16. Bulik CM, Reichborn-Kjennerud T. Medical morbidity in binge eating disorder. Int J Eat Disord. 2003;34(Suppl):S39–46. https://doi.org/10.1002/eat.10204.
17. Fairburn CG. Cognitive behavior therapy and eating disorders. New York: Guilford Press; 2008.
18. Grilo CM. Psychological and behavioral treatments for binge-eating disorder. J Clin Psychiatry. 2017;78(Suppl 1):20–4. https://doi.org/10.4088/JCP.sh16003su1c.04.

19. National Institute of Clinical Excellence (NICE). Eating disorders: recognition and treatment (NG69). 2017.
20. Wilson GT, Wilfley DE, Agras WS, Bryson SW. Psychological treatments of binge eating disorder. Arch Gen Psychiatry. 2010;67(1):94–101. https://doi.org/10.1001/archgenpsychiatry.2009.170.
21. McElroy SL. Pharmacologic treatments for binge-eating disorder. J Clin Psychiatry. 2017;78(Suppl 1):14–9. https://doi.org/10.4088/JCP.sh16003su1c.03.
22. Dalle Grave R, Cooper Z. Enhanced cognitive behavior treatment adapted for younger patients. In: Wade T, editor. Encyclopedia of feeding and eating disorders. Singapore: Springer; 2016. p. 1–8.
23. Dalle Grave R. Intensive cognitive behavior therapy for eating disorders. Hauppauge, NY: Nova; 2012.
24. Calugi S, Ricca V, Castellini G, Lo Sauro C, Ruocco A, Chignola E, et al. The eating disorder examination: reliability and validity of the Italian version. Eat Weight Disord. 2015;20(4):505–11. https://doi.org/10.1007/s40519-015-0191-2.
25. Fairburn CG, Cooper Z, O'Connor M. Eating disorder examination (EDE 16.0D). In: Fairburn CG, editor. Cognitive behavior therapy and eating disorders. New York: Guilford Press; 2008. p. 265–308.

Combining CBT-OB with Weight-Loss Drugs and Bariatric Surgery

14

CBT-OB has been designed to address the environmental, cognitive, emotional and behavioural factors hindering weight loss and weight maintenance. However, the treatment does not address the biological obstacles to weight loss (i.e., hunger, energy expenditure). For this reason, it may be advisable, in the subgroup of patients that have difficulties adopting the lifestyle modification needed to manage their obesity, to associate CBT-OB with weight-loss drugs or bariatric surgery, whose specific aim is to address the biological obstacles to weight loss and weight maintenance.

14.1 CBT-OB Combined with Weight-Loss Drugs

Phelan and Wadden were the first to propose associating a lifestyle modification intervention (based on BT-OB) with weight-loss drugs [1]. They suggested that combined treatment would result in significantly greater weight loss than either therapy alone because of the potentially complementary mechanisms of action of the two interventions. Indeed, weight-loss drugs act to modify internal signals that control hunger (the drive to eat) and satiation (fullness), while lifestyle modification helps patients to change external environmental stimuli (e.g., by grocery shopping from a list or recording food intake). Phelan and Wadden based their conclusion on the results of one study on fenfluramine (which was withdrawn from the market in 1997 because its intake was found to be associated with valvular heart disease [2]), suggesting that the effects of lifestyle modification would be potentiated by the addition of weight-control medication [3]. This has in fact been subsequently demonstrated by a trial in which adult patients with obesity were randomly assigned to receive either one of two forms of BT-OB lifestyle modification (one delivered by a primary care provider in 8 sessions of 10–15 min and one delivered in 30 group sessions), sibutramine alone (a drug withdrawn from the market in 2010 because it was found to be associated with a higher rate of cardiovascular events such as heart

R. Dalle Grave et al., *Treating Obesity with Personalized Cognitive Behavioral Therapy*, https://doi.org/10.1007/978-3-319-91497-8_14

attack and stroke [4]), or one of the two lifestyle modification programmes combined with sibutramine [5]. At 1 year, subjects who received combined therapy lost 2–2.5 times more weight than those receiving lifestyle modification or sibutramine alone, respectively.

Although fenfluramine and sibutramine have both since been withdrawn from the market, three weight medications are now licensed in Europe for the long-term treatment of obesity (i.e., orlistat, liraglutide and bupropion-naltrexone), while in USA two other drugs are also available (i.e., phentermine-topiramate and lorcaserin). These medicines, with the exception of orlistat, share a common strategy: to promote weight loss by manipulating hunger and satiety control in the central nervous system. Most of them are combinations of older medications that have been used for conditions other than obesity. Nevertheless, the mean loss of starting weight reported with these drugs beyond placebo is in the range of 3–4% for orlistat and lorcaserin, 3.7–5.2% for bupropion-naltrexone, about 5% for liraglutide and about 9% for phentermine-topiramate at full dosage. Continual use of the drug in question is required to achieve sustained weight loss [6], and the unique side effect profile of each drug must be carefully considered by a medical doctor expert in the pharmacological treatment of obesity when selecting the best agent for any given individual. Medication should be suspended in patients who do not respond with a weight loss of at least 5%, as there is no point in exposing the patient to the risks and costs of drug treatment when there is little possibility of long-term benefit [7].

Available weight-loss drugs can potentially be combined with CBT-OB to potentiate the effect of the treatment or to help patients to adopt the eating changes needed to lose a healthy amount of weight. This indication is in line with the 2013 AHA/ACC/TOS Obesity Guideline, which recommends that pharmacotherapy be considered if a patient has a BMI ≥30.0 or ≥27 and has been unable to lose weight or maintain weight loss through comprehensive lifestyle intervention [8]. Other appropriate candidates for obesity drug treatment are patients with BMI ≥30.0, or ≥27.0 with comorbidity, who have a history of being unable to lose weight or maintain weight loss and who have previously participated in a comprehensive lifestyle modification intervention; these patients may be offered the option to add pharmacotherapy at the time of initiation of a lifestyle intervention programme [8].

However, it is important to remember that there are several problems associated with drug treatment of obesity that have not yet been completely resolved. Firstly, available weight-loss drugs only produce a modest weight loss. The weight loss occurs in the first 6 months of treatment and then stops. Unfortunately, if the drug is suspended, the weight tends to be regained. This implies the need to implement drug treatment for obesity long term, but with the exception of orlistat—which has been tested in a 4-year study—the safety and efficacy of long-term weight-loss drug administration have not yet been demonstrated.

Furthermore, many patients do not like taking medicines continually, and an extended duration of treatment duration is likely to exacerbate the problems associated with the acceptability of drug treatment and therefore reduce patient compliance. In fact, the tolerability of the available weight-loss drugs is far from ideal, and all are associated with some side effects that in some cases are severe. Moreover, past experience—of the association between valvular disease and the use of fenfluramine, dexfenfluramine, and phentermine, discovered after many years of patients' use—dictates that caution is warranted when weight-loss drugs are involved. There is a need to set up an active system of surveillance to detect any potential severe side effects of these drugs.

Finally, the cost of weight-loss drugs is high and is generally not reimbursed by national health systems or insurance companies. This precludes the use of these drugs in a large proportion of the population, in particular those with a higher socioeconomic burden (in whom the prevalence of obesity is higher). Experience shows that if patients have to pay for their own weight-loss medication, especially if this represents an economic sacrifice, they will continue to do so if they see the benefit, but their compliance will invariably wane when their weight loss reaches a plateau. Indeed, it is difficult for them to see the need to continue spending money on a drug with the sole purpose of maintaining the weight lost.

14.1.1 Practical Suggestions on When and How to Combine Weight-Loss Drugs with CBT-OB

Helping patients to decide whether or not to associate a weight-loss drug with CBT-OB is not easy, but the patients should be actively involved. The therapist should illustrate the reasons for and against this course of action, educating them on the drugs' mechanisms of action, effects on weight loss and potential side effects. Together the therapist and patient should draw up and discuss a list of the pros and cons of starting pharmacological treatment, in order for them to reach a detailed informed decision. Patients should always be informed that the drug treatment should be used in conjunction with an intensive lifestyle intervention, as this approach approximately doubles weight loss. If the therapist conducting CBT-OB is not a medical doctor, he or she should only discuss with patients the option of and reasons for and against associating CBT-OB with weight-loss drugs and refer them to a physician for the final decision regarding prescription. This physician should be an expert in the use of weight-loss medication, familiar with CBT-OB, and motivate the patient to associate the weight-loss drug with lifestyle modification.

In general, there are three ways of combining pharmacological therapy with the CBT-OB described in this manual:

1. *At the beginning of CBT-OB*. Weight-loss medication can be considered in patients who report having failed to lose weight in their previous weight-loss attempts and do not think that they will be able do so by means of CBT-OB. If the drug is added at the beginning of the treatment, it may augment and enhance weight loss in the first 4–8 weeks—a predictor of long-term weight loss [9].
2. *After a certain period of the weight-loss phase of CBT-OB*. This option may be indicated if the weight lost during the weight-loss phase of CBT-OB is less than 0.5 kg per week for at least four consecutive weeks, and the patient seems unable to adequately address weight-loss obstacles via CBT-OB strategies and

procedures. In this case, combination treatment may help patients to improve their adherence to the diet by reducing hunger and increasing their sensation of satiety.

3. *In the maintenance phase of CBT-OB*. This may be a useful approach in patients who do not experience problems during the weight-loss phase but show difficulties in maintaining the weight lost by means of CBT-OB strategies and procedures. In such cases, adding a weight-loss drug in the weight-maintenance phase may help patients to maintain the long-term lifestyle changes and weight-maintenance mindset described in Chap. 9.

A detailed description of the specific weight-loss drugs is beyond the scope of this book. However, Table 14.1 shows a brief summary of the mechanisms of action, weight-loss effects, and side effects of the major weight-loss drugs with FDA approval for obesity. Non-medical therapists should defer advice on taking specific weight-loss drugs to the medical doctor who is treating the patient.

Vignette

The patient, a 45-year-old businessman with a BMI of 31.0, had experienced a progressive increase in body weight as an adult after starting work and giving up sport. He had previously attempted to lose weight several times, through many traditional prescriptive dietary regimes and also an individual programme based on BT-OB. In none of these weight-loss attempts was he ever able to change his eating behaviour and start the process of weight loss. Assessing with the therapist the reasons for the previous treatment failures, he reported that the main causes were excessive hunger and exposure to highly palatable foods at the restaurant that he had to attend daily for business purposes. Although the therapist informed the patient that CBT-OB suggests several strategies that would help him address eating in restaurants and social occasions, he was very sceptical about the likelihood of his success in changing his eating habits. At this point the therapist discussed with him the possibility of associating a weight-loss drug with CBT-OB in order to facilitate his adherence to caloric restriction in the first phase of the treatment. The therapist stressed the importance of adopting CBT-OB strategies and procedures to obtaining the best results from pharmacological treatment, both in terms of weight loss and improvements in the metabolic complications associated with obesity. The patient accepted the therapist's proposal, and, since he had prediabetes, he was prescribed liraglutide. He was able to adhere to CBT-OB actively and with great commitment and saw a healthy weight loss of 11% of his initial body weight. He reported that the drug reduced his appetite and thereby facilitated his application of CBT-OB strategies and procedures.

Table 14.1 Weight-loss drugs indicated for obesity with long-term Food and Drug Administration approval

Generic name of the drug	Mechanism of action	1-year weight change relative to placebo, mean, kg	Common side effects
Orlistat	Lipase inhibitor causing excretion of approximately 30% of ingested triglycerides in stool	60 mg, −2.5 kg 120 mg, −3.4 kg	Oily spotting, flatus with discharge, faecal urgency, fatty oily stool, increased defecation, faecal incontinence
Lorcaserin	Highly selective serotonergic 5-HT2C receptor agonist causing appetite suppression	−3.2 kg	Headache, dizziness, fatigue, nausea, dry mouth, cough, and constipation, in addition to back pain, cough, and hypoglycaemia in patients with type 2 diabetes
Liraglutide	Glucagon-like peptide 1 receptor agonist that promotes weight loss by suppression of food intake via central regulation of appetite and delayed gastric emptying	−5.4 kg	Nausea, diarrhoea, constipation, headache, vomiting, hypoglycaemia, decreased appetite, upset stomach, tiredness, dizziness, stomach pain, and changes in blood lipase levels
Phentermine/topiramate-ER	Noradrenergic + GABA-receptor activator, kainite/AMPA glutamate receptor inhibitor causing appetite suppression	7.5 mg/46 mg, −6.7 kg 15 mg/92 mg, −8.9 kg	Paraesthesia, dizziness, taste alterations, insomnia, constipation, dry mouth, elevated heart rate, memory or cognitive changes
Naltrexone HCl/bupropion HCl	Not entirely understood. Bupropion inhibits reuptake of dopamine and/or norepinephrine, interfering with the "reward pathway" induced by foods. Naltrexone blocks an opioid pathway that may slow weight loss	16 mg/360 mg, 4.6 32 mg/360 mg, −6.1 kg	Nausea, constipation, headache, vomiting, dizziness, trouble sleeping, dry mouth, and diarrhoea

14.2 CBT-OB Combined with Bariatric Surgery

The 2013 AHA/ACC/TOS Obesity Guideline, as described in Chap. 1, recommends bariatric surgery for individuals with a BMI ≥40.0 or BMI ≥35.0 with obesity-related comorbid conditions who are motivated to lose weight but who have not responded to lifestyle modification interventions (with or without pharmacotherapy) [8]. Since no trial is available to identify the optimal duration and weight-loss outcomes of non-surgical treatment prior to recommending bariatric surgery, the decision to proceed with surgery should be clinical and based on several factors such as patient motivation, treatment adherence, operative risk and optimisation of comorbid conditions [8].

The most frequently performed bariatric procedure in the world is the Roux-en-Y gastric bypass (RYGB; 45%), but sleeve gastrectomy (SG; 37%) and adjustable gastric banding are also viable options (AGB; 10%) [10]. In fact, recent data indicate that SG has overtaken RYGB as the most common intervention nowadays. SG is primarily a restrictive procedure, in which the surgeon, after oral placement of a gastroscope, uses this as a guide to staple the stomach into a banana shape, reducing the volume by around 75%. RYGB, on the other hand, is a procedure in which the surgeon creates a 15–30 mL gastric pouch via surgical stapling/transection and "rewiring" of the small intestine (in a Roux-en-Y configuration) so that a part of proximal small intestine receives gastric content before biliary secretions are added; this is designed to determine both gastric restriction and a reduction in absorption. However, it should be noted that the metabolic parameters (e.g., fasting blood glucose) of such patients tend to normalise before significant weight loss, suggesting that the mechanisms of action of these procedures involve other complex mechanisms (e.g., neuroendocrine, bile acids and microbiome alterations) [10].

Bariatric surgery is very effective in producing weight loss and, according to the report of the American College of Surgeon Bariatric Surgery Center Network, at 1-year follow-up the mean BMI loss is 15.34 for RYGB, 11.87 for SG and 7.05 for AGB [11]. However, weight-loss trajectories are highly variable [12], and about 50% of patients experience some weight regain by 2 years post-surgery [13]. Moreover, about a quarter of patients have regained a considerable proportion of their overall weight loss at 3 years post-surgery [12].

Indeed, bariatric surgery does not address the psychological factors that contribute to the adoption of maladaptive eating and physical activity habits (e.g., dysfunctional cognitive thoughts and assumptions, events and associated mood changes), and it is therefore possible that the variability in post-operative weight-loss outcomes may be partially dependent on cognitive and emotional mechanisms [14]. In fact, available data indicate that while the impact of frequent preoperative psychiatric disorders is inconclusive [15], post-operative binge eating, loss of eating control, uncontrolled eating/grazing and depression have a negative influence on adherence to dietary guidelines and weight-loss outcomes [16].

Nonetheless, available data suggest that enforcing and sustaining healthy lifestyle facilitates patients' adherence to therapy and therefore helps to prevent weight regain after bariatric surgery [17]. A recent systematic review and meta-analysis examined the effects of lifestyle modification programmes based on BT-OB delivered after bariatric surgery in terms of weight loss [18]. The main finding of this systematic review was that BT-OB had a positive effect on weight loss following bariatric surgery, as patients who received this intervention had significantly greater weight loss than those who received the usual care or no treatment. Furthermore, a meta-analysis conducted on the available RCTs suggested that weight loss was nearly 2% greater following behavioural lifestyle interventions compared with the usual interventions [18]. Hence, lifestyle modification programmes for weight management following bariatric surgery seem to increase weight loss, and psychological interventions based on CBT-OB or BT-OB have therefore been recommended for consideration as an adjunct to bariatric surgery [8]. That being said, these interventions are still not routinely offered in post-bariatric surgery programmes.

CBT programmes conducted before bariatric surgery, on the other hand, seem not to be so effective at improving the rate of weight loss. One study, for example, found no significant difference in the rate of weight loss or other outcomes between participants allocated to 10 weeks of CBT prior to bariatric surgery and those receiving to nutritional support or education [19]. In contrast, however, one study has found that six sessions of telephone-based CBT before bariatric surgery produced a significant improvement in eating psychopathology and depression in patients immediately after the intervention, in comparison to the standard preoperative care [14].

14.2.1 Practical Suggestions on When and How to Introduce CBT-OB in Bariatric Patients

Based on the above trial data and our clinical experience, the optimal period to introduce CBT-OB seems to be after bariatric surgery. However, no data is yet available on precisely when to implement it. There are two possible strategies, the first being to start CBT-OB in all patients 6 months after the intervention—when the acute effect of the biological gastrointestinal alterations on food intake tend to be mitigated and a subgroup of patient stops losing weight or starts to regain [12]. The second strategy is to propose CBT-OB only to the subgroup of patients displaying difficulties adhering to the dietary and physical activity recommendations of the bariatric team—if possible before significant weight regain has occurred. While the latter option may be less burdensome for healthcare providers, we are in favour of the former, because all bariatric surgery patients may benefit from the acquisition of strategies and procedures designed to improve eating and exercising habits and developing a weight-control mindset in the long term. Irrespective of the strategy adopted, we therefore advise integrating CBT-OB into the standard post-surgical treatment protocol, alongside the usual care. Patients should be informed in advance, preferably before the preoperative period, of the need to start CBT-OB after 6 months (or when they experience difficulties adhering to the eating and exercising habits required to manage obesity in the long term). They should be informed that at this point the acute biological effects on reducing food intake will tend to wane, and it will therefore be necessary for them to become more active in controlling when and what to eat. As in the Preparatory Phase of standard CBT-OB, patients should be educated on the goals and nature of the CBT-OB programme. The following general information should be provided, in addition to that described in Sect. 3.4.2:

- Bariatric surgery helps to reduce energy intake by restricting the size of the stomach (and some interventions also cause malabsorption) and producing changes in gastrointestinal hormones, bile acid production and microbiota composition. These changes seem to create an anorexigenic effect and reduce the rewarding effects of palatable food and impulsive eating. However, these effects, although persistent, tend to reduce in intensity with the passing of time. It is for this reason that the treatment involves CBT-OB. The CBT-OB programme is offered 6 months after the operation and is designed to help patients to develop specific skills and the mindset necessary to control weight in the long term.
- Several studies have shown that adding treatments similar to CBT-OB in the post-operative period improves the amount of weight loss achieved.

The content and the duration of CBT-OB after bariatric surgery are similar to those described in this book, without any specific adaptations. Hence the treatment can be delivered either individually or in a group, as described in Chap. 11. As described in Chap. 12, the intensive version of CBT-OB may be the best choice in certain patients. In particular, it may be indicated in the preoperative period in a subgroup of patients with severe obesity and complications, to reduce the risk associated with the surgical intervention. It should also be considered in the post-operative period in patients who are having difficulty implementing the lifestyle modifications necessary for achieving adequate weight loss, those with persistent weight-related disabilities or those with the recurrence or onset of eating disorder, which may compromise the long-term success of the surgical intervention.

Vignette

A 55-year-old man had a sleeve gastrectomy at the age of 54, when his weight was 181 kg. He lost 35 kg in the first 6 months after the operation but then started to eat highly palatable foods during the day and his body weight increased by about 10 kg. He also reported a worsening of his physical fitness and difficulty in walking more than 100 m. At the assessment interview, he reported having a habit of eating rapidly and discarding his meal plan in favour of tasty and energy-dense foods. The therapist and the patient agreed that a period of intensive CBT-OB could help to improve his physical condition and help him readopt the eating habits he needed to continue weight loss. In intensive CBT-OB unit, in addition to the standard procedures of the treatment, a CBT-OB dietician assisted the patient during some meals and trained him to eat slowly using the following strategies: cutting the food into small pieces, taking small bites, chewing for a long time before swallowing, focusing on the act of eating and appreciating the taste of each bite, having a break during the meal, filling in the Monitoring Record in real time and stopping eating as soon as he felt full. With this support, the patient started to eat regular meals (three per day) and snacks (two per day), and he also gradually increased his daily step count. Upon discharge, he continued his treatment with standard outpatient CBT-OB, planning the food to buy and eat in advance, eating consciously and walking about 10,000 steps per day. These improvements in his eating and physical activity habits were associated with a progressive weight loss, and 6 months after discharge from the unit he had lost 40 kg, which he kept off throughout the weight-maintenance phase until the final review.

References

1. Phelan S, Wadden TA. Combining behavioral and pharmacological treatments for obesity. Obes Res. 2002;10(6):560–74. https://doi.org/10.1038/oby.2002.77.
2. Connolly HM, Crary JL, McGoon MD, Hensrud DD, Edwards BS, Edwards WD, et al. Valvular heart disease associated with fenfluramine-phentermine. N Engl J Med. 1997;337(9):581–8. https://doi.org/10.1056/nejm199708283370901.
3. Craighead LW, Stunkard AJ, O'Brien RM. Behavior therapy and pharmacotherapy for obesity. Arch Gen Psychiatry. 1981;38(7):763–8.
4. James WP, Caterson ID, Coutinho W, Finer N, Van Gaal LF, Maggioni AP, et al. Effect of sibutramine on cardiovascular outcomes in overweight and obese subjects. N Engl J Med. 2010;363(10):905–17. https://doi.org/10.1056/NEJMoa1003114.
5. Wadden TA, Berkowitz RI, Womble LG, Sarwer DB, Phelan S, Cato RK, et al. Randomized trial of lifestyle modification and pharmacotherapy for obesity. N Engl J Med. 2005;353(20):2111–20. https://doi.org/10.1056/NEJMoa050156.
6. Kim S. Drugs to treat obesity: do they work? Postgrad Med J. 2016;92(1089):401–6. https://doi.org/10.1136/postgradmedj-2015-133388.
7. Yanovski SZ, Yanovski JA. Long-term drug treatment for obesity: a systematic and clinical review. JAMA. 2014;311(1):74–86. https://doi.org/10.1001/jama.2013.281361.
8. Jensen MD, Ryan DH, Apovian CM, Ard JD, Comuzzie AG, Donato KA, et al. 2013 AHA/ACC/TOS guideline for the management of overweight and obesity in adults: a report of the American College of Cardiology/American Heart Association Task Force on Practice Guidelines and The Obesity Society. J Am Coll Cardiol. 2014;63(25 Pt B):2985–3023. https://doi.org/10.1016/j.jacc.2013.11.004.
9. Unick JL, Neiberg RH, Hogan PE, Cheskin LJ, Dutton GR, Jeffery R, et al. Weight change in the first 2 months of a lifestyle intervention predicts weight changes 8 years later. Obesity (Silver Spring). 2015;23(7):1353–6. https://doi.org/10.1002/oby.21112.
10. Daigle CR, Schauer PR. Surgery for obesity. In: Brownell KD, Walsh BT, editors. Eating disorders and obesity: a comprehensive handbook. 3rd ed. New York: Guilford Press; 2017. p. 525–31.
11. Hutter MM, Schirmer BD, Jones DB, Ko CY, Cohen ME, Merkow RP, et al. First report from the American College of Surgeons Bariatric Surgery Center Network: laparoscopic sleeve gastrectomy has morbidity and effectiveness positioned between the band and the bypass. Ann Surg. 2011;254(3):410–20; discussion 20–2. https://doi.org/10.1097/SLA.0b013e31822c9dac.
12. Courcoulas AP, Christian NJ, Belle SH, Berk PD, Flum DR, Garcia L, et al. Weight change and health outcomes at 3 years after bariatric surgery among individuals with severe obesity. JAMA. 2013;310(22):2416–25. https://doi.org/10.1001/jama.2013.280928.
13. Magro DO, Geloneze B, Delfini R, Pareja BC, Callejas F, Pareja JC. Long-term weight regain after gastric bypass: a 5-year prospective study. Obes Surg. 2008;18(6):648–51. https://doi.org/10.1007/s11695-007-9265-1.

14. Cassin SE, Sockalingam S, Du C, Wnuk S, Hawa R, Parikh SV. A pilot randomized controlled trial of telephone-based cognitive behavioural therapy for preoperative bariatric surgery patients. Behav Res Ther. 2016;80:17–22. https://doi.org/10.1016/j.brat.2016.03.001.
15. Livhits M, Mercado C, Yermilov I, Parikh JA, Dutson E, Mehran A, et al. Preoperative predictors of weight loss following bariatric surgery: systematic review. Obes Surg. 2012;22(1):70–89. https://doi.org/10.1007/s11695-011-0472-4.
16. Sheets CS, Peat CM, Berg KC, White EK, Bocchieri-Ricciardi L, Chen EY, et al. Post-operative psychosocial predictors of outcome in bariatric surgery. Obes Surg. 2015;25(2):330–45. https://doi.org/10.1007/s11695-014-1490-9.
17. Busetto L, Dicker D, Azran C, Batterham RL, Farpour-Lambert N, Fried M, et al. Practical recommendations of the obesity management task force of the European Association for the Study of Obesity for the post-bariatric surgery medical management. Obes Facts. 2017;10(6):597–632. https://doi.org/10.1159/000481825.
18. Rudolph A, Hilbert A. Post-operative behavioural management in bariatric surgery: a systematic review and meta-analysis of randomized controlled trials. Obes Rev. 2013;14(4):292–302. https://doi.org/10.1111/obr.12013.
19. Gade H, Friborg O, Rosenvinge JH, Smastuen MC, Hjelmesaeth J. The impact of a preoperative cognitive behavioural therapy (CBT) on dysfunctional eating behaviours, affective symptoms and body weight 1 year after bariatric surgery: a randomised controlled trial. Obes Surg. 2015;25(11):2112–9. https://doi.org/10.1007/s11695-015-1673-z.

CBT-OB and Digital Technology

15

Over the last decade, there has been growing interest in using digital technology, namely, the Internet, computers, mobile devices such as smartphones and mobile software applications (apps) [1], for general health promotion and disease management. Several obesity-management tools are already available, and such technologies may offer a practical and reliable means of managing obesity. In addition, they are widespread, accessible, convenient and low-cost. In the foreseeable future, digital technology could be used to overcome difficulties in disseminating and scaling up effective lifestyle-modification treatments for obesity, such as CBT-OB. Digital delivery systems for treatments such as CBT-OB will make them available to a very large number of people, and digital technology may also conceivably be exploited in a second major strategy [2], specifically using modern technology to train therapists—a strategy which would considerably lower the barriers to widespread dissemination of efficacious, evidence-based treatments.

15.1 Using Technology to Deliver the Treatment

The majority of the research into using modern technology in the treatment of obesity has thus far focused on assessing the efficacy of treatments delivered by phone, but recently some studies have also evaluated the efficacy of digital treatments delivered via the Internet. In addition, we have begun to experiment with delivering CBT-OB sessions using video-chat technology.

15.1.1 Phone Treatments

The efficacy of phones as a delivery system for lifestyle-modification treatment for obesity has been tested in several studies. In 2007, a trial designed to compare the efficacy of phone delivery versus a traditional face-to-face clinical approach was

R. Dalle Grave et al., *Treating Obesity with Personalized Cognitive Behavioral Therapy*, https://doi.org/10.1007/978-3-319-91497-8_15

conducted. The major outcome measure adopted was achievement of 10% weight loss and weight maintenance [3]. Participants with obesity in both groups received a 3-month weight-loss programme, followed by a 4-month weight-maintenance programme, both delivered either by phone or in-person appointments. The median weight loss at 3 months was promising, at 10.6 kg and 12.7 kg for phone and face-to-face programmes, respectively, and at 26 weeks these figures were 12.8 kg and 12.5 kg, respectively. Authors concluded that using the phone to deliver the treatment was a viable alternative to the traditional weight-management clinic [3]. The validity of this conclusion was later confirmed by another randomised trial examining the efficacy of phone delivery versus an on-site approach in participants with obesity [4]. Each group received 18 sessions, and at 6 months those in the phone group had lost 7.7% of their initial weight, as compared to 8.9% in the face-to-face group. These findings suggest that phone-based treatment for obesity is approximately as effective as in-person treatment in terms of weight-loss outcomes [4].

Furthermore, another study has demonstrated the effectiveness of phone-based counselling in weight-loss maintenance [5]. Women with obesity who had lost an average of 10 kg during a 6-month run-in period were randomly assigned to receive a 1-year twice-monthly weight-maintenance programme delivered either by phone or on-site. Women in a third group received newsletters only. Participants in the two weight-maintenance interventions both regained only 1.2 kg during the year in comparison, with a significantly greater regain of 3.7 kg being reported for those in the newsletter group. Likewise, another study found excellent maintenance of weight loss at 2-year follow-up via an intervention delivered primarily by phone [6]. Hence, the available evidence suggests that a phone-delivered approach seems to be almost as effective as in-person delivery in terms of both weight loss and weight-loss maintenance.

15.1.2 Video-Chat Treatments

No study has yet been set up to evaluate the use of video-chat technology in the treatment of obesity. However, there are several reasons to indicate that this may be an effective means of delivering lifestyle-modification interventions to such patients. As mentioned, phone-based treatment has demonstrated comparable efficacy to traditional methods of delivery. Furthermore, smartphones and tablets are now fairly ubiquitous, and free video-chat apps (such as Skype and FaceTime) are readily accessible to all. It may be that the face-to-face interaction that they allow may render them even more effective than audio-only phone-based treatment for obesity.

Hence we have begun to test this approach with some patients who live some distance from our clinic and/or experience considerable difficulties in attending face-to-face sessions in person. We always ensure to conduct the Preparatory Phase in person, but we have found that thereafter some or all CBT-OB sessions can be easily administered via video chat. Although it is still too early to provide findings on efficacy, we can state that thus far adherence rates are similar to those we regularly see with traditional face-to-face CBT-OB. Moreover, patients' feedback has been positive. In the future, in addition to long-term efficacy data, it will be interesting to discover whether it is feasible to deliver the treatment purely via webchat, without the need for initial in-person preparatory sessions.

15.1.3 Digital Procedures

As described in detail above, self-monitoring of food intake and physical activity is a core procedure of CBT-OB (see Chap. 4), and smartphone apps may be exploited for this purpose too. With the widespread use of the Internet, many digital tools have been developed for monitoring dietary intake and physical activity. Early studies have shown that the use of mobile devices improves adherence to self-monitoring with respect to the traditional hardcopy food diary [7], despite a decline in self-monitoring rate. Hence, mobile monitoring associated with clinical feedback appears to be an effective approach.

For example, one recent study in a sample of patients awaiting treatment used smartphone-connected smart scales to promote daily weighing, alongside weekly e-mailed lessons and semiautomated feedback [8]. The adherence to daily weighing using the smart scale was high, and at 6 months participants in the daily weighing intervention had lost more than 5% of their initial body weight—significantly more than the waiting-list group, who received no such intervention. This suggests that CBT-OB self-monitoring of food intake, physical activity and body weight could be effectively implemented using digital technology. Indeed, this approach would not only facilitate the calculation of energy intake and expenditure, and real-time self-monitoring (which is sometimes difficult or embarrassing to do on paper Monitoring Records in social situations), but it is also likely to be particularly appreciated by the younger generations, who are more accustomed to using smartphones than writing on sheets of paper.

15.1.4 Digital Treatments

Well-designed digital treatments are already available for depression and most of the anxiety disorders, for problems such as insomnia [9] and for eating disorders [10]. Furthermore, in the field of obesity treatment, an Internet-based lifestyle-modification weight-management programme has demonstrated efficacy within a primary care setting (with a mean weight loss of 6% over the 3-month programme) [11]. Another study showed how a 12-week, Internet-based weight-loss intervention can be successfully implemented in a workplace setting; participating employees with overweight or obesity saw a clinically significant weight loss of 5 kg from baseline to 6 months [12]. Moreover, participant engagement with the intervention website was high, as was adherence to self-monitoring of weight, caloric intake and physical activity. An Internet-based intervention has also been compared with an on-site weight-loss programme, both using the same 24-session intervention, in adults with obesity [13]. The participants in the Internet programme lost around

5 kg in 6 months, as compared to the 8 kg lost by those who received on-site treatment. In conclusion, it appears that successful Internet programmes, which provide weekly e-mail feedback, can result in a weight loss of nearly two-thirds the magnitude of those achieved by traditional on-site behavioural programmes, with the added advantages of low cost and easy accessibility and management.

That being said, little is known about the use of the Internet during the weight-maintenance period. Some studies have demonstrated the benefit of Internet-delivered programmes in reducing the number of patients who regained weight. However, when compared with the face-to-face intervention, only the latter reduced the amount of weight regained [14]. Despite these promising results, it is not yet clear how best to implement digital treatments. To date they have been applied to different settings in different ways. In most cases they have been associated with some form of support, but the person charged with delivering it has had heterogeneous qualifications and training (being termed, respectively, a "guide," "coach," "facilitator," "therapist" or "clinician") [1]. This makes it very difficult to interpret and integrate the findings of such research. With a view to clarifying the situation, a new form of classification has recently been proposed, featuring three main categories [1]:

1. *Autonomous digital treatment.* A programme-led intervention in which the intervention is delivered with no external support.
2. *Supported digital treatment.* A programme-led intervention in which the intervention is delivered with support from a non-specialist practitioner.
3. *Blended digital treatment.* A programme-led intervention in which the intervention is under the supervision of a clinician or a clinician-led intervention in which a clinician-led treatment incorporates a digital intervention.

Autonomous and supported digital interventions are designed principally to deliver the intervention in community settings, while the blended digital approach is mainly suited to clinical settings [1]. Providing a digital treatment without support ("autonomous digital treatment") is the most scalable form of treatment, although available data in other fields of health treatment indicate that the provision of support improves outcomes. However, the support does not necessarily need to be provided by a clinician ("blended digital treatment"), and non-specialist practitioners ("supported digital treatment," also termed "guided self-help") may be involved. Indeed, the main role of such "facilitators" is to promote a user's engagement in treatment and to enhance their adherence to the digital intervention—a role that does not require extensive training or supervision. Due to a favourable balance between cost and potential efficacy, guided self-help may be particularly useful for individuals from low- and middle-income backgrounds [1].

Nonetheless, there is little data yet available on the best way to design digital intervention software. While the early digital healthcare interventions in treatment were no more than printed self-help guides delivered via the Internet, the latest generations, delivered by specific website or smartphone apps, have dedicated much more attention to appearance and ease of use; they now tend to include interactive features such as learning exercises, self-monitoring tools, progress reports, downloadable documents, audio and video files, audio and video feedback, avatars, quizzes, chat forums and games [1]. It is foreseeable that these, in the forthcoming widespread application of virtual reality-based procedures and artificial intelligence-informed communication, have the potential to make the digital treatment even more powerful and effective.

For the moment, in absence of robust data about the efficacy of digital treatments and on the best way to deliver them, it is our opinion that these should only be implemented in research settings such as our own. If their clinical utility is scientifically demonstrated, as it is hoped it will be, evidence-based digital approaches can then be disseminated in real-world clinical practice. If and when that occurs, it will be essential to develop accurate systems for evaluating, regulating and promoting these interventions for an appropriate use of this new treatment technology.

15.2 Using Modern Technology to Train Therapists

One of the most important challenges to overcome in the treatment of obesity is the dissemination of evidence-based treatments such as CBT-OB. Indeed, even in the more advanced Western countries, these treatments are mainly used in research settings, and very few therapists apply them in standard clinical practice. Most clinicians continue to "prescribe" patient diet and exercise using the traditional biomedical approach, but it is crucial that more attention is paid to cognitive behavioural barriers to adherence to lifestyle modification (see Sect. 1.1.1), if the ongoing obesity "epidemic" is to be countered successfully.

The greatest obstacle to the widespread implementation of CBT-OB, for example, is that this approach is not usually taught in either graduate or post-graduate courses for medical doctors, dieticians, psychologists or physical trainers. It is also clear that the traditional methods of promoting evidence-based lifestyle-modification treatments—such as scientific papers, 1- or 2-day workshops and treatment manuals—are not sufficient to enable a clinician to acquire the necessary skills for applying such approaches effectively. Although this book has been designed to illustrate in detail how to treat clinical cases in the real world, it can only go so far. In order to equip the clinician with the tools needed to implement this effective treatment, new forms of training are required.

This was why we focused our efforts on developing the first Certificate of Professional Training in Eating Disorders and Obesity to offer intensive training in CBT-OB and CBT-E for eating disorders. Now established in Italy, this 1-year course uses an interactive approach to learning. It includes didactic features such as observation of simulated sessions and role-playing to help therapists acquire the knowledge and skills necessary for them to practice CBT-OB and CBT-E. The course is attended by professionals from different backgrounds (e.g., physicians, psychiatrists, psychologists, dieticians and nurses), and several role-playing sessions are dedicated to the practice and administration of the treatment within a multidisciplinary team—as recommended at intensive levels of care. To date, more than

500 professionals have thus been trained in CBT-OB and CBT-E, and several CBT-OB-/CBT-E-trained teams have consequently been set up in Italy.

Unfortunately, this face-to-face approach does not overcome the obstacle of training scalability and dissemination of the intervention, as only few therapists can attend a 1-year course, for logistic and financial reasons. One promising solution to this problem is "web-centred training," a technology, developed at the Oxford Centre for Research on Eating Disorders (CREDO), for training therapists in CBT-E for eating disorders and in behavioural activation (BA) for depression. Web-based training has the advantage that it can reach a large number of therapists simultaneously, conceivably when it is convenient for them [15]. The training website describes and illustrates the treatment in great detail and includes features to help trainees to learn both the main strategies and procedures of the intervention and the skills needed to apply them. The web-centred training approach is highly scalable, as it may be used alone or accompanied by support from a non-specialist (guided training). A recent proof-of-concept study of web-centred training in CBT-E for eating disorders has shown that the therapists who completed the training programme (84.3% of 102) benefit from a substantial increase in their competency scores, indicative of a good level of skill in this regard [10].

While no web-based training has been yet developed for CBT-OB, the data from that designed for training in CBT-E is promising. If confirmed by future studies, it will indicate that this form of low-cost digital training has the potential to overcome the major obstacles to the widespread dissemination of evidence-based treatments, including those promoting the treatment of obesity through lifestyle modification. It is therefore hoped that such approaches are carefully evaluated and promoted with a view to potentiating our response to the obesity crisis worldwide.

References

1. Fairburn CG, Patel V. The impact of digital technology on psychological treatments and their dissemination. Behav Res Ther. 2017;88:19–25. https://doi.org/10.1016/j.brat.2016.08.012.
2. Fairburn CG, Patel V. The global dissemination of psychological treatments: a road map for research and practice. Am J Psychiatry. 2014;171(5):495–8. https://doi.org/10.1176/appi.ajp.2013.13111546.
3. Donnelly JE, Smith BK, Dunn L, Mayo MM, Jacobsen DJ, Stewart EE, et al. Comparison of a phone vs clinic approach to achieve 10% weight loss. Int J Obes. 2007;31(8):1270–6. https://doi.org/10.1038/sj.ijo.0803568.
4. Digenio AG, Mancuso JP, Gerber RA, Dvorak RV. Comparison of methods for delivering a lifestyle modification program for obese patients: a randomized trial. Ann Intern Med. 2009;150(4):255–62.
5. Perri MG, Limacher MC, Durning PE, Janicke DM, Lutes LD, Bobroff LB, et al. Extended-care programs for weight management in rural communities: the treatment of obesity in underserved rural settings (TOURS) randomized trial. Arch Intern Med. 2008;168(21):2347–54. https://doi.org/10.1001/archinte.168.21.2347.
6. Appel LJ, Clark JM, Yeh HC, Wang NY, Coughlin JW, Daumit G, et al. Comparative effectiveness of weight-loss interventions in clinical practice. N Engl J Med. 2011;365(21):1959–68. https://doi.org/10.1056/NEJMoa1108660.

7. Burke LE, Conroy MB, Sereika SM, Elci OU, Styn MA, Acharya SD, et al. The effect of electronic self-monitoring on weight loss and dietary intake: a randomized behavioral weight loss trial. Obesity (Silver Spring). 2011;19(2):338–44. https://doi.org/10.1038/oby.2010.208.
8. Steinberg DM, Tate DF, Bennett GG, Ennett S, Samuel-Hodge C, Ward DS. The efficacy of a daily self-weighing weight loss intervention using smart scales and e-mail. Obesity (Silver Spring). 2013;21(9):1789–97. https://doi.org/10.1002/oby.20396.
9. Andersson G, Titov N. Advantages and limitations of Internet-based interventions for common mental disorders. World Psychiatry. 2014;13(1):4–11. https://doi.org/10.1002/wps.20083.
10. Fairburn CG, Allen E, Bailey-Straebler S, O'Connor ME, Cooper Z. Scaling up psychological treatments: a countrywide test of the online training of therapists. J Med Internet Res. 2017;19(6):e214. https://doi.org/10.2196/jmir.7864.
11. Tate DF, Jackvony EH, Wing RR. A randomized trial comparing human e-mail counseling, computer-automated tailored counseling, and no counseling in an Internet weight loss program. Arch Intern Med. 2006;166(15):1620–5. https://doi.org/10.1001/archinte.166.15.1620.
12. Ross KM, Wing RR. Implementation of an Internet weight loss program in a worksite setting. J Obes. 2016;2016:9372515. https://doi.org/10.1155/2016/9372515.
13. Harvey-Berino J, West D, Krukowski R, Prewitt E, VanBiervliet A, Ashikaga T, et al. Internet delivered behavioral obesity treatment. Prev Med. 2010;51(2):123–8. https://doi.org/10.1016/j.ypmed.2010.04.018.
14. Wing RR, Tate DF, Gorin AA, Raynor HA, Fava JL. A self-regulation program for maintenance of weight loss. N Engl J Med. 2006;355(15):1563–71. https://doi.org/10.1056/NEJMoa061883.
15. Centre for Research on Eating Disorders at Oxford (CREDO). Therapist training: scalable methods for training therapists. http://www.credo-oxford.com/3.1.html.

Appendix A: The CBT-OB Monitoring Record

Day .... Daily calorie goal ....

A. ENERGY INTAKE					
Time	**Food and drink consumed**	**Calories**	*	**Place**	**Comments and contexts**
	Daily energy intake				

B. ENERGY EXPENDITURE			
			Calories
Steps	Number		
Formal exercise	Type	Minutes	
Formal exercise	Type	Minutes	
Basal metabolic rate			
Diet-induced thermogenesis (about 10% of the total calories consumed)			
		Daily energy expenditure	

C. ENERGY BALANCE				
	-		=	
Daily energy intake		**Daily energy expenditure**		**Energy balance**

R. Dalle Grave et al., *Treating Obesity with Personalized Cognitive Behavioral Therapy*, https://doi.org/10.1007/978-3-319-91497-8

Appendix B: The Personal Formulation Template

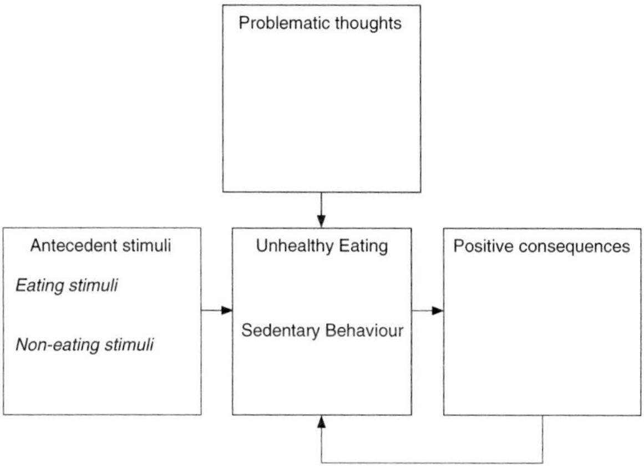

Appendix C: Menus and Food Groups

1.1 Menus

This section provides two example menus with respective calorie contents of 1200 and 1500/day. The following items are displayed in the menu scheme:

- Meals (breakfast, mid-morning snack, lunch, mid-afternoon snack, dinner)
- Food groups (see below)
- Portion size (with reference to the food group)

The therapist should educate the patients that to increase the variety of the foods consumed without adjusting the calories, gram-for-gram substitutions can be made within specific food groups.

1200 kcal menu

Meals and snacks	Food group	Portion size	kcal
Breakfast	Milk, yoghurt and cheese	0.5 portion	45
	Wholemeal bread	0.5 portion	90
Snack	Fruit	1 portion	80
Lunch	Whole-wheat pasta/brown rice	1 portion	280
	Vegetable	1 portion	45
	Olive oil	1 portion	90
Snack	Fruit	1 portion	80
Dinner	Meat/fish/pulses	1.5 portion	285
	Vegetable	1 portion	45
	Olive oil	1 portion	90
	Wholemeal bread	0.5 portion	90

1500 kcal menu

Meals and snacks	Food group	Portion size	kcal
Breakfast	Milk, yogurt and cheese	1 portion	90
	Wholemeal bread	1 portion	180
Snack	Fruit	1 portion	80
Lunch	Whole-wheat pasta/brown rice	1 portion	280
	Vegetable	1 portion	45
	Olive oil	1 portion	90
	Whole bread	1 portion	90

Meals and snacks	Food group	Portion size	kcal
Snack	Milk, yogurt and cheese	0.5 portion	45
Dinner	Meat/fish/pulses	1.5 portion	285
	Vegetable	1 portion	45
	Olive oil	1 portion	90
	Wholemeal bread	1/2 portion	90
	Fruit	1 portion	80

Food Groups

For ease of use, CBT-OB distinguishes five main food groups, which include foods grouped together because they provide similar amounts of the key nutrients of that food group, plus a sixth that includes foods with high energy density (e.g. seasonings and sweets) and alcohol:

1. Bread, cereal, rice and pasta
2. Meat, poultry, fish, eggs and pulses
3. Milk, yogurt and cheese
4. Vegetables
5. Fruit
6. Seasonings, sweets and alcohol

In the food group tables, a reference food for each group and its recommended portion size is indicated. Patients are educated that, to vary the foods consumed in meals, they should make gram-for-gram substitutions according to the information provided in each table, taking into account their individual preferences.

Bread, cereal, rice and pasta group	
Reference food 1: wholemeal bread	*Portion size: 80 g 180 kcal*
Possible substitutions	
2 regular slices of white bread (60 g)	3 packets of restaurant breadsticks (40 g)
5 tablespoons of cornflakes (50 g)	2 small or 1 medium potato (200 g)
1 small packet of crackers (40 g)	1 small portion of pasta or rice (50 g)
6 cracker slices (40 g)	2 slices of cooked polenta (200 g)
Reference food 2: whole-wheat pasta/brown rice	*Portion size: 90 g 280 kcal*
1 medium dish of pasta (80 g–1 cup)	2 medium potatoes (320 g)
1 medium dish of rice (80 g–1 cup)	3 slices of cooked polenta (350 g)
1 small portion of ravioli or tortellini (90 g)	3 regular slices of white bread (100 g)
1 portion of potato gnocchi (210 g)	4 regular slices of brown bread (130 g)
1 portion of baked lasagne or cannelloni (170 g)	5 packets of restaurant breadsticks (60 g)

Meat, poultry, fish, eggs and pulses group	
Reference food: chicken breast	*Portion size: 190 g 190 Kcal*
Possible substitutions	

Meat, poultry, fish, eggs and pulses group	
½ dish of leg of lamb (180 g)	1/2 mullet (230 g)
4 or 5 slices of turkey (180 g)	1/2 dish of cuttlefish (280 g)
½ dish of lamb fillet (180 g)	1/2 mackerel (110 g)
1 tin of beef in jelly (280 g)	1 sole or sea bass (230 g)
1 dish of cured beef (130 g)	1 small salmon fillet (100 g)
1 dish of lean ham (120 g)	2 handfuls of dried beans (60 g)
2 fillets of cod or plaice (260 g)	1 dish of fresh beans (140 g)
1 sea bream (200 g)	1 dish of fresh peas (370 g)
1/2 dish of octopus (330 g)	2 handfuls of dried lentils (70 g)

Milk, yoghurt and cheese group	
Reference food: skimmed milk	*Portion size: 250 g 90 kcal*
Possible substitutions	
1 glass of partially skimmed milk (200 g)	2 pots of low-fat fruit yoghurt (250 g)
1 cup of whole milk (140 g)	2 tablespoonfuls of parmesan cheese (20 g)
2 pots of skimmed milk yoghurt (250 g)	

Vegetable group	
Reference food: vegetable	*Portion: 200–250 g 45 kcal*
Possible substitutions	
1 small dish of asparagus (150 g)	1 small dish of broccoli (170 g)
1 small dish of beetroot (240 g)	1 small dish of cauliflower (180 g)
1 small dish of carrots (130 g)	1 bowl of cucumber (320 g)
1 small dish of artichokes (200 g)	1 small dish of onions (180 g)
1 small dish of fennel (500 g)	1 small dish of lettuce (240 g)
1 small dish of mushrooms (160 g)	1 small dish of yellow peppers (150 g)
1 small dish of eggplant (240 g)	1 bowl of radishes (350 g)
1 small dish of salad tomatoes (260 g)	1 small dish of pumpkin (250 g)
1 small dish of turnips (250 g)	1 bowl of rocket (160 g)
1 small dish of courgette (400 g)	

Fruit group	
Reference food: peeled apple	*Portion size: 150 g 80 kcal*
Possible substitutions	
4 or 5 apricots (280 g, whole)	1 medium apple (150 g, pulp; 170 g whole)
1/4 fresh pineapple (200 g, pulp)	2 slices of melon (240 g, pulp)
2 slices of pineapple (120 g, pulp)	2 small pears (230 g, pulp; 300 g, whole)
1 slice of watermelon (500 g)	2 peaches (290 g, pulp; 350 g, whole)
2 medium oranges (230 g, pulp; 310 g, whole)	2–3 peach pieces in syrup (140 g)
1 medium banana (120 g, pulp; 200 g, whole)	4 prunes (40 g, pulp; 55 g, whole)
4 clementines (220 g, pulp; 260 g, whole)	1 small bunch of grapes (130 g)
2 or 3 kiwi fruits (180 g, pulp; 240 g, whole)	1 tablespoon of jam (25–30 g)
2 tangerines (110 g, pulp; 130 g, whole)	1 small dish of cherries (210 g, whole)
3 walnuts (12 g)	11 green olives in brine (55 g)
7 almonds (14 g)	7 black olives in brine (35 g)
10 peanuts (15 g)	

Seasonings, sweets and alcohol group	
Reference food 1: extra virgin olive oil	*Portion size*: *10 g* *90 kcal*
Possible substitutions	
1 tablespoon of peanut, corn, rapeseed, soy or sunflower oil	1 tablespoon of other seed oil 1 tablespoon of olive oil
Reference food 2: plain cake	*Portion size*: *60–70 g* *260 kcal*
Possible substitutions	
6–8 plain biscuits (50 g) 1 cream or jam brioche (50 g) 2 chocolates (40 g) 1 small slice of fruit tart (60–70 g) 1 choc ice (80 g)	2 balls of ice cream (80–90 g; coffee or fruit, flavour) 1 small pack of popcorn (60 g) 1 small slice of panettone (70 g) Almond nougat (60 g)
Reference food 3: wine	*Portion size*: *150 g* *110 kcal*
Possible substitutions	
1 can of beer (330 ml) 1 glass of red or white wine (130 g)	1 small glass of liqueur (40 g)

Appendix D: The Weight-Loss Obstacles Questionnaire

Instructions: The following questions refer to the past seven days only. Please read each question carefully. Please answer all the questions.

PROCEDURES

1. Did you fill in your Monitoring Records every day? ☐ yes ☐ no
If not, how many days did you miss?________ What was the reason?
____
____
____

2. Did you count calories every day? ☐ yes ☐ no
If not, how many days did you miss?________ What was the reason?
____
____
____

3. Did you do your physical activity every day? ☐ yes ☐ no
If not, how many days did you miss?________ What was the reason?
____
____
____

4. Did you use the step counter every day? ☐ yes ☐ no
If not, how many days did you miss?________ What was the reason?
____
____
____

5. Did you check your weight once a week? ☐ yes ☐ no
If not, how many days did you check your weight?________ What was the reason?
____
____
____

6. Did you stick to your calorie limit every day? ☐ yes ☐ no
If not, how many days did you go over the limit?________ What was the reason?
____
____
____

7. Did you do at least 10,000 steps every day? ☐ yes ☐ no
If not, how many days did you miss?________ What was the reason?
____
____
____

BEHAVIOURS

8. Did youe at betweenyour planned mealsand snacks? ☐ yes☐ no
If yes, how many times did you eat between meals? ________ What was the reason?
____
____
____

9. Did you overeat at mealtimes? ☐ yes☐ no
If so, how many times?________ What was the reason?
____
____
____

10. Did youskip anymeals? ☐ yes☐ no
If so, how many times?________ What was the reason?
____
____
____

11. Did you have any episodes of binge eating (i.e.being unable to stop yourself eating a large amount of food)? ☐ yes☐ no
If so, how many times?________ What was the reason?
____
____
____

12. Did youeat at night? ☐ yes☐ no
If so, how many times?________ What was the reason?
____
____
____

13. Did you avoid eatingcertain food groups on some days? ☐ yes☐ no
If so, how many times?________ What was the reason?
____
____
____

14. Did youdrink too much alcohol? ☐ yes☐ no
If so, how many times?________ What was the reason?
____
____
____

ATTITUDES

15. How satisfiedare you with your weight loss so far?

0	1	2	3	4	5	6	7	8	9	10
Not at all										Extremely

16. How able do you think you are to lose weight?

0	1	2	3	4	5	6	7	8	9	10
Not at all										Extremely

17. How motivated are youto lose weight?

0	1	2	3	4	5	6	7	8	9	10
Not at all										Extremely

SOCIAL SUPPORT

How often have you received support from significant others?

18. In times of crisis

0	1	2	3	4	5	6	7	8	9	10
Never										All the time

19. In creating an environment that facilitates change

0	1	2	3	4	5	6	7	8	9	10
Never										All the time

20. In applying the programme procedures

0	1	2	3	4	5	6	7	8	9	10
Never										All the time

How often have you received criticism from significant others?

21. On your body weight

0	1	2	3	4	5	6	7	8	9	10
Never										All the time

22. On your eating behaviour

0	1	2	3	4	5	6	7	8	9	10
Never										All the time

23. On your level of physical activity

0	1	2	3	4	5	6	7	8	9	10
Never										All the time

Appendix E: The Weight and Primary Goals Questionnaire

Questions on your weight goal:

1. What is your dream weight? ___________
   (The weight you would reach in an ideal world, even though you understand that this is probably unattainable)
2. What is your desired weight? ___________
   (The weight you think you should and probably will achieve during the treatment)
3. What is your acceptable weight? ___________
   (The highest weight you think you would be able to accept)?

Questions on your desired weight (the weight you wrote in question 2):

4. In the past,was your desired weight different? □ yes□ no
   If so, why? ____
5. How long have you been at your desired weight in your life?
   - □ Less than 1 year
   - □ Between 1 and 3 years
   - □ Between 3 and 5 years
   - □ More than 5 years
6. How hard do you think it will be to remain at your desired weight?
   □ Very □ A lot □ A little □ Not very
7. How important is it for you to achieve your desired weight?
   □ Very □ A lot □ A little □ Not very
8. How would you feel if you did not reach your desired weight?
   ____
   ____

Questions on your primary goals for losing weight:

Instructions: Please put an X in the box you think most appropriate for each statement.

1 = Totally disagree; **2** = Disagree; **3** = Slightly disagree;

4 = Slightly agree; **5** = Agree; **6** = Totally agree

9. Why do you want to reach your desired weight?

	1	2	3	4	5	6
To improveyour physicalappearance						
To reduce the size of some parts of your body						
To reducing your clothing size						
To have a greater choice of clothes						
To reach the weight advised by the doctor						
To go back to the weight you had at an important time in your life						
To go back to the weight you achieved in a previous weight loss attempt						
To reach your ideal weight, according to the ideal weight table						
To have the same weight as other people your age						
To have the same weight as friends or family members						
To have the same weight as famous people						
To improve your health						
To improve your physical fitness						
To improve the quality of your free time						
To improve your sex life						
To be more sexually attractive to others						
To getattention from others						
To get a promotion						
To get a new job						
To improve your social life						
To stop being stigmatised						
To improve your interpersonal relationships						
To improve your self-esteem						
To feel better psychologically						
To be able to have a baby						
To be around for your children						

Of the primary goals that you scored "5" or "6" in question 9:

10. Which is the most important?______________________________

11. Which necessarily require weight loss?______________________________

12. Which do not necessarily require weight loss?______________________________

13. How would it feel if you did not achieve these goals?______________________________

____

Appendix F: The Body Image Inventory

Instructions: The following questions refer to the past 4 weeks (28 days). Please read each question carefully and respond to ALL questions. Thank you.

How many times in the last 28 days…	Never	1–5 days	6–12 days	13–15 days	16–22 days	23–27 days	Every day
Questions on body concerns:							
Have you been dissatisfied with your body?							
Have you had critical thoughts about your body?							
Have you been worried about the size of some parts of your body?							
Have you been preoccupied with your body?							
Have you had contempt for your body?							
Have you felt disgust for your body?							
Have you been ashamed of your body?							
Have you felt embarrassed about your body?							
Have you judged yourself poorly because of your body?							
Questions on body avoidance:							
Have you worn clothes that hide your body?							
Have you avoided physical intimacy situations to avoid judgment about your body?							
Have you avoided wearing clothes that reveal your shape?							
Have you avoided places where it is necessary to expose your body?							

How many times in the last 28 days…	Never	1–5 days	6–12 days	13–15 days	16–22 days	23–27 days	Every day
Have you avoided weighing yourself?							
Have you avoided looking at yourself in a mirror?							
Questions on body checking:							
Have you weighed yourself?							
Have you studied the appearance of your body in the mirror?							
Have you measured the circumferences of some parts of your body?							
Have you pinched your body folds to see how much fat there is?							
Have you compared the shape of your body to that of others?							
Have you tried on some clothes to see if they are tight?							
Have you asked for reassurance from others about your shape and weight?							
Questions on feeling fat:							
Have you felt fat?							

MIX
Papier aus verantwortungsvollen Quellen
Paper from responsible sources
FSC® C105338

If you have any concerns about our products,
you can contact us on
ProductSafety@springernature.com

In case Publisher is established outside the EU,
the EU authorized representative is:
Springer Nature Customer Service Center GmbH
Europaplatz 3, 69115 Heidelberg, Germany

Printed by Libri Plureos GmbH
in Hamburg, Germany